# Explainable Artificial Intelligence for Biomedical Applications

# RIVER PUBLISHERS SERIES IN BIOMEDICAL ENGINEERING

*Series Editors*

**DINESH KANT KUMAR**
*RMIT University,*
*Australia*

The "River Publishers Series in Biomedical Engineering" is a series of comprehensive academic and professional books which focus on the engineering and mathematics in medicine and biology. The series presents innovative experimental science and technological development in the biomedical field as well as clinical application of new developments.

Books published in the series include research monographs, edited volumes, handbooks and textbooks. The books provide professionals, researchers, educators, and advanced students in the field with an invaluable insight into the latest research and developments.

Topics covered in the series include, but are by no means restricted to the following:

- Biomedical engineering
- Biomedical physics and applied biophysics
- Bio-informatics
- Bio-metrics
- Bio-signals
- Medical Imaging

For a list of other books in this series, visit www.riverpublishers.com

# Explainable Artificial Intelligence for Biomedical Applications


**Editors**

**Utku Kose**

Suleyman Demirel University, Turkey

**Deepak Gupta**

Maharaja Agrasen Institute of Technology, India

**Xi Chen**

Meta, USA



River Publishers

Routledge
Taylor & Francis Group
NEW YORK AND LONDON

**Published 2023 by River Publishers**
River Publishers
Alsbjergvej 10, 9260 Gistrup, Denmark
www.riverpublishers.com

**Distributed exclusively by Routledge**
605 Third Avenue, New York, NY 10017, USA
4 Park Square, Milton Park, Abingdon, Oxon OX14 4RN

*Explainable Artificial Intelligence for Biomedical Applications / Utku Kose, Deepak Gupta and Xi Chen.*



Routledge is an imprint of the Taylor & Francis Group, an informa business

ISBN 978-87-7022-849-7 (hardback)
ISBN 978-87-7004-050-1 (paperback)
ISBN 978-10-0381-058-2 (online)
ISBN 978-1-032-62935-3 (ebook master)

# Contents

**Preface** xiii

**Foreword** xvii

**Acknowledgement** xix

**List of Contributors** xxi

**List of Figures** xxv

**List of Tables** xxxiii

**List of Abbreviations** xxxv

**1 Gastric Cancer Detection using Hybrid-based Network and SHAP Analysis** 1
*Varanasi L. V. S. K. B. Kasyap, D. Sumathi, and Karthika Natarajan*
1.1 Introduction . . . . . 2
1.2 XAI Approaches . . . . . 4
1.2.1 Model agnostic vs. model specific . . . . . 5
1.2.2 Local and global methods . . . . . 5
1.2.3 Pre-model, in-model, and post-model . . . . . 5
1.2.4 Visualization or surrogate methods . . . . . 6
1.2.5 Approaches . . . . . 6
1.3 Materials and Methods . . . . . 7
1.3.1 Data processing and augmentation . . . . . 7
1.3.2 Multi-scale network (MSN) module . . . . . 8
1.3.3 Inner network (In-Net) module . . . . . 8
1.3.4 Slice-based classification (SC-Net) module . . . . . 9
1.3.5 Implementation of the proposed network . . . . . 9

1.4 Experiments and Results . . . . . . . . . . . . . . . . . . . . 10
1.4.1 BOT gastric dataset . . . . . . . . . . . . . . . . . 10
1.4.2 Results . . . . . . . . . . . . . . . . . . . . . . . . 11
1.5 Conclusion. . . . . . . . . . . . . . . . . . . . . . . . . 13
References . . . . . . . . . . . . . . . . . . . . . . . . . . 13

**2 LIME Approach in Diagnosing Diseases – A Study on Explainable AI 17**
*Iyyanki Muralikrishna and Prisilla Jayanthi*
2.1 Introduction . . . . . . . . . . . . . . . . . . . . . . . . 17
2.2 XAI Model for Predicting Heart Attack. . . . . . . . . . . . 19
2.3 XAI for Opthalmology . . . . . . . . . . . . . . . . . . . . 22
2.4 LIME – Local Interpretable Model-Agnostic Explanations. . 23
2.4.1 LIME approach for predicting COVID-19 . . . . . . 24
2.4.2 Prediction of thyroid using LIME approach. . . . . . 25
2.4.3 LIME method – air pollutant industries. . . . . . . . 25
2.4.4 Binary classification of breast cancer – LIME method 26
2.5 Multiclassification of ECG Signals using GRAD-CAM . . . 27
2.6 Conclusion. . . . . . . . . . . . . . . . . . . . . . . . . 28
Acknowledgments . . . . . . . . . . . . . . . . . . . . . . . 29
References . . . . . . . . . . . . . . . . . . . . . . . . . . 29

**3 Explainable Artificial Intelligence (XAI) in the Veterinary and Animal Sciences Field 33**
*Amjad Islam Aqib, Mahreen Fatima, Afshan Muneer, Khazeena Atta, Muhammad Arslan, C-Neen Fatima Zaheer, Sadia Muneer and Maheen Murtaza*
3.1 Introduction . . . . . . . . . . . . . . . . . . . . . . . . 34
3.2 Mechanism of Explainable Artificial Intelligence in Biomedical Application . . . . . . . . . . . . . . . . . . 36
3.3 XAI in Diagnosis, Prevention, and Treatment. . . . . . . . . 37
3.4 XAI in Dairy Farming. . . . . . . . . . . . . . . . . . . . 39
3.5 XAI in Poultry Farming . . . . . . . . . . . . . . . . . . . 42
3.5.1 Poultry drones . . . . . . . . . . . . . . . . . . . . 43
3.5.2 Avian illness detection models . . . . . . . . . . . . 44
3.5.3 Models for detecting behavioral disorders . . . . . . 44
3.6 Conclusion. . . . . . . . . . . . . . . . . . . . . . . . . 49
References . . . . . . . . . . . . . . . . . . . . . . . . . . 50

4 **Interpretable Analysis of the Potential Impact of Various Versions of Corona Virus: A Case Study** **57**
*Pawan Whig and Ashima Bhatnagar Bhatia*
4.1 Introduction . . . . . . . . . . . . . . . . . . . . . . . . . 58
4.2 Modeling using Machine Learning . . . . . . . . . . . . . . . 60
4.2.1 Multiclass classification . . . . . . . . . . . . . . . . . 61
4.2.2 Multi-output regression models with multiple models . . . . . . . . . . . . . . . . . . . . . . . 63
4.2.3 Different expert models . . . . . . . . . . . . . . . . . 64
4.2.4 Hybrid models . . . . . . . . . . . . . . . . . . . . . 64
4.3 Sentimentality Analysis . . . . . . . . . . . . . . . . . . . 65
4.3.1 Sentiment analysis techniques . . . . . . . . . . . . . 66
4.3.2 Sentiment analysis across languages . . . . . . . . . 67
4.4 Case Study Discussion . . . . . . . . . . . . . . . . . . . . 67
4.5 Model Interpretation . . . . . . . . . . . . . . . . . . . . . 74
4.5.1 Results and discussion . . . . . . . . . . . . . . . . . 74
4.6 Conclusion and Future Scope . . . . . . . . . . . . . . . . . 75
Acknowledgements . . . . . . . . . . . . . . . . . . . . . . . . 75
References . . . . . . . . . . . . . . . . . . . . . . . . . . . . 75

5 **XAI in Biomedical Applications** **79**
*K. K. Kırboğa and E. U. Küçüksille*
5.1 Introduction . . . . . . . . . . . . . . . . . . . . . . . . . 79
5.2 Main Text . . . . . . . . . . . . . . . . . . . . . . . . . . 80
5.2.1 Main biomedical goals of XAI . . . . . . . . . . . . . 80
5.2.2 Use of XAI in Biomedical Studies . . . . . . . . . . . 83
5.3 Limitations and Future Direction . . . . . . . . . . . . . . . 93
5.4 Conclusion . . . . . . . . . . . . . . . . . . . . . . . . . . 94
References . . . . . . . . . . . . . . . . . . . . . . . . . . . . 95

6 **What Makes Survival of Heart Failure Patients? Prediction by the Iterative Learning Approach and Detailed Factor Analysis with the SHAP Algorithm** **101**
*A. Çifci, M. İlkuçar, and İ. Kırbaş*
6.1 Introduction . . . . . . . . . . . . . . . . . . . . . . . . . 102
6.2 Related Works Using Heart Failure Dataset . . . . . . . . . . 103
6.3 Materials and Methods . . . . . . . . . . . . . . . . . . . . 105
6.3.1 Heart failure dataset . . . . . . . . . . . . . . . . . . 105
6.3.2 Overview of artificial neural networks . . . . . . . . 105

6.4 Results . . . . . 110
6.5 Conclusion . . . . . 117
References . . . . . 118

**7 Class Activation Mapping and Deep Learning for Explainable Biomedical Applications** **123**
*Prasath Alias Surendhar S., R. Manikandan, and Ambeshwar Kumar*
7.1 Introduction . . . . . 124
7.2 Background Study . . . . . 127
7.3 Discussion . . . . . 132
7.4 Conclusion . . . . . 136
References . . . . . 137

**8 Pragmatic Study of IoT in Healthcare Security with an Explainable AI Perspective** **145**
*Adrija Mitra, Yash Anand, and Sushruta Mishra*
8.1 Introduction . . . . . 145
8.2 Objective . . . . . 147
8.3 Motivation . . . . . 147
8.4 Standards for Cybersecurity . . . . . 148
8.5 Comparison of Existing Relevant Models . . . . . 149
8.5.1 Secure explainable intelligent model for smart healthcare under block-chain framework . . . . . 150
8.5.2 Secure IoT healthcare with access control based on explainable deep learning . . . . . 155
8.6 Comparative Analysis of the Models . . . . . 160
8.7 Using explainable AI in IoT security . . . . . 162
8.8 Conclusion . . . . . 164
References . . . . . 164

**9 Chest Disease Identification from X-rays using Deep Learning** **167**
*M. Hacibeyoglu and M.S. Terzi*
9.1 Introduction . . . . . 168
9.2 Deep Learning . . . . . 170
9.2.1 Convolutional neural networks . . . . . 171
9.2.2 Dataset . . . . . 176
9.2.3 Experimental study . . . . . 179
9.3 Conclusion . . . . . 180
References . . . . . 184

**10 Explainable Artificial Intelligence Applications in Dentistry: A Theoretical Research** **189**
*B. Aksoy, M. Yücel, H. Sayın, O.K.M. Salman, M. Eylence, and M.M. Özmen*
10.1 Introduction . . . . . . . . . . . . . . . . . . . . . . . . . . 189
10.1.1 An overview of the dentistry . . . . . . . . . . . . 190
10.1.2 Imaging techniques in the dentistry . . . . . . . . 191
10.1.3 Problem solving with artificial intelligence in dentistry images . . . . . . . . . . . . . . . . . . 192
10.2 Imaging Techniques using X-rays . . . . . . . . . . . . . . 193
10.3 CBCT Imaging . . . . . . . . . . . . . . . . . . . . . . . . 195
10.4 Artificial Intelligence Techniques in Dental Applications . . . . . . . . . . . . . . . . . . . . . . . . . 197
10.4.1 Explainable artificial intelligence . . . . . . . . . . 198
10.4.2 The importance of artificial intelligence and explainable artificial intelligence in dental practices . . . . . . . . . . . . . . . . . . . . . . 200
10.5 Academic Studies in the Dentistry . . . . . . . . . . . . . . 201
10.6 Conclusion . . . . . . . . . . . . . . . . . . . . . . . . . . 203
References . . . . . . . . . . . . . . . . . . . . . . . . . . . . . 204

**11 Application of Explainable Artificial Intelligence in Drug Discovery and Drug Design** **213**
*Najam-ul-Lail, Iqra Muzammil, Muhammad Aamir Naseer, Iqra Tabussam, Sidra Muzmmal and Aqsa Muzammil*
11.1 Introduction . . . . . . . . . . . . . . . . . . . . . . . . . . 214
11.1.1 Drug discovery . . . . . . . . . . . . . . . . . . . 214
11.1.2 Explainable artificial intelligence . . . . . . . . . . 214
11.2 Deep Learning and Machine Learning . . . . . . . . . . . . 217
11.2.1 Support vector machines . . . . . . . . . . . . . . 219
11.2.2 Random forests . . . . . . . . . . . . . . . . . . . 220
11.2.3 *K*-nearest neighbor . . . . . . . . . . . . . . . . . 220
11.2.4 Naïve Bayes approach . . . . . . . . . . . . . . . 220
11.2.5 Restricted Boltzmann machine . . . . . . . . . . . 221
11.2.6 Deep belief networks . . . . . . . . . . . . . . . . 221
11.2.7 Conventional neural networks . . . . . . . . . . . 221
11.2.8 Advantages of deep learning . . . . . . . . . . . . 222
11.2.9 Limitations of deep learning . . . . . . . . . . . . 222
11.2.10 Neurosymbolic models . . . . . . . . . . . . . . . 222
11.2.11 Advances in XAI . . . . . . . . . . . . . . . . . . 225

11.2.12 Different XAI approaches that aid in drug discovery . . . . . 226
11.2.13 Limitations of XAI in drug discovery . . . . . . . 232
11.3 Conclusion . . . . . . . . . . . . . . . . . . . . 232
References . . . . . . . . . . . . . . . . . . . . . . 233

**12 Automatic Segmentation of Spinal Cord Gray Matter from MR Images using a U-Net Architecture 245**
*R. Polattimur and E. Dandil*
12.1 Introduction. . . . . . . . . . . . . . . . . . . . 246
12.2 Materials and Methods . . . . . . . . . . . . . . . 250
12.2.1 Spinal cord dataset . . . . . . . . . . . . . . 250
12.2.2 Dataset organization and image pre-processing . . 252
12.2.3 U-Net . . . . . . . . . . . . . . . . . . . . 252
12.3 Experimental Results. . . . . . . . . . . . . . . . 254
12.4 Conclusions and Discussions. . . . . . . . . . . . . 258
Acknowledgements . . . . . . . . . . . . . . . . . . . 260
References . . . . . . . . . . . . . . . . . . . . . . 260

**13 XAI for Drug Discovery 265**
*Ilhan Uysal and Utku Kose*
13.1 Introduction. . . . . . . . . . . . . . . . . . . . 265
13.2 Main Text. . . . . . . . . . . . . . . . . . . . . 268
13.2.1 The working principle of explainable artificial intelligence . . . . . . . . . . . . . . . . . 269
13.2.2 Current methods in the scope of explainable artificial intelligence . . . . . . . . . . . . . 270
13.2.3 Approaches in XAI with drug discovery . . . . . . 273
13.3 Conclusion . . . . . . . . . . . . . . . . . . . . 280
References . . . . . . . . . . . . . . . . . . . . . . 281

**14 Explainable Intelligence Enabled Smart Healthcare for Rural Communities 289**
*Soumyadeep Chanda, Rohan Kumar, Aditya Kumar Singh, and Sushruta Mishra*
14.1 Introduction. . . . . . . . . . . . . . . . . . . . 289
14.2 Relevant Models for Smart Rural Healthcare . . . . . . 291
14.2.1 An interpretable emergency ambulance response model . . . . . . . . . . . . . . . . . 291
14.2.2 An explainable farmer health insurance model. . . 295

14.2.3 A bridge between NGO and hospitals model. . . . 298
14.3 An Explainable AI Approach to Smart Rural Healthcare . . 303
14.4 Conclusion . . . . . . . . . . . . . . . . . . . . . . . . . . 304
References . . . . . . . . . . . . . . . . . . . . . . . . . . . 305

**15 Explainable Artificial Intelligence in Drug Discovery for Biomedical Applications 309**
*Godwin M. Ubi, Edu N. Eyogor, Hannah E. Etta, Nkese D. Okon, Effiom B. Ekeng, and Imabong S. Essien*
15.1 Introduction. . . . . . . . . . . . . . . . . . . . . . . . . . 310
15.2 Methodology . . . . . . . . . . . . . . . . . . . . . . . . . 311
15.2.1 Tramadol drug . . . . . . . . . . . . . . . . . . . 312
15.2.2 Cannabinol drug . . . . . . . . . . . . . . . . . . 318
15.2.3 Sildenafil (Viagra) drug. . . . . . . . . . . . . . . 319
15.2.4 Praziquantel drug . . . . . . . . . . . . . . . . . . 325
15.3 Discussion . . . . . . . . . . . . . . . . . . . . . . . . . . 329
15.4 Conclusion . . . . . . . . . . . . . . . . . . . . . . . . . . 330
Acknowledgements . . . . . . . . . . . . . . . . . . . . . . . 331
References . . . . . . . . . . . . . . . . . . . . . . . . . . . 331

**16 XAI in the Hybrid Classification of Brain MRI Tumor Images 337**
*S. Akça, F. Atban, Z. Garip, and E. Ekinci*
16.1 Introduction. . . . . . . . . . . . . . . . . . . . . . . . . . 338
16.2 Materials and Methods . . . . . . . . . . . . . . . . . . . . 340
16.2.1 Dataset . . . . . . . . . . . . . . . . . . . . . . . 340
16.2.2 Method . . . . . . . . . . . . . . . . . . . . . . . 340
16.3 Results . . . . . . . . . . . . . . . . . . . . . . . . . . . . 343
16.3.1 Performance metrics and confusion matrix . . . . 343
16.3.2 *K*-fold cross-validation . . . . . . . . . . . . . . . 345
16.3.3 Results of simulation . . . . . . . . . . . . . . . . 345
16.3.4 Discussions . . . . . . . . . . . . . . . . . . . . . 346
16.4 Conclusion . . . . . . . . . . . . . . . . . . . . . . . . . . 349
References . . . . . . . . . . . . . . . . . . . . . . . . . . . 349

**17 Comparative Analysis of Breast Cancer Diagnosis Driven by the Smart IoT-based Approach 353**
*Bhavya Mittal, Pranshu Sharma, Sushruta Mishra, and Sibanjan Das*
17.1 Introduction. . . . . . . . . . . . . . . . . . . . . . . . . . 354
17.1.1 Objective . . . . . . . . . . . . . . . . . . . . . . 356

17.2 Analysis of Computational Techniques for Breast Cancer Diagnosis using IoT . . . . . . . . . . . . . . . . . . . . . . . . 357
17.2.1 Smart breast cancer diagnosis using machine learning . . . . . . . . . . . . . . . . . . . . 357
17.2.2 A deeper analysis of how deep learning is a step ahead of machine learning . . . . . . . . . . . . . . 360
17.2.3 Breast cancer diagnosis using deep learning and IoT . . . . . . . . . . . . . . . . . . . . 362
17.2.4 Challenges of breast cancer diagnosis using modern techniques . . . . . . . . . . . . . . . . . . . 365
17.2.5 Future scope and application . . . . . . . . . . . . 365
17.3 Conclusion . . . . . . . . . . . . . . . . . . . . . . . . . . . 370
Acknowledgements . . . . . . . . . . . . . . . . . . . . . . . . . 371
References . . . . . . . . . . . . . . . . . . . . . . . . . . . . . 371

**Index** **375**

**About the Editors** **379**

# Preface

In the 21st century, so far, biomedical applications have been in a great momentum, thanks to the use of advanced technology. Here, the use of artificial intelligence models has a remarkable role to advance the outputs in terms of different tasks such as medical inferencing, diagnosis, and treatment planning. When it is evaluated from the variety of successful tasks, artificial intelligence is already an effective decision support tool for doctors, medical staff, and researchers. That situation is associated with intense developments, which are done often in the intersection of artificial intelligence and biomedical. Even early applications of intelligent systems were done for biomedical problems at first. So, more steps were taken for improving capabilities of artificial intelligence in analyzing biomedical data and solving the corresponding cases. As a result, current intelligent system applications are often associated with comparing machine and human limitations. It is known that today's intelligent systems ensure competitive findings when compared with human touches. Especially difficult tasks such as early diagnosis, prognosis, precision treatment, and drug design often receive revolutionary and promising results from the side of artificial intelligence.

Although technological developments are excellent for artificial intelligence usage in biomedical, there is the issue that today's intelligent systems go beyond the human capabilities. That means we are no longer able to track the mechanisms shaping the output results by analyzing the input variables. As long as deep learning models or hybrid machine learning formations require many parameters for success, it is almost impossible to have interpretable reasons for how these models can create a relation between input data and output decisions. At this point, it is not possible to detect failure and success points of intelligent systems. Being known as black box, such type of intelligent systems cannot be used directly without understanding their safety level. So, such black-box systems should not be accepted as trustworthy until some solutions may be used to solve the issue. Nowadays, explainable artificial intelligence (XAI) is a trendy solution to ensure explainability for black-box models, which are associated with especially deep learning. Of course, the interpretability in white-box machine learning techniques is now more important when alternative solutions for trustworthy intelligent systems are thought.

The objective of this edited book is to provide the latest advancements in terms of XAI in biomedical applications. Intense consideration was given to employ the most recent research results by covering as much different topics as possible under the umbrella of biomedical field. A remarkable focus was also given to have alternative reviews for present and future state of XAI applications in the context of biomedical problems. Because there are also different solution methods for achieving explainability, the book had a careful selection for informing the audience about the variety of XAI methods. Not only including the XAI but also recalling the interpretable methods, the book hosts a total of 17 chapters targeting XAI use cases in specific problem areas. Contributions by each chapter are as follows.

Chapter 1 focuses on the diagnosis of gastric cancer by using a hybrid-network-based model. In detail, the exact mechanism of the model was analyzed, thanks to the SHAP analysis in the context of XAI research.

Chapter 2 considers another XAI method, LIME, to examine the disease diagnosis. It provides a general overview and examines the research flows in terms of applying and understanding the LIME method for diagnosis cases.

Chapter 3 ensures a review work by considering the XAI usage in veterinary and animal science field. It comes with a remarkable content by touching the animal sciences and showing the need for XAI from the veterinaries' perspective and the corresponding research topics.

Chapter 4 aims to examine a recent massive health issue: the corona virus. In this context, it provides an interpretable analysis for the potential impact of different versions of corona virus.

Chapter 5 comes with a deep review of XAI usage in biomedical applications. It hosts detailed explanations for different XAI methods and solutions with perspectives on present and future potentials.

Chapter 6 targets its research way in the survival of heart failure patients. As associated with the XAI, it considers the prediction capabilities of iterative learning by running factor analysis with the SHAP method.

Chapter 7 considers another important XAI method, CAM, for the research on deep learning for image-based data. In detail, it provides a general overview for the CAM usage and also discusses the use cases in alternative XAI solutions as well.

Chapter 8 provides a remarkable perspective on the usage of IoT in healthcare applications. The coverage of the chapter is with establishing the security with the XAI perspective.

Chapter 9 is another work associated with medical image data. It generally considers the chest disease identification from X-rays and focuses on the usage of deep learning.

Chapter 10 ensures another remarkable review of XAI, by considering dentistry as the target area. As it is critical to have the XAI touch in especially image data, the chapter achieves a timely theoretical examination for the literature of artificial intelligence applied in dentistry.

Chapter 11 hits a critical research topic, drug discovery, in the view of XAI solutions. In this context, it ensures a deep review of the research efforts for explainable drug discovery and design applications, which are supported by XAI.

Chapter 12 considers an automatic segmentation method for the spinal cord gray matter from MR image data. It employs the remarkable U-Net model for the problem solution.

Chapter 13 provides another review of drug discovery, by considering the XAI usage. It mostly considers alternative use cases of XAI for ensuring successful and trustworthy drug discovery efforts.

Chapter 14 considers a massive perspective in the context of smart healthcare services. At this point, it provides a recent view on XAI usage in the applications regarding the rural community.

Chapter 15 comes with an alternative review for XAI usage in drug discovery research. By giving an importance to the molecular inputs, it is another chapter to hit that critical research topic from the perspective of XAI.

Chapter 16 is based on research regarding classification of brain tumor images through a hybrid deep/machine learning model and alternative machine learning techniques. In detail, it considers the use of Grad-CAM for XAI purposes.

Chapter 17 recalls the IoT-based applications and focuses on the breast cancer diagnosis. In detail, it provides a remarkable comparative work.

As it may be seen, the book rises over different research orientations to understand more about the scope of XAI for better, trustworthy biomedical applications. We believe that all chapters will be useful for researchers, professionals, and degree students for understanding essentials of XAI, and the application ways for biomedical problems.

As the editors, we would like to thank all respectful authors for their valuable contributions. Our special thanks go to Prof. Omer Deperlioglu (from Afyon Kocatepe University, Turkey) for his kind foreword. Finally, we are grateful to the readers and looking forward to receiving their feedback for the book. In this context, any ideas for further projects are welcome, too.

*Editors*
**Dr. Utku Kose**
**Dr. Deepak Gupta**
**Dr. Xi Chen**

# Foreword

In the field of biomedical, artificial intelligence has a great role in technological advancements. The use of intelligent algorithms allows us to improve known results and solve the most competitive problems associated with tasks such as diagnosis, treatment, and drug discovery. The latest research shows that the effective use of deep learning models achieves better findings when compared with humans. It is good to have automated solutions for saving time, saving costs, and building careful decision support for the human side. However, more advanced use of artificial intelligence causes them to be black box because we need more parameters to be optimized for better findings. That is a problem as we do not have any idea about inside mechanisms of such intelligent systems and we should still trust artificial intelligence in risky biomedical cases. Although there is a strong relation between artificial intelligence and biomedical, black-box state is a threating factor for the future advancements. As a chance, the scientific audience was not silent for this and XAI (explainable artificial intelligence) was introduced in order to integrate explainability components for tracking input–output relations.

According to me, XAI should be among essential requirements for building trustworthy intelligent systems. That is more critical when we think about using intelligent systems for biomedical cases. When we examine the literature, it may be seen that different medical data types can be analyzed through different methods such as CAM, LIME, and SHAP. As long as we take the support from mathematical and logical background for creating observable data relations, the XAI literature will host many alternative methods. That is just a matter of time according to human requirements for safe smart tools. So, there is a need for intense reviews of XAI-biomedical research, regarding the latest advancements and even future perspectives.

This edited book titled as *Explainable Artificial Intelligence (XAI) for Biomedical Applications* is a timely contribution as the field of biomedical needs a direct focus on how we can run XAI in different biomedical topics. As we know, there is a great variety of research topics in the context of biomedical field. From that perspective, this book comes with a remarkable collection of 17 chapters including different solution tasks such as diagnosis, image analysis, and data discovery. It is great to see that the book also hosts critical reviews and targets specific problem areas such as dentistry, animal sciences, and IoT use cases. It is also nice to see that the chapters were carefully gathered to discuss different, recent XAI methods used in biomedical problem areas. Each chapter has pure language to reflect the necessary knowledge to the target audience. I believe the book will be a valuable reference for not only researchers but also degree students.

As my final words, I would like to express my sincere thanks to the valuable editors: Dr. Utku Kose, Dr. Deepak Gupta, and Dr. Xi Chen. Without their efforts, such a timely contribution would not be possible. All the best for a "healthy future" with safe employment of artificial intelligence!

**Dr. Omer Deperlioglu**
*Afyon Kocatepe University, Turkey*
deperlioglu@aku.edu.tr

# Acknowledgement

As the editors, we would like to thank all valuable River Publishers staff, and especially Junko Nakajima, Rajeev Prasad, and Nicki Dennis for their kind support for realizing such a timely book project.

*Editors*
**Dr. Utku Kose**
**Dr. Deepak Gupta**
**Dr. Xi Chen**

# List of Contributors

**Akça, S.,** *Sakarya University of Applied Sciences, Turkey*

**Aksoy, B.,** *Isparta University of Applied Sciences, Turkey*

**Anand, Yash,** *Kalinga Institute of Industrial Technology, India*

**Aqib, Amjad Islam,** *Cholistan University of Veterinary and Animal Sciences, Pakistan*

**Arslan, Muhammad,** *Cholistan University of Veterinary and Animal Sciences, Pakistan*

**Atban, F.,** *Sakarya University of Applied Sciences, Turkey*

**Atta, Khazeena,** *University of Veterinary and Animal Sciences, Pakistan*

**Bhatia, Ashima Bhatnagar,** *Vivekananda Institute of Professional Studies, Pakistan*

**Chanda, Soumyadeep,** *Kalinga Institute of Industrial Technology, India*

**Çifci, A.,** *Burdur Mehmet Akif Ersoy University, Turkey*

**Dandıl, E.,** *Bilecik Seyh Edebali University, Turkey*

**Das, Sibanjan,** *Kalinga Institute of Industrial Technology, India*

**Ekeng, Effiom B.,** *University of Calabar, Nigeria*

**Ekinci, E.,** *Sakarya University of Applied Sciences, Turkey*

**Essien, Imabong S.,** *University of Calabar, Nigeria*

**Etta, Hannah E.,** *University of Calabar, Nigeria*

**Eylence, M.,** *Isparta University of Applied Sciences, Turkey*

**Eyogor, Edu N.,** *University of Calabar, Nigeria*

**Fatima, Mahreen,** *Cholistan University of Veterinary and Animal Sciences, Pakistan*

**Garip, Z.,** *Sakarya University of Applied Sciences, Turkey*

**Hacibeyoglu, M.,** *Necmettin Erbakan University, Turkey*

**İlkuçar, M.,** *Muğla Sıtkı Koçman University, Turkey*

**Jayanthi, Prisilla,** *KG Reddy College of Engineering and Technology, India*

**Kasyap, Varanasi L. V. S. K. B.,** *VIT-AP University, India*

**Kırbaş, İ.,** *Burdur Mehmet Akif Ersoy University, Turkey*

**Kırboğa, K. K.,** *Bilecik Seyh Edebali University, Turkey*

**Kose, Utku,** *Suleyman Demirel University, Turkey*

**Küçüksille, E. U.,** *Suleyman Demirel University, Turkey*

**Kumar, Ambeshwar,** *Dayananda Sagar University, India*

**Kumar, Rohan,** *Kalinga Institute of Industrial Technology, India*

**Manikandan, R.,** *SASTRA Deemed University, India*

**Mishra, Sushruta,** *Kalinga Institute of Industrial Technology, India*

**Mitra, Adrija,** *Kalinga Institute of Industrial Technology, India*

**Mittal, Bhavya,** *Kalinga Institute of Industrial Technology, India*

**Muneer, Afshan,** *Cholistan University of Veterinary and Animal Sciences, Pakistan*

**Muneer, Sadia,** *University of Agriculture, Pakistan*

**Muralikrishna, Iyyanki,** *Administrative Staff College of India, India*

**Murtaza, Maheen,** *Cholistan University of Veterinary and Animal Sciences, Pakistan*

**Muzammil, Aqsa,** *Islamia University, Pakistan*

**Muzammil, Iqra,** *University of Veterinary and Animal Sciences, Pakistan*

**Muzmmal, Sidra,** *Islamia University, Pakistan*

**Najam-ul-Lail,** *University of Veterinary and Animal Sciences, Pakistan*

**Naseer, Muhammad Aamir,** *University of Agriculture, Pakistan*

**Natarajan, Karthika,** *VIT-AP University, India*

**Okon, Nkese D.,** *University of Calabar, Nigeria*

**Özmen, M. M.,** *Isparta University of Applied Sciences, Turkey*

**Polattimur, R.,** *Bilecik Seyh Edebali University, Turkey*

**Salman, O. K. M.,** *Isparta University of Applied Sciences, Turkey*

**Sayın, H.,** *Isparta University of Applied Sciences, Turkey*

**Sharma, Pranshu,** *Kalinga Institute of Industrial Technology, India*

**Singh, Aditya Kumar,** *Kalinga Institute of Industrial Technology, India*

**Sumathi, D.,** *VIT-AP University, India*

**Surendhar S., Prasath Alias,** *Aarupadai Veedu Institute of Technology, India*

**Tabussam, Iqra,** *University of Agriculture, Pakistan*

**Terzi, M. S.,** *Necmettin Erbakan University, Turkey*

**Ubi, Godwin M.,** *University of Calabar, and Biggmade Scientific Research Academy, Nigeria*

**Uysal, Ilhan,** *Burdur Mehmet Akif Ersoy University, Turkey*

**Whig, Pawan,** *Vivekananda Institute of Professional Studies, Pakistan*

**Yücel, M.,** *Isparta University of Applied Sciences, Turkey*

**Zaheer, C-Neen Fatima,** *University of Agriculture, Pakistan*

# List of Figures

| | | |
|---|---|---|
| **Figure 1.1** | XAI model. | 4 |
| **Figure 1.2** | XAI taxonomy. | 5 |
| **Figure 1.3** | The architecture of the MSN module. | 8 |
| **Figure 1.4** | The gastric images and non-gastric cancer images, along with the corresponding generated heat maps. | 10 |
| **Figure 1.5** | The architectural framework of the proposed deep learning model. | 11 |
| **Figure 1.6** | Diagnostic performance of the proposed model at various magnification rates in training and validation phases. | 12 |
| **Figure 2.1** | XAI relationship with AI.. | 18 |
| **Figure 2.2** | Various methods of XAI. | 19 |
| **Figure 2.3** | The flowchart of the proposed algorithm – ANFIS-GA. | 20 |
| **Figure 2.4** | ML life-cycle in conjunction with XAI. | 21 |
| **Figure 2.5(a)** | Explanations generated by LIME. | 21 |
| **Figure 2.5(b)** | Explanations generated by SHAP. | 22 |
| **Figure 2.6** | (a) Original image. (b) Eye-tracker. (c) GRAD-CAM. (d) SIDU. | 23 |
| **Figure 2.7** | The output of the prediction of COVID-19 data of eight states. | 24 |
| **Figure 2.8** | Local explanation of the LIME method. | 24 |
| **Figure 2.9** | Explanation and binary regression for COVID. | 25 |
| **Figure 2.10** | Interpretation of LIME. | 26 |
| **Figure 2.11** | Local explanation.. | 26 |
| **Figure 2.12** | Interpretation of air pollution using LIME.. | 27 |
| **Figure 2.13** | Interpretation of the prediction of breast cancer. | 28 |
| **Figure 2.14** | Multiclassification of ECG using LIME. | 29 |

**Figure 3.1** Scope of explainable artificial intelligence in different fields NLP(natural language process) for classification and text summarization, Engineering could be used to find cause and prediction of any project , in medical and defence could be sed for CT scan brain and lungs tumor diagnosis and in threat monitoring respectively. . . . . . . . . . . . . . . 35
**Figure 3.2** Maintaining milk quality by XAI: XAI machines has many operational programs in livestock management such as monitoring dairy management increasing milk production, production on the farm and diagnosis diseases. . . . . . . . . . . . . . . . . . . 40
**Figure 3.3** Milking platform Automatic milking system(AMS): In addition to milk yield and composition, the frequency and intervals of milking determine the SCC and bacteriological characteristics of the milk, which are influenced by many factors. In addition, AMS equipment allows large amounts of data to be recorded about individual cows and herd performance. . . . . . . . . . . . . . . . . . . . . . 41
**Figure 3.4** Detecting feeding behavior through the intelligence method: A time sequence model and audio analysis can be used to detect changes in eating vocalizations based on differences between eating and normal vocalizations of poultry.. . . . . . . . . . . . . . . . 44
**Figure 4.1** Different versions of corona viruses. . . . . . . . . . 58
**Figure 4.2** Modification in SARS-CoV-2. . . . . . . . . . . . . 59
**Figure 4.3** Flowchart of the machine learning model. . . . . . . 60
**Figure 4.4** Multiclass classification. . . . . . . . . . . . . . . . 61
**Figure 4.5** One vs all model. . . . . . . . . . . . . . . . . . . . 62
**Figure 4.6** Chained multi-output regression. . . . . . . . . . . . 63
**Figure 4.7** Hybrid models. . . . . . . . . . . . . . . . . . . . . 65
**Figure 4.8** Various sentiment analysis techniques. . . . . . . . . 66
**Figure 4.9** Sentiment analysis representation. . . . . . . . . . . 68
**Figure 4.10** Sentiment analysis case study. . . . . . . . . . . . . 68
**Figure 4.11** Number of tweet counts by dates. . . . . . . . . . . 70
**Figure 4.12** Frequency of tweets by hour. . . . . . . . . . . . . . 71
**Figure 4.13** Frequency of tweets by country. . . . . . . . . . . . 71
**Figure 4.14** Positive tweet analysis using word cloud. . . . . . . 72
**Figure 4.15** Negative tweet analysis using world cloud.. . . . . . 72

**Figure 4.16** Comparison of positive tweets using various classifiers.. . . . . . . . . . . . . . . . . . . . . 73
**Figure 4.17** Comparison of negative tweets using various classifiers.. . . . . . . . . . . . . . . . . . . . . 73
**Figure 5.1** XAI methods and use in the biomedical field. . . . . 81
**Figure 5.2** The experiment with image ablation (upper) and word ablation (below). The first row of image ablation displays visual explanations of the word hydrant, while the second row displays masked regions with high relevance scores.. . . . . . . . . . 85
**Figure 5.3** (a) Attention, Grad-CAM, guided Grad-CAM (G.Grad-CAM), and LRP image explanations of the words hydrant (first row) and grass (second row). (b) For each word in the expected caption, the linguistic explanations of LRP. Blue and red colors, respectively, indicate negative and positive relevance scores.. . . . . . . . . . . . . . . . . . . . . . . . . . 86
**Figure 5.4** In a Venn diagram, an overview of challenges and future potential is presented [26].. . . . . . . . . . . 86
**Figure 5.5** An overview of the interpretability of mathematical structures. (a) Easy-to-understand modeling, such as linear models, helps improve interpretability. (b) Feature extraction. In comprehensions that require mathematical knowledge, the data and parameters in the model are transformed and selectively selected. (c) Sensitivity. It serves to explain how different data are represented differently. In the figure, the transformation of bird to duck can be traced using clustering [26]. . . . . . . . . . . . . . . . . . . . . 87
**Figure 5.6** (a1) With the TCAV [27] method, a hyperplane CAV that separates the target concepts from each other can be found. (a2) The CAV accuracies applied to different layers and the content of the concepts involved in deep and shallow layers are shown. (b) SVCCA finds the concept of the subspace most meaningful and contains the most information. (c) t-SNE organizes dog images in a meaningful way.. . . . . . . . . . . . . . . . . . 88
**Figure 5.7** Biological quality metrics' importance in determining each gene–gene connection's functional significance was revealed. . . . . . . . . . . . . . . . . . . . 89

**Figure 5.8** The stack-ensemble model's breakdown plots for (a) Summit County, Utah, and (b) Union County, Florida. . . . . . . . . . . . . . . . . . . . . . . . 90
**Figure 5.9** The impact of (a) smoking, (b) poverty, (c) elevation, (d) white population, (e) Hispanic population, and (f) PM2.5 on the prediction of LBC mortality rates vary by location. Stack-ensemble models' "breakdown plots" were used to calculate the contribution of risk factors in each county.. . . . . . . . . . . . . . 91
**Figure 5.10** A wound classification model may be created with DNN, transfer learning, and an explainable AI tool. . 93
**Figure 6.1** Block diagram of our framework.. . . . . . . . . . . 107
**Figure 6.2** ANN structure. . . . . . . . . . . . . . . . . . . . . . . 109
**Figure 6.3** A node structure. . . . . . . . . . . . . . . . . . . . . 109
**Figure 6.4** Transfer functions. (a) Sigmoid. (b) Hyperbolic tangent. (c) ReLu.. . . . . . . . . . . . . . . . . . . . 110
**Figure 6.5** Flowchart of the modeling development process. . . 111
**Figure 6.6** Validation and training graph for network structure with hidden layer node number 1. . . . . . . . . . . 113
**Figure 6.7** ANN training performance graphics. (a) Accuracy. (b) Loss function. (c) Validation. . . . . . . . . . . . 114
**Figure 6.8** Feature importance based on SHAP values. (a) Mean absolute SHAP values. (b) SHAP summary plot for ANN model trained on the heart failure dataset. . . . 115
**Figure 6.9** SHAP waterfall plot for ANN model trained on the heart failure dataset.. . . . . . . . . . . . . . . . . . 116
**Figure 7.1** Relationship between explainable Machine learning and Deep Learning. . . . . . . . . . . . . . . . . . . 127
**Figure 8.1** IoT in healthcare market size, by component, 2014–2025 (USD Billion) (data missing). . . . . . . 146
**Figure 8.2** Working of block-chain. . . . . . . . . . . . . . . . . . 151
**Figure 8.3** Framework for IoT block-chain system. . . . . . . . 153
**Figure 8.4** Interface of the block-chain-based IoT healthcare system. . . . . . . . . . . . . . . . . . . . . . . . . . . 154
**Figure 8.5** Framework of access control system based on deep learning. . . . . . . . . . . . . . . . . . . . . . . 158
**Figure 9.1** A CNN architecture composed of input, one convolutional layer, one pooling layer, and one fully connected layer and output.. . . . . . . . . . . . . . . 172
**Figure 9.2** A sample kernel of size 3 × 3. . . . . . . . . . . . . 172
**Figure 9.3** Convolution process and feature maps.. . . . . . . . . 173

**Figure 9.4** Activation functions for CNN. . . . . . . . . . . . . . 174
**Figure 9.5** Max pooling and average pooling. . . . . . . . . . . 175
**Figure 9.6** Loss functions for CNN. . . . . . . . . . . . . . . . . 175
**Figure 9.7** Optimizers for CNN. . . . . . . . . . . . . . . . . . . 176
**Figure 9.8** Multi-label images in each of the 14 pathology classes. . . . . . . . . . . . . . . . . . . . . . . . 177
**Figure 9.9** The developed CNN model. . . . . . . . . . . . . . 180
**Figure 9.10** The architecture of the developed CNN model. . . . 181
**Figure 9.11** Performance criteria. . . . . . . . . . . . . . . . . . 181
**Figure 9.12** Training loss and accuracy convergence graphic.. . . 182
**Figure 9.13** The results of developed CNN on the basis of disease classes. . . . . . . . . . . . . . . . . . . . 182
**Figure 9.14** The comparison of the developed CNN with VGG-16 and ResNet-152. . . . . . . . . . . . . . . 183
**Figure 9.15** The comparison of the developed CNN with studies in the literature. . . . . . . . . . . . . . . . 183
**Figure 10.1** Periapical and panographic radiography images.. . . 191
**Figure 10.2** X-ray image of the hand of Wilhelm Conrad Rontgen's wife, Anna Bertha, captured by himself.. . . . . . . . 194
**Figure 10.3** Sample of a head X-ray.. . . . . . . . . . . . . . . . 195
**Figure 10.4** Example X-ray images. (a) Spinal cord. (b) Tooth. (c) Hand. . . . . . . . . . . . . . . . . . . . . . . 195
**Figure 10.5** Artificial intelligence sub-branches. . . . . . . . . . 198
**Figure 10.6** Example of GRAD-CAM model.. . . . . . . . . . . 200
**Figure 11.1** Drug discovery without explainable artificial intelligence.. . . . . . . . . . . . . . . . . . . . . . 218
**Figure 11.2** Drug discovery with explainable artificial intelligence.. . . . . . . . . . . . . . . . . . . . . . 218
**Figure 11.3** The framework of artificial intelligence. . . . . . . . 220
**Figure 11.4** Uses of explainable artificial intelligence in drug discovery. . . . . . . . . . . . . . . . . . . . . . . 226
**Figure 12.1** (a) MR image obtained from the axial plane of the cervical region of the spinal cord. (b) GM and WM regions of the spinal cord with 4× zooming of the cross-sectional area.. . . . . . . . . . . . . . . . . 246
**Figure 12.2** The methodology of the proposed U-Net deep learning architecture for spinal cord GM segmentation on MR images. . . . . . . . . . . . . 250
**Figure 12.3** Spinal cord GM MR images obtained from four different data centers (sites) in the SCGMC dataset and ground truth masks of four different raters. . . . 251

**Figure 12.4** (a) GM MR images of the spinal cord in SCGMC dataset and (a1) their ground truth masks, (b) GM MR images of the spinal cord with crop and resizing after image pre-processing and (b1) their ground truth masks. . . . . . . . . . . . . . . . . . . . . . . . 253
**Figure 12.5** The architecture of the U-Net deep learning network used in this study for automatic segmentation of the spinal cord GM.. . . . . . . . . . . . . . . . . . . . . 254
**Figure 12.6** Graph of change of training/validation accuracy and training/validation loss values of U-Net model for 100 epochs. . . . . . . . . . . . . . . . . . . . . . . . 256
**Figure 12.7** Some successfully segmented MR slices in the dataset using the U-Net deep learning architecture in this study. (a) MR image. (b) Ground truth. (c) U-Net segmentation.. . . . . . . . . . . . . . . . . 257
**Figure 12.8** Some slices of the spinal cord GM region that was not fully segmented in experimental studies. . . . . . 259
**Figure 13.1** The relationship between artificial intelligence, machine learning, deep learning, and explainable artificial intelligence. . . . . . . . . . . . . . . . . . . . 267
**Figure 13.2** Resolution process of XAI systems. . . . . . . . . . 269
**Figure 13.3** Comparison between CAM and MultiCAM. . . . . . 271
**Figure 13.4** The LIME method. . . . . . . . . . . . . . . . . . . 271
**Figure 13.5** The SHAP method. . . . . . . . . . . . . . . . . . . 272
**Figure 13.6** Approaches in XAI with drug discovery. . . . . . . . 274
**Figure 13.7** The feature attribution methods. . . . . . . . . . . . 275
**Figure 13.8** The instance-based methods. . . . . . . . . . . . . . 276
**Figure 13.9** The graph-convolution-based methods.. . . . . . . . 277
**Figure 13.10** The uncertainty estimation method. . . . . . . . . . 279
**Figure 14.1** Analysis of rural healthcare monitoring. . . . . . . . 293
**Figure 14.2** Flow diagram of emergency ambulance response model. . . . . . . . . . . . . . . . . . . . . . 294
**Figure 14.3** Comparison between the types of illness and days spent in hospital. . . . . . . . . . . . . . . . . . . . . 297
**Figure 14.4** Shortage of medical staff in rural areas. . . . . . . . 297
**Figure 14.5** Digitization in rural India. . . . . . . . . . . . . . . 299
**Figure 14.6** Graph comparing the treatment of urban and rural residents. . . . . . . . . . . . . . . . . . . . . . . 300
**Figure 14.7** Graph showing Indian ambulance service market size, by region, and by value. . . . . . . . . . . . . . 301
**Figure 14.8** Flow diagram for the working of the toll-free number model. . . . . . . . . . . . . . . . . . . . . . . 302

| | | |
|---|---|---|
| **Figure 14.9** | Generating insights using XAI and clinical expertise. | 304 |
| **Figure 15.1** | Showing chemical structure of Tramadol drug.. | 312 |
| **Figure 15.2** | Showing interactions of major and minor genes with tramadol drug via XAI. | 313 |
| **Figure 15.3** | Showing alternatives drugs interactions with same major and minor genes as tramadol via XAI.. | 314 |
| **Figure 15.4** | Protein structure of CYP206 major gene.. | 314 |
| **Figure 15.5** | Protein structure of OPKR1 major gene. | 314 |
| **Figure 15.6** | Protein structure of OPRM1 major gene.. | 315 |
| **Figure 15.7** | Chemical structure of Endomorphin – 2 drug as alternative to tramadol drug. | 315 |
| **Figure 15.8** | Chemical structure of Risperidine drug as alternative to tramadol drug. | 315 |
| **Figure 15.9** | Chemical structure of Carfentanil drug as alternative to tramadol drug. | 316 |
| **Figure 15.10** | Chemical structure of cannabinol drug.. | 316 |
| **Figure 15.11** | Showing interactions of major and minor genes with cannabinol drug via XAI. | 316 |
| **Figure 15.12** | Showing alternatives drugs interactions with same major and minor genes as cannabinol via XAI.. | 317 |
| **Figure 15.13** | Protein structure of CD5 major gene.. | 317 |
| **Figure 15.14** | Protein structure of CNR1 minor gene.. | 318 |
| **Figure 15.15** | Protein structure of CNR2 minor gene.. | 318 |
| **Figure 15.16** | Chemical structure of Sildenafil drug. | 319 |
| **Figure 15.17** | Showing interactions of major and minor genes with Sildenafil drug via XAI.. | 320 |
| **Figure 15.18** | Showing alternatives drugs interactions with same major and minor genes as Sildenafil drug via XAI. | 320 |
| **Figure 15.19** | Protein structure of NOS1 major gene. | 321 |
| **Figure 15.20** | Protein structure of CYP34A major gene. | 322 |
| **Figure 15.21** | Protein structure of PRKG1 major gene. | 322 |
| **Figure 15.22** | Protein structure of ALDH7A1 major gene. | 323 |
| **Figure 15.23** | Protein structure of PDE4B major gene. | 323 |
| **Figure 15.24** | Protein structure of NOS3 major gene. | 324 |
| **Figure 15.25** | Chemical structure of Tadalafil drug. | 324 |
| **Figure 15.26** | Chemical structure of Verdanafil drug. | 325 |
| **Figure 15.27** | Chemical structure of Praziquantel drug.. | 325 |
| **Figure 15.28** | Showing interactions of major and minor genes with Praziquantel drug via XAI. | 326 |
| **Figure 15.29** | Showing alternatives drugs interactions with same major and minor genes as Praziquantel drug via XAI. | 327 |

| | | |
|---|---|---|
| **Figure 15.30** | Protein structure of DNAI2 major gene. | 327 |
| **Figure 15.31** | Protein structure of EPGN major gene.. | 327 |
| **Figure 15.32** | Protein structure of FBRS major gene. | 328 |
| **Figure 15.33** | Protein structure of ALGI1 major gene. | 328 |
| **Figure 15.34** | Chemical structure of GDP - mannose drug. | 328 |
| **Figure 15.35** | Chemical structure of MgATP drug. | 328 |
| **Figure 15.36** | Chemical structure of uridine diphosphate drug. | 329 |
| **Figure 16.1** | Brain tumor dataset classes. (a) Glioma. (b) Meningioma. (c) Pituitary. (d) Healthy.. | 341 |
| **Figure 16.2** | Glinoma class images. (a) Axial. (b) Coronal. (c) Sagittal. | 341 |
| **Figure 16.3** | Proposed VGG-16 architecture.. | 342 |
| **Figure 16.4** | Implementing Grad-CAM for glioma class label. | 343 |
| **Figure 16.5** | Grad-CAM for brain MRI images. (a) Glinomo class images. (b) Block 3 Conv 5 layer Grad-CAM-glinoma. (c) Glinoma tumor Grad-CAM heat map. (d) Meningioma class images. (e) Block 3 Conv 5 layer Grad-CAM-meningioma. (f) Meningioma tumor Grad-CAM heat map. (g) Pituitary class images. (h) Block 3 Conv 5 layer Grad-CAM-pituitary. (i) Pituitary tumor Grad-CAM heat map.. | 344 |
| **Figure 16.6** | Five-fold cross-validation. | 345 |
| **Figure 16.7** | Accuracy for each model. (a) LR. (b) Linear SVM. (c) KNN. (d) DT. (e) RF. (f) AdaBoost. (g) Gaussian NB. (h) Bernoulli NB. (i) MLP.. | 346 |
| **Figure 16.8** | Confusion matrix for ML algorithms. (a) LR. (b) Linear SVM. (c) KNN. (d) DT. (e) RF. (f) AdaBoost. (g) Gaussian NB. (h) Bernoulli NB. (i) MLP. | 348 |
| **Figure 17.1** | Stages in diagnosis of breast cancer using machine learning.. | 355 |
| **Figure 17.2** | Architecture model for breast cancer classification. | 358 |
| **Figure 17.3** | A classic machine learning based system. | 359 |
| **Figure 17.4** | Mean value cases.. | 360 |
| **Figure 17.5** | Worst feature cases.. | 361 |
| **Figure 17.6** | Breast cancer diagnosis with deep learning. | 362 |
| **Figure 17.7** | CNN algorithm in deep learning for breast cancer diagnosis. | 363 |
| **Figure 17.8** | CNN architecture.. | 364 |
| **Figure 17.9** | Images (data) for the diagnosis.. | 364 |
| **Figure 17.10** | Negative and positive images of a patient's data.. | 365 |

# List of Tables


**Table 1.1** Pipeline of the In-Net module. . . . . . . . . . . . . . 9
**Table 1.2** Comparison of the patch-based ACA in various models. . . . . . . . . . . . . . . . . . . . . . 11
**Table 1.3** Comparison of the slice-based ACA in various models. . . . . . . . . . . . . . . . . . . . . . 12
**Table 2.1** List of pollutant industries in Tamil Nadu (2021). . . 27
**Table 4.1** Statistical analysis of data. . . . . . . . . . . . . . . . 72
**Table 6.1** Description of each feature.. . . . . . . . . . . . . . . 106
**Table 6.2** Correlation matrix for features.. . . . . . . . . . . . . 108
**Table 6.3** Test accuracy rates for hidden layer nodes.. . . . . . . 113
**Table 6.4** Test confusion matrix. . . . . . . . . . . . . . . . . . 114
**Table 6.5** Comparison of results on the heart failure dataset. . . . . . . . . . . . . . . . . . . . . . . . . 117
**Table 10.1** Research trends on artificial intelligence in dentistry by years.. . . . . . . . . . . . . . . . . . . . 201
**Table 12.1** Hardware specifications of the computer used for experimental studies in this study. . . . . . . . . . . 255
**Table 12.2** Results of DSC, JSI, TPR, TNR, and PPV metrics obtained for the proposed U-Net deep learning model on MR slices in the test set for 100 epochs in experimental studies. . . . . . . . . . . . . . . . . . 258
**Table 12.3** Comparison of DSC scores obtained on the SCGMC dataset. . . . . . . . . . . . . . . . . . . 260
**Table 14.1** Comparison of the current and the proposed model.. . . . . . . . . . . . . . . . . . . . . 292
**Table 15.1** Major and minor genes affected by Tramadol and alternative drugs. . . . . . . . . . . . . . . . . . . . 313
**Table 15.2** Major and minor genes affected by Cannabinol and alternative drugs. . . . . . . . . . . . . . . . . . . . 319
**Table 15.3** Major and minor genes affected by Sildenafil and alternative drugs. . . . . . . . . . . . . . . . . . . . 321

**Table 15.4** Major and minor genes affected by Praziquantel and alternative drugs. . . . . . . . . . . . . . . . . . . . . . 326
**Table 16.1** Comparison of performance metrics of ML algorithms. . . . . . . . . . . . . . . . . . . . . . . . . 347
**Table 17.1** Comparison of various machine techniques. . . . . . 366
**Table 17.2** Comprehensive review of the machine techniques.. . 368

# List of Abbreviations

| | |
|---|---|
| **ACA** | Average classification accuracy |
| **AD** | Alzheimer's disease |
| **Ada-WHIPS** | Adaptive weighted high-importance path particles |
| **ADMET** | Absorption, distribution, metabolism, excretion, toxicity |
| **ADT** | Android development tools |
| **AES** | Advanced Encryption Standard |
| **AF** | Atrial fibrillation |
| **AG** | Atrophic gastritis |
| **AI** | Artificial intelligence |
| **AIM** | Artificial intelligence in medicine |
| **ALS** | Amyotrophic lateral sclerosis |
| **ANFIS** | Adaptive neuro fuzzy inference system |
| **ANN** | Artificial neural Networks |
| **AUC** | Area under the curve |
| **BC** | Block-chain |
| **BPH** | Benign prostatic hyperplasia |
| **BPL** | Below the poverty line |
| **C** | Convolutional layer |
| **CAD** | Computer-aided diagnostics |
| **CAM** | Class activation mapping |
| **CART** | Classification and regression tree |
| **CASP** | Computer-aided synthetic planning |
| **CAV** | Concept activation vector |
| **CBCT** | Cone beam computed tomography |
| **CBN** | Cannabinol |
| **CEM** | Contrastive explanation method |
| **CFS** | Correlation-based feature selection |
| **CIA** | Confidentiality integrity availability |
| **CNN** | Convolutional neural network |
| **CNS** | Central nervous system |
| **COVID-19** | Corona virus disease 2019 |
| **CPK** | Creatinine phosphokinase |

| | |
|---|---|
| **CSPs** | Cloud service providers |
| **CT** | Computed tomography |
| **DAE** | Deep auto-encoder |
| **DBNs** | Deep belief networks |
| **DeepLIFT** | Deep learning important features |
| **DL** | Deep learning |
| **DLM** | Deep learning models |
| **DMTA** | Design-test-make-analyze |
| **DNN** | Deep neural network |
| **DRL** | Deep restoration learning |
| **DSA** | Digital signature algorithm |
| **DSC** | Dice similarity coefficient |
| **DT** | Decision tree |
| **DVT** | Dental volumetric tomography |
| **ECFP** | Extended connectivity fingerprints |
| **ECG** | Electrocardiogram |
| **ECOC** | Error-correcting output codes |
| **ED** | Erectile dysfunction |
| **EF** | Ejection fraction |
| **EMR** | Electronic medical record |
| **ENT** | Ear–nose–throat |
| **ESPs** | Edge service providers |
| **f** | Function in the proposed model |
| **FCN** | Fully convolutional neural |
| **FDA** | Food and Drug Administration |
| **FI** | Furcation involvement |
| **FIS** | Fuzzy inference system |
| **FN** | False negative |
| **FOV** | Field of view |
| **FP** | False positive |
| **G.Grad-CAM** | Guided Grad-CAM |
| **GA** | Genetic algorithm |
| **GAN** | Generative adversarial networks |
| **GAP** | Global average pooling |
| **GBM** | Gradient-boosting machine |
| **GC** | Gastric cancer |
| **GCN** | Graph convolutional network |
| **GIB** | Graph information bottleneck |
| **GLM** | Generalized linear model |
| **GM** | Gray matter |

| | |
|---|---|
| **GMP** | Global max pooling |
| **GNN** | Graph neural network |
| **GNNExplainer** | GNN explainer |
| **GP** | Gaussian process |
| **GPU** | Graphics processing units |
| **Grad-CAM** | Gradient-weighted class activation mapping |
| **H & E** | Hematoxylin-eosin |
| **HIPAA** | Health Insurance Portability and Accountability Act |
| **ICTs** | Information and communication technologies |
| **IDE** | Integrated development platform |
| **IIoT** | Industrial Internet of Things |
| **IM** | Intestinal metaplasia |
| **In-Net** | Inner network |
| **IoMT** | Internet of Medical Things |
| **IoT** | Internet of Things |
| **JSI** | Jaccard similarity index |
| **KG** | Knowledge graph |
| **KNN** | *K* nearest neighbors |
| ***k*-NN** | *k*-nearest neighbor |
| **LCs** | Lightweight clients |
| **LIMA** | Local insights model agnostic |
| **LIME** | Local interpretable model-agnostic explanation |
| **LR** | Linear regression |
| **LRP** | Layer layer-wise relevance propagation |
| **LSHTM** | London school of hygiene and tropical medicine |
| **LSTM** | Long short-term memory |
| **M** | Max pool layer |
| **MAE** | mean absolute error |
| **MF** | Membership function |
| **MIA** | Medical image analysis |
| **ML** | Machine learning |
| **MLP** | Multilayer perceptron |
| **MMP** | Matched molecular pair |
| **MR** | Magnetic resonance |
| **MRI** | Magnetic resonance imaging |
| **MS** | Multiple sclerosis |
| **MSE** | Mean squared error |
| **MSN** | Multi-scale network |
| **N** | Count of explanatory variables |
| **NB –** | Naive Bayes |

| | |
|---|---|
| **NIH** | National Institutes of Health |
| **NLP** | Natural language processing |
| **NN** | Neural network |
| **NO** | Nitric oxide |
| **NYHA** | New York Heart Association |
| **OPS** | Octopus poultry safe |
| **OvA** | One-vs-All |
| **OvO** | One-vs-One |
| **OvR** | One-vs-Rest |
| **PAH** | Pulmonary arterial hypertension |
| **PCA** | Principal component analysis |
| **PDE** | Phosphodiesterol type 5 |
| **PDP** | Partial dependence plot |
| **P-HNN** | Progressive holistically nested network |
| **PmHM** | Public and medical health management |
| **PPMI** | Parkinson's progression markers initiative |
| **PPV** | Positive predictive value |
| **PSC** | Protein sequence composition |
| **QSAR** | Quantitative structure–activity relationship |
| **RBF** | Radial basis functions |
| **RBM** | Restricted Boltzmann machine |
| **ReLU** | Rectified linear unit |
| **RF** | Random forest |
| **RFID** | radio frequency identification |
| **RMSE** | Root mean squared error |
| **RNN** | Recurrent neural networks |
| **ROC** | Receiver operating characteristic curve |
| **RSA** | Rivest, Shamir, and Adleman |
| **SACM** | Secure access control mechanism |
| **SCGMC** | Spinal cord gray matter segmentation challenge |
| **SC-Net** | Slice-based classification |
| **SGD** | Stochastic gradient descent |
| **SHAP** | Shapley additive explanations |
| **SIB** | Swiss Institute of Bioinformatics |
| **SIDU** | Similarity distance and uniqueness |
| **SIR** | Susceptible infected recovered |
| **SMILES** | Simplified molecular input line entry systems |
| **SNR** | Signal-to-noise ratio |
| **SVM** | Support vector machine |
| **TD3** | Twin delayed deep deterministic |

| | |
|---|---|
| **THC** | Tetrahydrocannabinol |
| **TN** | True negative |
| **TNR** | True negative rate |
| **TP** | True positive |
| **TPR** | True positive rate |
| **t-SNE** | t-Distributed stochastic neighbor embedding |
| **VADER** | Valence aware dictionary and sentiment reasoner |
| **WHO** | World Health Organization |
| **WLE** | White light endoscopic |
| **WM** | White matter |
| **x** | The available variable |
| **x'** | The selected variable |
| **XAI** | Explainable artificial intelligence |
| **XGBoost** | Extreme gradient boosting |

# 1

# Gastric Cancer Detection using Hybrid-based Network and SHAP Analysis

**Varanasi L. V. S. K. B. Kasyap, D. Sumathi, and Karthika Natarajan**

VIT-AP University, India
Email: varanasi.20bce7315@vitap.ac.in; sumathi.research28@gmail.com; bharathikarthika@gmail.com

## Abstract

Gastric cancer is one of the most widely reported problems in the world, causing high modality rates in recent times. Gastroscopy is an efficient method that is widely used to analyze gastric problems. The advent of deep learning helps doctors to detect gastric cancer in the early stages. The performance of the existing methods in detecting gastric cancer from the images is not accurate. This study proposes a novel deep-learning framework that can be used to detect gastric cancer from gastric slice images. The proposed method is based on a patch-based analysis of the given input image. Specifically, the model selects and extracts the features from the images in the training phase and evaluates the genuine risk of the patients. This is one of the novel contributions of the proposed work. The bag-of-features technique is applied to the extracted features in the proposed network for the selected patches for better analysis. Experimental results prove that the proposed framework can detect gastric cancer from the images effectively and efficiently. The model is robust enough to detect the minute lesions that can cause the gastric tumor in the further stages. The dataset used in this analysis is publicly available, and the results achieved by this model are higher than the other conventional models that use the same dataset. The proposed framework gives higher accuracy scores compared with existing frameworks.

## 1.1 Introduction

Stomach cancer, often known as gastric cancer (GC), is a type of cancer. When cells in the stomach's lining grow out of control, they develop into tumors that can infiltrate healthy tissues and spread to other body regions. Global data show that GC is the second most common cause of cancer-related fatalities and the fourth most prevalent malignancy worldwide [1]. Environmental and genetic factors, among others, play a complex role in the onset and development of GC, and their effects on these processes have not yet been fully understood. Even after receiving a full course of treatment that includes surgery, chemotherapy, and radiotherapy, the five-year survival percentage for advanced GC is still less than 30% [2], whereas the five-year survival rate for early GC can be over 90%, sometimes even having a curative impact [3]. The incidence and development of GC is a complicated process involving numerous mechanisms, steps, and stages. Several transitional phases include the precancerous state, namely "normal gastric mucosa – chronic non-atrophic gastritis – atrophic gastritis – intestinal metaplasia – dysplasia – gastric cancer," as per the observations of Correa's currently more widely accepted pattern of human GC [4]. Atrophic gastritis (AG) and intestinal metaplasia (IM) are two conditions that are thought to be precancerous lesions that are strongly linked to GC [5]. AG and IM are more likely to turn into GC if not treated promptly. Their early detection and prompt treatment have significant practical implications for the prevention and treatment of GC.

Examination of GC could be done with the help of various sources, namely imaging tests, pathological images, and endoscopy. To initiate, stomach cancer has to be detected successfully via endoscopy. The surface structure can be precisely analyzed by image-enhanced endoscopic techniques, including narrow-band imaging [6] and linked color imaging [7]. According to the studies, the precision of gastrointestinal tumor diagnosis [8] could be augmented by the deployment of endoscopic techniques. However, research states that even endoscopy examinations lead to still missed 10% of upper gastrointestinal malignancies [9]. Even if two experts participated, there would be missed diagnoses in an endoscopic unit [10]. The cause was that accurate gastroscopy image diagnosis requires years of practice to develop. Next, the gold standard for tumor diagnosis is histological image recognition. Diagnostic mistakes and a heavy workload for pathologists have been brought on by the dearth of pathologists [11]. Lastly, imaging tests are crucial in assessing the lymph node metastases of stomach cancer. An imaging evaluation's primary focus is on the lesions' morphological characteristics. For instance, the perigastric adipose tissue is so dense that it resembles lymph nodes. Doctors may make errors in diagnosis due to inexperience and missing diagnoses. The accuracy of the diagnosis will eventually decline, particularly in several cases [12].

Artificial intelligence (AI) is exploding in medicine due to the growing demand for detection, categorization, and segmentation or delineation of more accurate margins. After various findings in this recent scenario, the universal ground truth is that AI makes machines think like humans. One of the most crucial components of AI is machine learning. Deep learning is more accurate and flexible than standard machine learning techniques like support vector machines and Bayesian networks, and it is also easier to adapt to other fields and applications. Although AI-based technologies have shown impressive outcomes in the medical field, they have not been widely used in clinics. The main reasons are the black-box technique's unique feature and other factors, including high computing costs. It results from the inability to clearly represent the knowledge for a particular task carried out by a deep learning model, despite the underlying statistical principles. Simpler AI techniques, such as linear regression and decision trees, are self-explanatory since the model parameters allow one to visualize the classification decision border in a few dimensions. However, they do not possess the complexity needed for activities like classifying 3D and the majority of 2D medical images. Trust can be built among the patients only when the medical diagnosis done by the doctor is found to be open, clear, and explicable. It should ideally be able to fully explain the reasoning behind a certain choice to all parties concerned. Deploying deep learning models in the healthcare sector is challenging as the black box models need more interpretations. A model in AI needs to act as an aid for medical professionals, and, in addition, it should also permit the human expert to review the choices and exercise judgment. It has been understood from various articles that AI is used in various applications. This has drastically changed over the past 10 years due to advancements in machine learning (ML) and the broad industrial adoption of ML, which were made possible by more powerful machines, better learning algorithms, and easier access to enormous amounts of data [13]. Deep learning (DL) techniques [14] began to rule accuracy metrics around 2012, through which better results are obtained within the stipulated time. As a result, many real-world issues are now being solved using machine learning models in various industries, from fashion, education, and finance [15] to medicine and healthcare. Explainability is essential for the safe and trustworthy use of AI and a vital facilitator for its practical application.

By dispelling misconceptions about AI, end users can develop trust by seeing what a model considers while making a choice. For users who do not use deep learning, such as the majority of medical professionals, it is even

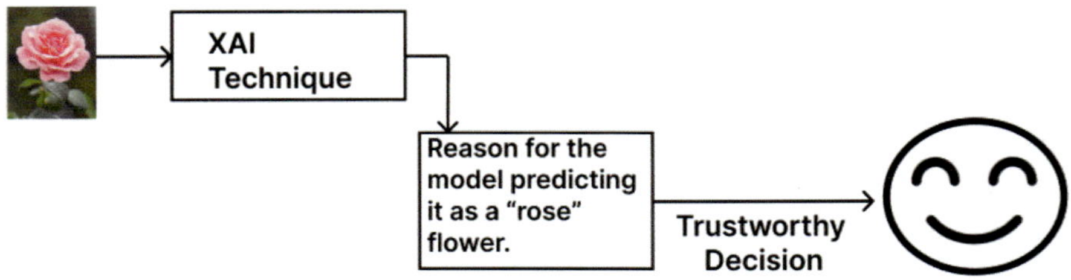


**Figure 1.1** XAI model.

more crucial to display the domain-specific attributes used in conclusion. Machine learning algorithms' output and outcomes can now be understood and trusted by human users when those are obtained through a set of procedures and techniques known as explainable artificial intelligence (XAI). An AI model, its anticipated effects, and potential biases are all described in terms of explainable AI. It contributes to defining model correctness, fairness, transparency, and outcomes in decision-making supported by AI. A business must establish trust and confidence when putting AI models into production. A model to be established could adopt a suitable approach to AI development by deploying AI explainability.

Figure 1.1 depicts the way of working that XAI performs. An association could be made between explainability and uncertainty. Uncertainty is a key problem since deep learning classifiers typically cannot respond "I am not sure" in ambiguous situations and instead return the class with the highest probability, even if by a small margin. Recent research has examined uncertainty combined with the issue of explainability to highlight the instances where a model is unclear and, as a result, make the models more defensible to users unfamiliar with deep learning.

Understanding the deep learning models is complex as they are not transparent since it is impossible to gain knowledge directly from the neurons' weights. It has been shown in the study [16] that determining the significance of a neuron for a certain task is not solely dependent on the size, specificity, or influence of activations on networks. The researchers of an earlier study [17] thoroughly review explainable artificial intelligence (AI) terminology, ideas, and use scenarios. The next section describes the taxonomy of XAI approaches.

## 1.2 XAI Approaches

Figure 1.2 shows the taxonomy of XAI techniques that could be deployed. Various techniques, such as model agnostic versus model specific, a

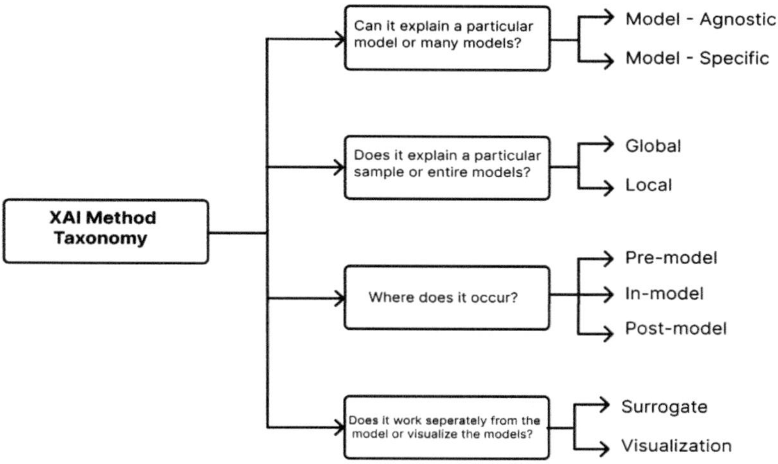


**Figure 1.2** XAI taxonomy.

comparison of local and global methods, pre-model, in-model, and post-model specifications, and an overview of surrogate and visualization methods are discussed.

### 1.2.1 Model agnostic vs. model specific

Model-specific interpretation techniques are built around the exclusive model's parameters. Model agnostic approaches are not restricted to a certain model architecture and are typically applicable in *post-hoc* analysis. These techniques lack direct access to the structural or internal model weights.

### 1.2.2 Local and global methods

Local methods pertain to the single instance or single outcome of the model. Global approaches concentrate on the inside of a model by utilizing the whole understanding of model, training, and related data. It aims to provide a general explanation for the model's behavior. This strategy seeks to identify the features contributing much toward improving the model's performance. It is also known as feature engineering.

### 1.2.3 Pre-model, in-model, and post-model

Pre-model techniques are autonomous and can be applied to any model architecture. Some popular examples of these techniques include principal component analysis (PCA) [18] and t-distributed stochastic neighbor embedding (t-SNE) [19]. In-model methods are interpretability techniques that are built into the model itself. Some techniques are used after creating a model; hence, they are called post-model techniques. These techniques can produce insightful conclusions regarding a model's precise lessons acquired during training.

### 1.2.4 Visualization or surrogate methods

Surrogate methodologies use an ensemble of many models to examine other black-box models. Decisions that come out of the surrogate model are analyzed and compared with the decision obtained through the black-box model.

### 1.2.5 Approaches

Two well-known local explanation methods that can be used to explain any given black-box classifier are local interpretable model-agnostic explanation (LIME) and Shapley additive explanations (SHAP). These techniques learn a local interpretable model (like a linear model) around each prediction, explaining each prediction of every classifier in a comprehensible and accurate way. LIME and SHAP, in particular, estimate feature attributions on individual instances, which reflect each feature's contribution to the black box prediction. The next section describes in detail SHAP.

#### 1.2.5.1 Shapley additive explanations (SHAP)

Among the popular model agnostic techniques available, Shapley additive explanations (SHAP) could be used to analyze the results. It explains how a machine learning model's predictions turned out. Shapley values are applied. The model characteristics are given weights known as Shapley values. It demonstrates how each feature affected the outcomes of the predictions. It establishes how features affect the outcomes of predictions. In the earlier study [20], researchers developed SHAP-a technique through the game theoretically ideal Shapley values to explain specific predictions. A popular strategy from cooperative game theory with desirable features is Shapley values. A data instance's feature values participate in a coalition as players. The average marginal contribution of a feature value overall potential coalition is known as the Shapley value. SHAP explanations guarantee a fair assessment of features and the contribution of output features as SHAP values [21]. In the financial industry, SHAP is frequently utilized for various projects, as mentioned in previous studies [22, 24]. Oikawa et al. [25]

proposed a multistage detection network to detect gastric cancer using pathological images. In the first stage of the network, handcrafted features were used as both pixel and geometric features. Support vector machine (SVM) is used in this study to differentiate the cancerous pathological images and non-cancerous images. The false-positive rate of this network is 18.7%. Xu et al. [26] presented a CNN (convolutional neural network) based approach to segment the histopathological images and classify them based on the epithelial and stromal regions of the input image. The images are separated into patches and analyzed. Wang et al. [27] predicted gastric cancer using advanced CNN methods based on lymph node images. However, this task is laborious and computationally expensive. Ueyama et al. [28] constructed a CNN-based network to detect gastric cancer from the narrow band histopathological images. This approach is high-speed, but the accuracy is comparatively low compared with other methods. Zheng et al. [29] designed a CNN model based on transfer learning with VGG-19 as primary architecture and achieved an accuracy of 91% in detecting gastric cancer based on white light endoscopic (WLE) images. Hirasawa et al. [30] curated a dataset of 3584 gastric cancer endoscopic images and built a database. The images in the data have 512 × 512 pixel resolution focused more on the affected area. The description of each image is also given. The whole dataset is made with 69 different patient data. Lee et al. [31] presented a dataset containing 367 ulcer patch images and 255 normal images for ulcer detection using white light endoscopy. Song et al. [32] introduced an AI-based system for predicting gastric cancer from histopathological images. The average specificity achieved by the model is 86%.

## 1.3 Materials and Methods

### 1.3.1 Data processing and augmentation

The dataset used for this study is taken from the King's Hospital, Oxford. The dataset is available for the public in the name of BOT gastric slice data. The dataset contains original gastric slice images of resolution 1024 × 1024. Since the dataset is in high-dimensional form, images have to reduce for the lower forms for better analysis. The images are scaled down to the resolution of 224 × 224 using random projection techniques. The features in the images are not lost in this process. These small patch images of 224 × 224 are split into training, testing, and validation data in the ratio of 70:20:10, respectively. The whole dataset contains 960 gastric cancer images and 571 non-cancerous images. The images are processed using the augmentation techniques like

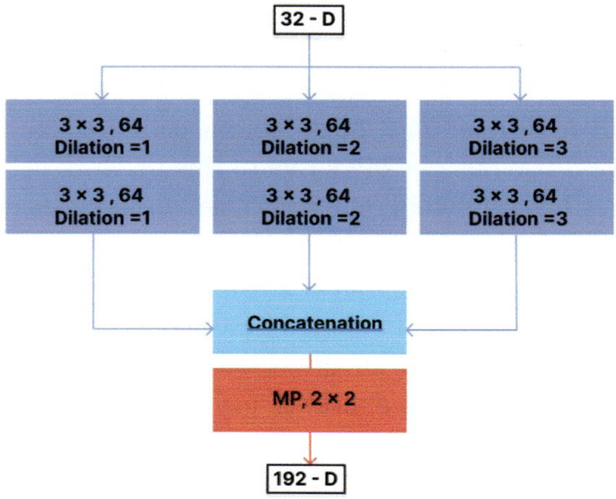


**Figure 1.3** The architecture of the MSN module.

cropping, rotation, and shearing to increase the count of images. After the image augmentation, the images in the dataset are 14,581 cancerous images and 11,721 non-cancerous images.

### 1.3.2 Multi-scale network (MSN) module

For the shallow layers in the networks, a greater number of feature maps are present for the deep layers where object information at different scales is present. The single convolutional layer is unable to detect the multi-scale targets simultaneously. Hence, a multi-scale network is proposed in this study for the shallow layer to overcome the problem. The architecture of the proposed network is shown in Figure 1.3.

The dilated convolutional layer is adopted in the network to amplify the receptive field of the network. This enables the network to run simultaneously to extract the multi-scale features. The extracted features with various dilation rates are conjugated and max pooled for the adjacent layer.

### 1.3.3 Inner network (In-Net) module

A recent study shows that the densely connected networks improve the feature extraction and performance of the network. The features extracted by the three different MSN modules are conjected for longer features in the deeper layers. The main focus of the In-Net module is to perform a better fusion of the extracted features at the deeper layers. The pipeline of the In-Net module

**Table 1.1** Pipeline of the In-Net module.

| Layer | Type | Dilation rate | Kernel size, number |
|---|---|---|---|
| 1 | C | 2 | $3 \times 3$, 1024 |
| 2 | C | 2 | $1 \times 1$, 512 |
| 3 | C | 2 | $3 \times 3$, 1024 |
| 4 | M | – | $2 \times 2$ |
| 5 | C | 1 | $3 \times 3$, 1024 |
| 6 | C | 1 | $1 \times 1$, 512 |
| 7 | C | 1 | $3 \times 3$, 1024 |

is given in Table 1.1. In contrast to the shallow layers, the feature maps at the deeper layers are small. Therefore, a single convolutional layer is capable of feature extraction. For feature fusion, a $1 \times 1$ kernel-sized convolutional layer in between two $3 \times 3$ kernel-sized convolutional layers is placed.

### 1.3.4 Slice-based classification (SC-Net) module

The proposed deep learning framework is based on image patches. The SC-Net module is built to classify the gastric slice image by probabilistic determination. For testing the proposed method, each gastric slice image is cropped to 81 smaller pieces of $224 \times 224$ pixels as the input image for the deep learning network. The result of patch-based classification is exemplified by the heat map shown in Figure 1.4. The colors of the heat map in Figure 1.4 represent the possibility of the gastric image being normal or cancerous. The lower the color value in the image is, the higher the chance of gastric cancer. The results may not be accurate if the whole image is taken and analyzed. The analysis performed is on the pixel level. The features selected and extracted at the training are observed at the pixels. The pixel-level classification gives an accurate analysis of gastric slice images. The lowest 10 scores are used for possibility calculation to attenuate the proposed framework. The label of the image (gastric/non-gastric) is determined by comparing the possibility with the pre-defined threshold value. In this study, the threshold value is set to 0.34.

### 1.3.5 Implementation of the proposed network

The proposed network is developed using the PyTorch and Keras toolboxes. The model is trained on the five different GPUS (GeoForce FTX 3500 X, 12 GB RAM) with a batch size of 128 and a learning rate of 0.001. Adam is used in support of the stochastic gradient descent with 100 epochs at training. The framework integrated with all the modules is given in Figure 1.5.

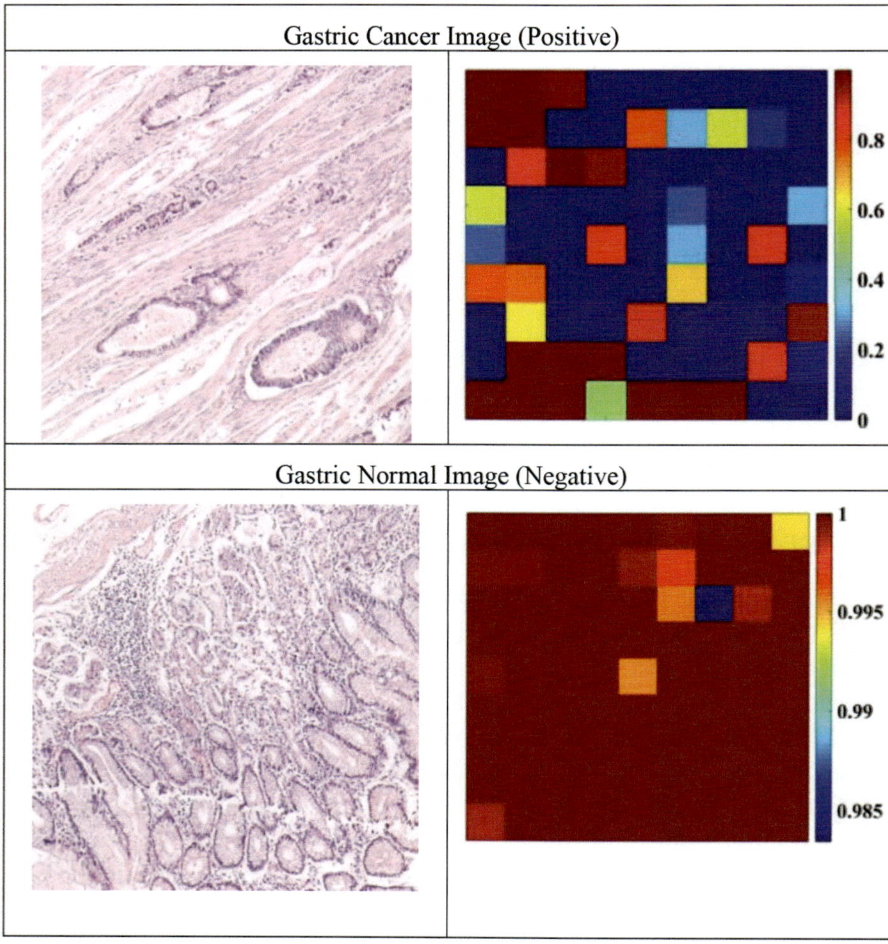


**Figure 1.4** The gastric images and non-gastric cancer images, along with the corresponding generated heat maps.

## 1.4 Experiments and Results

### 1.4.1 BOT gastric dataset

The dataset is curated by the King's Hospital, Oxford. This dataset is properly used in this study after processing and augmentation. The gastric slice images in the dataset are the hematoxylin–eosin (H&E) stained with a magnification factor of 0.3×. Gastric cancer-affected areas are partly provided in the dataset with a description. The predicted pixel positions are manually compared with the given description giving accurate results.

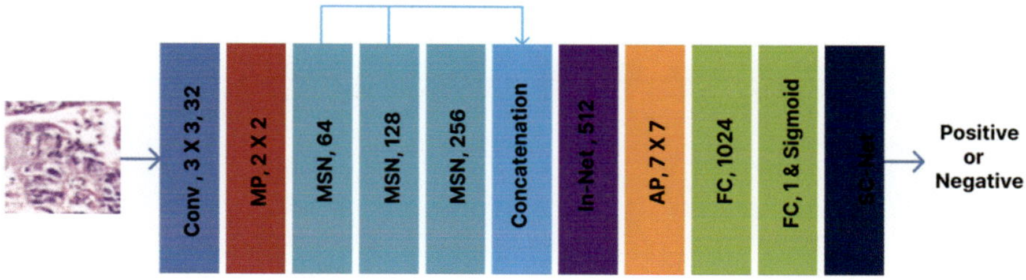


**Figure 1.5** The architectural framework of the proposed deep learning model.

**Table 1.2** Comparison of the patch-based ACA in various models.

| Model | ACA |
|---|---|
| AlexNet [] | 92.36% |
| ResNet [] | 91.51% |
| DenseNet | 91.34% |
| VGG-19 | 90.97% |
| Inception | 90.59% |
| Proposed model (this work) | **97.43%** |

### 1.4.2 Results

The average classification accuracy (ACA) of the testing images is considered the evaluation metric. The existing works are compared with the proposed model.

#### 1.4.2.1 Patch-based classification

In this section, the proposed model is compared with existing works like AlexNet [12], ResNet [13], DenseNet [14], VGG-19 [15], and Inception [16] on slice-based testing datasets. The obtained results are given in Table 1.2. The results show that the proposed network achieves high performance, i.e., an accuracy of 97.43%. This is 5% more than the high-performance network. The proposed network has fewer layers when compared to the existing networks. The existing methods alleviate the problem of overfitting, which is not there in the proposed network.

#### 1.4.2.2 Slice-based classification

The gastric slice images are tested with 2945 cancerous images and 1349 non-cancerous images. The proposed SC-Net module in the proposed model is compared with other benchmarking networks, and the results are presented in Table 1.3. The slice-based classification accuracy of the proposed network is significantly higher than the existing methods.

**Table 1.3** Comparison of the slice-based ACA in various models.

| Model | ACA |
|---|---|
| AlexNet [] | 95.45% |
| ResNet [] | 95.72% |
| DenseNet | 96.43% |
| VGG-19 | 97.27% |
| Inception | 98.65% |
| Proposed model | **99.82%** |

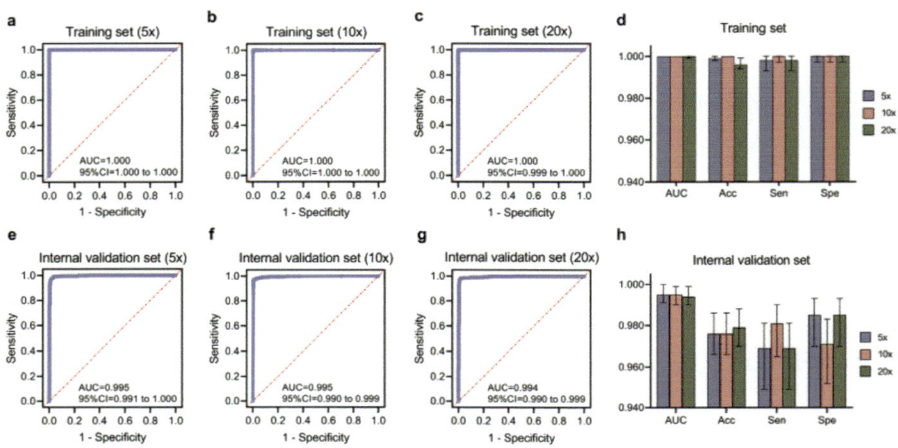


**Figure 1.6** Diagnostic performance of the proposed model at various magnification rates in training and validation phases.

Internal validation of the model achieved the AUC score of 0.995. The AUC score of the model highly relies on the magnification rate of the images. The differences in the accuracy at different magnification rates were statically significant. The results are given in Figure 1.6.

### 1.4.2.3 SHAP analysis

The (Shapley additive explanation) SHAP analysis framework is adopted in the proposed framework because of its diversified properties. In this framework, the prediction variability is distributed among available covariates. The contribution of explanatory variable prediction at each point is assessed as the underlying model. The SHAP analysis results in the Shapley values demonstrating the model predictions as the binary variable linear combination that describes the presence of the covariate in the proposed model or not. The SHAP algorithm estimates the prediction $p(x)$ linear function of binary variables where $z$ belongs to $\{0,1\}^N$ and the quantities belong to a real number, defined in eqn (1.1).

$$p(N') = \varphi_0 + \sum_{i=1}^{N} \varphi_i N'_i \tag{1.1}$$

where $N$ is the count of explanatory variables.

Eqn (1.2) shows the properties of the local accuracy, consistency, and missingness obtained at each variable:

$$\varphi_i(p,x) = \sum_{z'x'} \frac{|N'||(M - |x'| - 1)|}{N!} |p(x') - (z')|. \tag{1.2}$$

In the function $f$ in the proposed model, $x$ is the available variable and $x'$ will be the selected variable. The Shapley variables differ in the mean at the $i$th variable.

## 1.5 Conclusion

In this study, a novel deep-learning framework is presented for detecting gastric cancer. In this framework, different architectures were adopted at shallow and deep layers, i.e., MSN-module and In-Net module. The proposed framework is evaluated on BOT gastric dataset, and the results show that the model is robust and effective. The model also outperforms well-existed frameworks with fewer layers. The average classification accuracy of the model at the pixel level is 99.82%. This work can be improved further by integrating white light endoscopic images based prediction and the H&E-stained images for finer and early predictions at the root levels of the tumor.

## References

[1] F. Bray, J. Ferlay, I. Soerjomataram, R. L. Siegel, L. A. Torre, and A. Jemal, "Global Cancer Statistics 2018: GLOBOCAN Estimates of Incidence and Mortality Worldwide for 36 Cancers in 185 Countries," Ca-Cancer J. Clin. 68(6), 394–424 (2018). [CrossRef]

[2] K. D. Miller, R. L. Siegel, C. C. Lin, A. B. Mariotto, J. L. Kramer, J. H. Rowland, K. D. Stein, R. Alteri, and A. Jemal, "Cancer Treatment and Survivorship Statistics, 2016," Ca-Cancer J. Clin. 66(4), 271–289 (2016). [CrossRef]

[3] H. Katai, T. Ishikawa, K. Akazawa, Y. Isobe, I. Miyashiro, I. Oda, S. Tsujitani, H. Ono, S. Tanabe, T. Fukagawa, S. Nunobe, Y. Kakeji, and A. Nashimoto, "Five-year survival analysis of surgically resected

gastric cancer cases in Japan: a retrospective analysis of more than 100,000 patients from the nationwide registry of the Japanese Gastric Cancer Association(2001-2007)," Gastric Cancer 21(1), 144–154 (2018). [CrossRef].

[4] P. Correa and M. B. Piazuelo, "Natural history of helicobacter pylori infection," Dig. Liver Dis. 40(7), 490–496 (2008). [CrossRef]

[5] Y. H. Park and N. Kim, "Review of atrophic gastritis and intestinal metaplasia as a premalignant lesion of gastric cancer," J. Cancer Prev. 20(1), 25–40 (2015). [CrossRef]

[6] Sumiyama K (2017) Past and current trends in endoscopic diagnosis for early stage gastric cancer in Japan. Gastric Cancer 20(Suppl 1):20–27. https://doi.org/10.1007/s10120-016-0659-4

[7] Shinozaki S, Osawa H, Hayashi Y, Lefor AK, Yamamoto H (2019) Linked color imaging for the detection of early gastrointestinal neoplasms. 12:1756284819885246. https://doi.org/10.1177/1756284819885246

[8] Dohi O, Majima A, Naito Y, Yoshida T, Ishida T, Azuma Y, Kitae H, Matsumura S, Mizuno N, Yoshida N (2020) Can image-enhanced endoscopy improve the diagnosis of Kyoto classification of gastritis in the clinical setting? 32(2):191–203. https://doi.org/10.1111/den.13540244(5):512–524. https://doi.org/10.1002/path.5028.

[9] Cooper LA, Demicco EG (2018) PanCancer insights from The Cancer Genome Atlas: the pathologist's perspective. 244(5):512–524. https://doi.org/10.1002/path.5028.

[10] Toyoizumi H, Kaise M, Arakawa H, Yonezawa J, Yoshida Y, Kato M, Yoshimura N, Goda K, Tajiri H (2009) Ultrathin endoscopy versus high-resolution endoscopy for diagnosing superficial gastric neoplasia. Gastrointest Endosc 70(2):240–245. https://doi.org/10.1016/j.gie.2008.10.064.

[11] Xu Y, Jia Z, Wang L, F Z YA (2017) Large scale tissue histopathology image classification, segmentation, and visualization via deep convolutional activation features. BMC Bioinform 18(1):281. https://doi.org/10.1186/s12859-017-1685-x.

[12] Gao Y, Zhang ZD, Li S, Guo YT, Wu QY, Liu SH, Yang SJ, Ding L, Zhao BC, Li S, Lu Y (2019) Deep neural network-assisted computed tomography diagnosis of metastatic lymph nodes from gastric cancer. Chin Med J 132(23):2804–2811. https://doi.org/10.1097/cm9.0000000000000532.

[13] Jordan, M.I.; Mitchell, T.M. Machine learning: Trends, perspectives, and prospects. Science 2015, 349, 255–260. [CrossRef]

[14] LeCun, Y.; Bengio, Y.; Hinton, G. Deep learning. Nature 2015, 521, 436–444. [CrossRef] [PubMed]

[15] Khandani, A.E.; Kim, A.J.; Lo, A.W. Consumer credit-risk models via machine-learning algorithms. J. Bank. Financ. 2010, 34, 2767–2787. [CrossRef].

[16] Meyes, R.; de Puiseau, C.W.; Posada-Moreno, A.; Meisen, T. Under the Hood of Neural Networks: Characterizing Learned Representations by Functional Neuron Populations and Network Ablations. arXiv 2020, arXiv:2004.01254.

[17] Arrieta, A.B.; Díaz-Rodríguez, N.; Del Ser, J.; Bennetot, A.; Tabik, S.; Barbado, A.; García, S.; Gil-López, S.; Molina, D.; Benjamins, R.; et al. Explainable Artificial Intelligence (XAI): Concepts, taxonomies, opportunities and challenges toward responsible AI. Inf. Fusion 2020, 58, 82–115. [CrossRef].

[18] Doraikannan, Sumathi, Prabha Selvaraj, and Vijay Kumar Burugari. "Principal component analysis for dimensionality reduction for animal classification based on LR." Int. J. Innov. Technol. Explor. Eng 8.10 (2019).

[19] Maaten, L.V.D.; Hinton, G. Visualizing data using t-SNE. J. Mach. Learn. Res. 2008, 9, 2579–2605.

[20] Scott M. Lundberg and Su-In Lee. 2017. A unified approach to interpreting model predictions. In Proceedings of the 31st International Conference on Neural Information Processing Systems (NIPS'17). Curran Associates Inc., Red Hook, NY, USA, 4768–4777.

[21] Molnar, C. (2020). Interpretable machine learning. Lulu.com.

[22] Bhatt, U., Xiang, A., Sharma, S., Weller, A., Taly, A., Jia, Y., Ghosh, J., Puri, R., Moura, J. M., and Eckersley, P. (2020). Explainable machine learning in deployment. In ACM FAT, pages 648–657.

[23] Bracke, P., Datta, A., Jung, C., and Sen, S. (2019). Machine learning explainability in finance: an application to default risk analysis.

[24] Mokhtari, K. E., Higdon, B. P., and Bas¸ar, A. (2019). Interpreting financial time series with shap values. In Proceedings of the 29th Annual International Conference on Computer Science and Software Engineering, pages 166–172

[25] Oikawa K, Saito A, Kiyuna T, Graf HP, Cosatto E, Kuroda M. Pathological Diagnosis of Gastric Cancers with a Novel Computerized Analysis System. J Pathol Inform. 2017 Feb 28;8:5. doi: 10.4103/2153-3539.201114. PMID: 28400994; PMCID: PMC5359998.

[26] Xu J, Luo X, Wang G, Gilmore H, Madabhushi A. A Deep Convolutional Neural Network for segmenting and classifying epithelial and stromal regions in histopathological images. Neurocomputing. 2016 May 26;191:214-223. doi: 10.1016/j.neucom.2016.01.034. Epub 2016 Feb 17. PMID: 28154470; PMCID: PMC5283391.

[27] Wang X, Chen Y, Gao Y, et al. Predicting gastric cancer outcome from resected lymph node histopathology images using deep learning. Nat Commun 2021;12 (1):1637.

[28] Ueyama H, Kato Y, Akazawa Y, Yatagai N, Komori H, Takeda T, Matsumoto K, Ueda K, Hojo M, Yao T, Nagahara A, Tada T. Application of artificial intelligence using a convolutional neural network for diagnosis of early gastric cancer based on magnifying endoscopy with narrow-band imaging. J Gastroenterol Hepatol 2021; 36: 482–489 [PMID: 32681536 DOI: 10.1111/jgh.15190].

[29] Zheng W, Zhang X, Kim JJ, Zhu X, Ye G, Ye B, et al. High accuracy of convolutional neural network for evaluation of Helicobacter pylori infection based on endoscopic images: preliminary experience. Clin Transl Gastroenterol. 2019;10(12):e00109.

[30] Lee JH, Kim YJ, Kim YW, Park S, Choi YI, Park DK, Kim KG, Chung JW. Spotting malignancies from gastric endoscopic images using deep learning. Surg Endosc 2019; 33: 3790–3797 [PMID: 30719560 DOI: 10.1007/s00464-019-06677-2].

[31] Bergholt MS, Zheng W, Lin K, Ho KY, Teh M, Yeoh KG, Yan So JB, Huang Z. In vivo diagnosis of gastric cancer using Raman endoscopy and ant colony optimization techniques. Int J Cancer 2011; 128: 2673–2680 [PMID: 20726002 DOI: 10.1002/ijc.25618].

[32] Song Z, Zou S, Zhou W, et al. Clinically applicable histopathological diagnosis system for gastric cancer detection using deep learning. Nat Commun 2020;11 (1):4294.

# 2

# LIME Approach in Diagnosing Diseases – A Study on Explainable AI

**Iyyanki Muralikrishna[1] and Prisilla Jayanthi[2]**

[1]Former Director R&D JNTU Hyderabad, India; UC Berkeley, USA
[2]Faculty Associate, Ecole Centrale School of Engineering, Mahindra University, Hyderabad, India
Email: iyyanki@gmail.com; prisillaj28@gmail.com

## Abstract

In present medical decisions, the use of artificial intelligence (AI) systems is based on trust and transparency. Explainable AI (XAI) is an emerging field that happens to throw light on "black box" machine learning (ML) models in human understandable language. XAI is a solution to several scientific problems that need deep explanation and interpretation. XAI solutions with quantitative and qualitative analyses have proved the efficiency for many clinical problems. This chapter focuses on few algorithms of XAI, namely ANFIS-GA, LIME, GRAD-CAM, and SIDU. In this study, these algorithms were implemented on various cases such as heart attack prediction, eye fundus, thyroid, COVID-19, and air pollutant.

## 2.1 Introduction

In the recent era of technology development, AI has been paving its way in the field of medicine. The healthcare industry is flooded with the algorithms of intelligence and is surrounded with automatic and huge machines that run with AI algorithms. The growing digitalization of healthcare in the framework of Industry 4.0 provides a tremendous amount of data. Hence, the transparency of the health processes is increased by this tremendous data; it accelerates the flow of information through the industry and provides a valuable asset to build predictive models. Let us understand the concept of

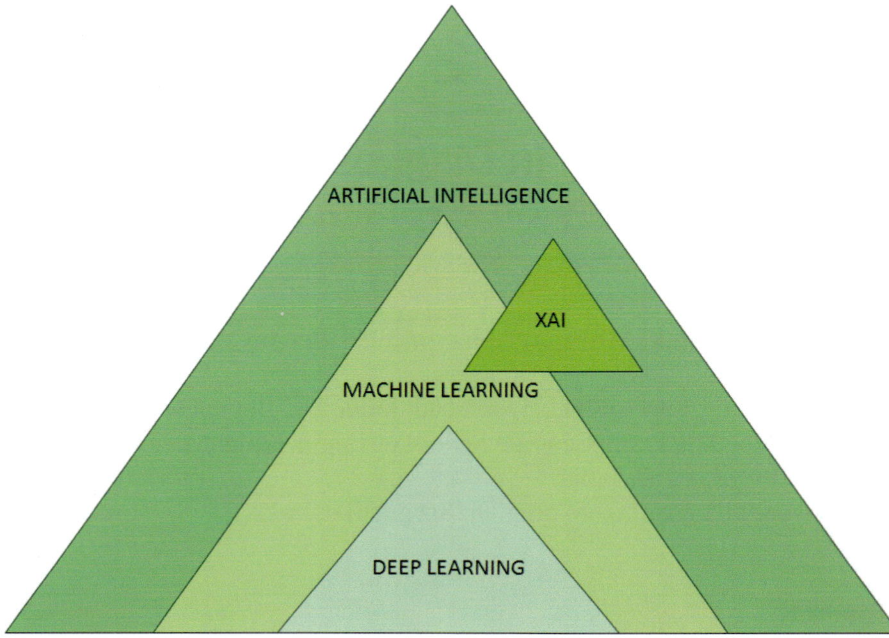


**Figure 2.1** XAI relationship with AI.

AI in healthcare industry. AI is the process of simulating human intelligence by the machine and ML is a subset of AI. Well-known ML algorithms have been implemented in medical field, which includes regression models, Naïve Bayes, *K*-nearest neighbors (KNN), support vector machine (SVM), decision tree (DT), and random forest (RF) [1]. Apart from ML approaches, several studies have used DL models for medical applications. The DL algorithm can learn representations of raw data without feature engineering. Typical DL methods include artificial neural networks (ANNs), convolutional neural networks (CNNs), deep neural networks (DNNs), and recurrent neural networks (RNNs) [2]. Explainable artificial intelligence (XAI) is a subset of AI and ML but not DL (Figure 2.1) [3].

The goal of XAI is to make sure that AI programs are transparent in the purpose they serve and how they work. XAI has become more crucial for the medical and healthcare studies using DL models [4]. XAI has a common goal and objective for data science engineers trying to move forward with the progress of AI. Explainability [5] and interpretability [6] provide transparency by allowing data scientists to screen data and analyze algorithmic outcomes for unacceptable outcomes. Hence, XAI [7] was a solution to trust and transparency in medical advice and therapeutic decisions. One among the five

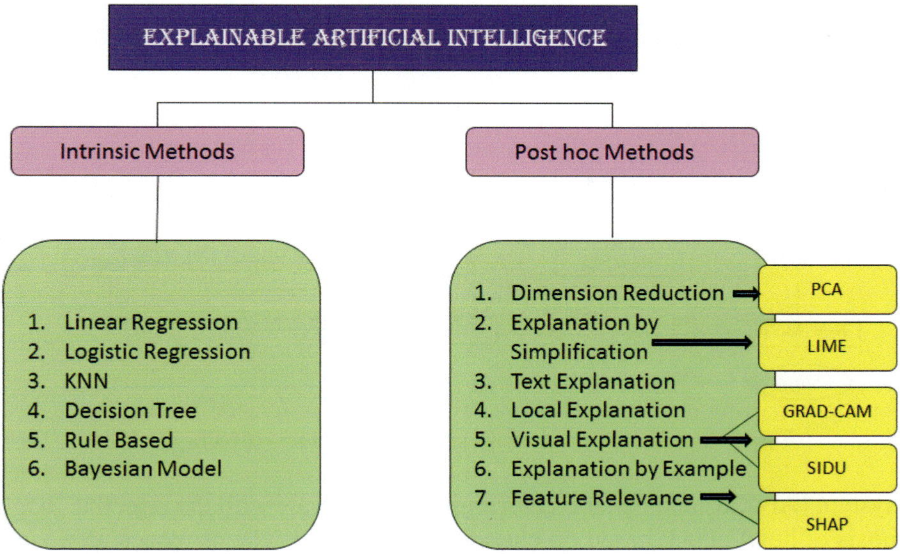


**Figure 2.2** Various methods of XAI.

major principles is trust, which is characterized in AI system. The remaining four principles are resiliency, lack of bias, reproducibility, and accountability.

XAI has two methods, namely intrinsic and *post-hoc* method. Intrinsic methods include linear/logistic regression, KNN, decision tree, rule based, and Bayesian model. While, *post-hoc* methods include Shapley additive explanations (SHAP), principal component analysis (PCA), gradient weighted class activation mapping (GRAD-CAM), similarity distance and uniqueness (SIDU), and local interpretable model-agnostic explanations (LIME) [3]. According to *post-hoc* explainability methods (Figure 2.2), the following come under this category: dimension reduction, text, visual, local explanation, explanation by example, explanation by simplification, and feature relevance.

XAI programs are designed to concentrate on the development of several systems by addressing few issues in two areas: (1) classifying event in heterogeneous and multimedia data and (2) constructing decision policies for an autonomous system for simulating missions. In this chapter, the authors discussed few algorithms of XAI, namely ANFIS-GA, LIME, GRAD-CAM, and SIDU.

## 2.2 XAI Model for Predicting Heart Attack

Aghamohammadi et al. [8], in their research work, proposed an effective classification algorithm with the combination of adaptive neuro fuzzy inference

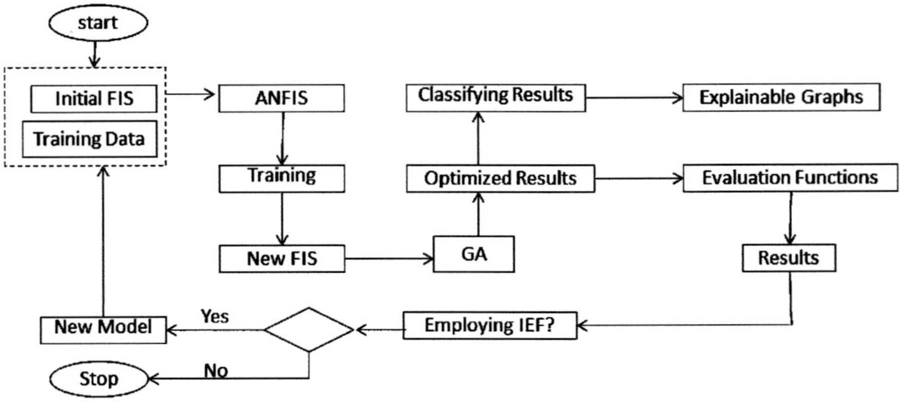


**Figure 2.3** The flowchart of the proposed algorithm – ANFIS-GA [8].

system (ANFIS) and genetic algorithm (GA). It deals with the effective diagnosis of heart attack based on classification method. The proposed approach (Figure 2.3) reads the patient data to predict the patient who may be at a risk of having heart attack. The model is trained on the dataset fed into it using a neural network to determine fuzzy parameters. Later, the membership functions (MFs) generated by the fuzzy inference system (FIS) are optimized by genetic algorithm (GA). The possibility of heart attack can be classified into five stages: no risk, slight risk, average risk, high risk, and very high risk. The explainable interface of the system provides trustworthy, safe, and transparent predictions for the medical diagnosis. Finally, the system's reliability is evaluated using the metrics called sensitivity, specificity, precision, accuracy, and root mean squared error (RMSE).

Similarly, XAI algorithms were implemented for predicting heart diseases [9], diabetes [10], EMG hand gesture classification [11], and different types of pain (chest, headache, spine, shoulder, and surgical/postoperative pain) [12].

## Case-2

Dave [13] implemented XAI-based approach for healthcare applications using the heart disease dataset. The proposed XAI model is depicted in Figure 2.4, and the techniques LIME and SHAP give more explanation. XGBoost (eXtreme Gradient Boosting) algorithm [14] was implemented for performance with the speed. XGBoost trained the dataset that consisted of 13 attributes. XAI techniques (circle 3) provide explanations along with prediction results in Figure 2.4. Contrastive explanation method (CEM) is another XAI method that gives local explanations for a black-box model. CEM is the

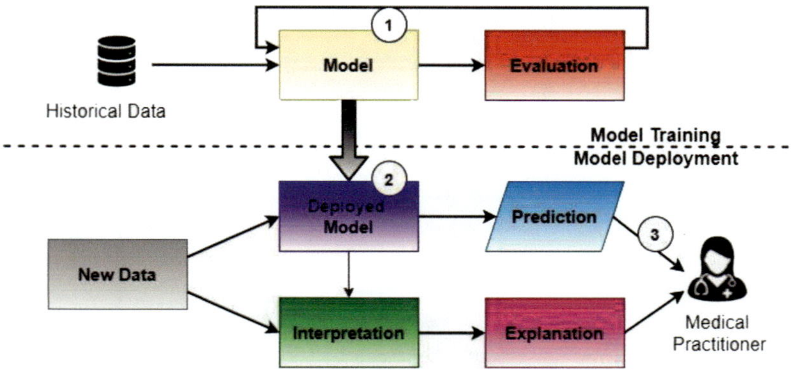


**Figure 2.4** ML life-cycle in conjunction with XAI [13].

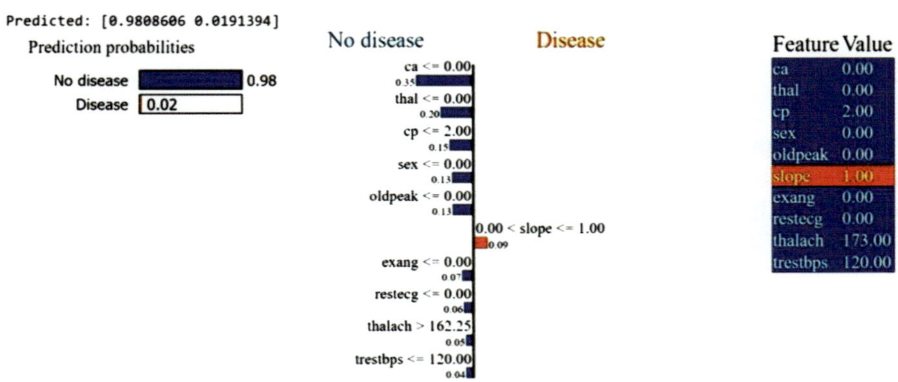


**Figure 2.5 (a)** Explanations generated by LIME.

best approach for classification models used to improve the accuracy of ML model for the cases of misclassified instances.

Figure 2.5(a) shows LIME output. The prediction probabilities trained by the XGBoost model is shown on the left side of the figure for the two classes "No disease" (98%) and "Disease" (2%). The middle part provides the features along with their weights that impact the probability of prediction. The actual value of a feature for any specific local instance is represented on the right side.

In Figure 2.5(b), it visualizes the feature effects on the prediction at different values. The following color represents the value of the feature (blue – low, purple – median value, and red – high).

Consider for the attribute "ca" (Figure 2.5(b)), the blue dots indicate the SHAP value is negative, while the red and purple dots represent the SHAP

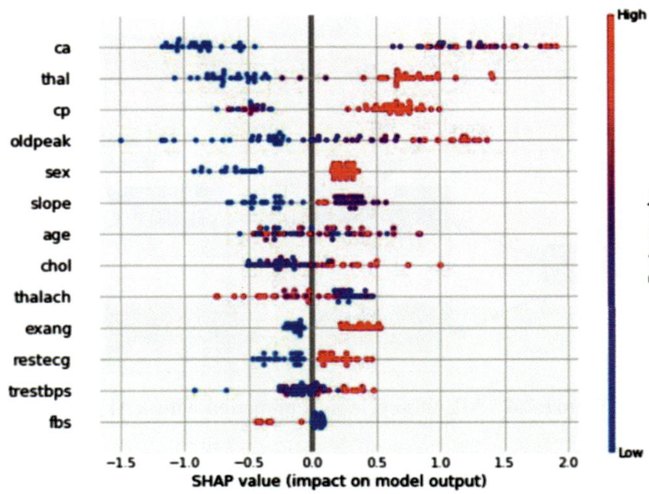


**Figure 2.5(b)** Explanations generated by SHAP.

values are positive. This signifies that when no vessels are blocked, chances of disease are low but when the number of vessels blocked increases, the chances of having a disease increase.

## 2.3 XAI for Opthalmology

In the present medical field [15], many ophthalmology practitioners are using AI and its subfields ML and DL to revolutionize vision care. Kok [16] states that several XAI models have been attracted to address the issues of interpretability and explainability of the black-box models in healthcare. Thereby, the authors proved that black-box model behavior can be explained using feature-based XAI techniques, SHAP and LIME.

Muddamsetty et al. [17], in their research work, discussed two models of XAI, namely SIDU and GRAD-CAM for eye fundus.

**GRAD-CAM:**

This technique is a class-discriminative localization one, which generates visual explanations without requiring retraining. In Figure 2.6, the generated heatmaps in the third and fourth columns by the GRAD-CAM and SIDU demonstrate how the visual explanation methods are closely aligning with human experts.

**SIDU:**

This method generates heatmaps (Figure 2.6(d)) based on two steps: similarity difference and uniqueness. It was proved via quantitative and qualitative

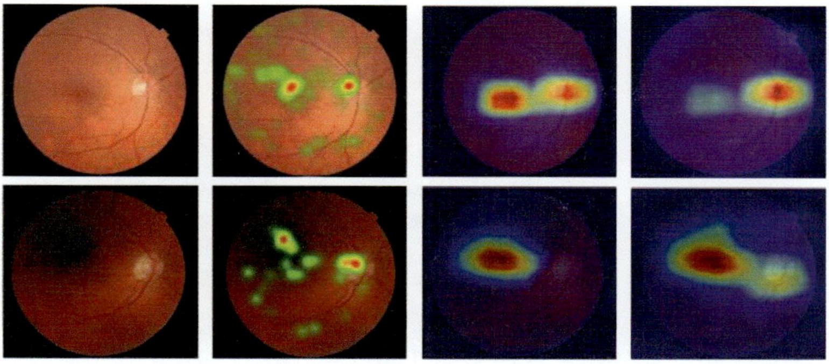

**Figure 2.6** (a) Original image. (b) Eye-tracker. (c) GRAD-CAM. (d) SIDU [17].

experiments for both general and critical medical data, and the SIDU method outperforms state-of-the-art. The ability of localizing ROI in the clinical eye fundus images makes SIDU a better approach to provide transparent explanation and audit model output.

## 2.4 LIME – Local Interpretable Model-Agnostic Explanations

LIME is an approach to gain transparency on what is happening inside the algorithm. It takes the black-box ML model and identifies the relationship between the input and output. ML model interpretation is significant in handling big datasets and complex data types. The metrics like accuracy, $r^2$ score, ROC AUC curves, and precision–recall curves do not provide confidence on model reliability to ML practitioner.

The accuracy and interpretability of the model can be predicted and interpreted by using the python libraries such as LIME, SHAP, interpret, etc.

LIME works using the following steps:

- LIME reads an individual sample and generates a fake dataset and later permutes the fake dataset.
- It computes distance metrics (or similarity metric) between permuted fake data and original observations.
- It predicts on this new permuted fake data using the complex model.

LIME has three core modules that are used on different kinds of datasets:

- lime_tabular – generates explanations for structured datasets.
- lime_text – generates explanations for text datasets.
- lime_image – generates explanations for image datasets.

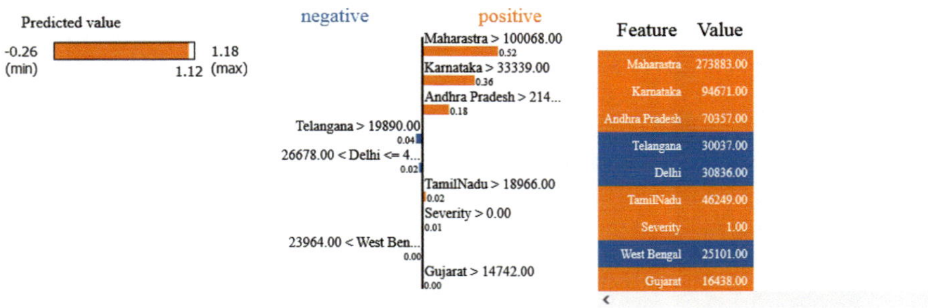


**Figure 2.7** The output of the prediction of COVID-19 data of eight states.

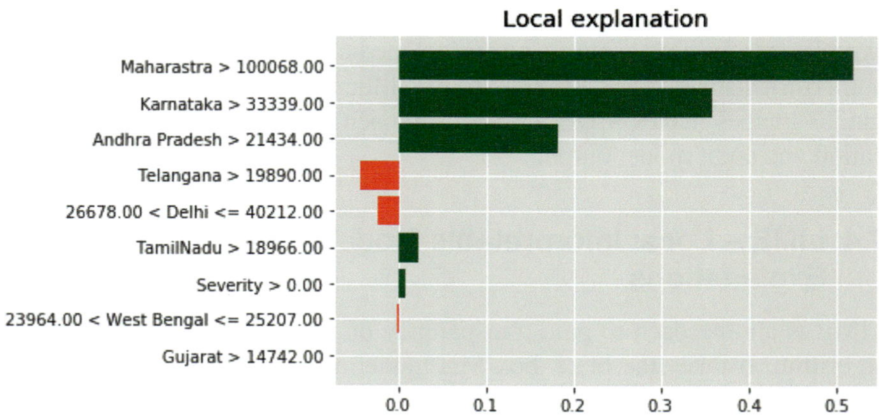


**Figure 2.8** Local explanation of the LIME method.

The authors have implemented the LIME method using lime_tabular module on the datasets of COVID, thyroid, and air pollutant industries.

## 2.4.1 LIME approach for predicting COVID-19

COVID-19 dataset was obtained from MOHFW (www.mohfw.gov.in) for eight states of India; the data were collected from the month of September to December 2021. The numbers of cases considered were from Maharashtra, Karnataka, Andhra Pradesh, Telangana, Delhi, Tamil Nadu, Gujarat, and West Bengal. The term "severity" indicates 1 for more number of cases in the state and 0 for less number of cases. The output of the LIME method is shown with prediction interpretation (Figure 2.7) and local explanation (Figure 2.8).

Gabbay [18] proposed ML models (Figure 2.9) with a LIME-based explainable model on COVID-19 data that provides prediction explainability.

| Feature | Value |
|---|---|
| pneumonia | 1.00 |
| immsupr | 0.00 |
| copd | 0.00 |
| age_group | 7.00 |
| HSD | 10.00 |
| diabetes | 1.00 |
| contact_other_covid | 0.00 |
| obesity | 0.00 |
| pregnancy | 0.00 |
| other_disease | 1.00 |
| renal_chronic | 1.00 |
| sex | 1.00 |
| symptoms_month | 1.00 |
| asthma | 0.00 |
| cardiovascular | 1.00 |
| hypertension | 0.00 |
| tobacco | 0.00 |
| entry_month | 1.00 |

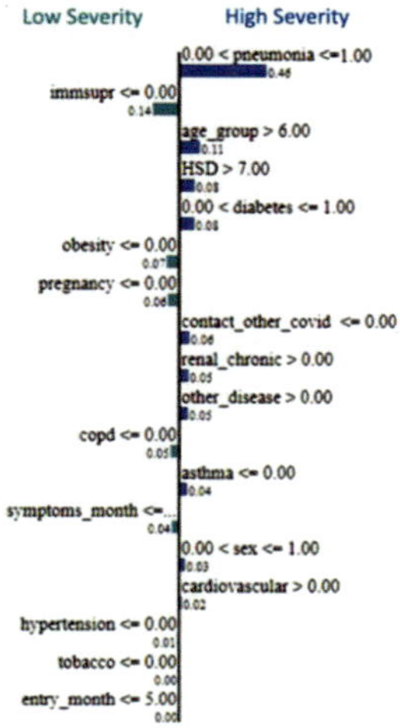


| | B | Sig. |
|---|---|---|
| sex | .345 | .000 |
| pneumonia | 3.196 | .000 |
| age_group | .127 | .000 |
| pregnancy | .481 | .394 |
| diabetes | .258 | .009 |
| copd | .257 | .341 |
| asthma | -.818 | .034 |
| immsupr | .812 | .007 |
| hypertension | .072 | .481 |
| other_disease | .278 | .282 |
| cardiovascular | .278 | .213 |
| obesity | .319 | .001 |
| renal_chronic | .272 | .272 |
| tobacco | -.135 | .380 |
| Constant | -4.049 | .000 |

**Figure 2.9** Explanation and binary regression for COVID [18].

The experimental results proved that the model produced 80% prediction accuracy for the dataset. Later, integration of the explainable ML models into a mobile app was proposed to enable the usage of the models by all medical staff globally.

### 2.4.2 Prediction of thyroid using LIME approach

For this study, the thyroid dataset was obtained from Gandhi Hospital, Secunderabad, India. The output of interpretation (Figure 2.10) and local explanation (Figure 2.11) indicates that the attributes T4 and Tsh play a significant role to determine the thyroid. The term "result" represents whether the patient has thyroid (1) or not (0).

### 2.4.3 LIME method – air pollutant industries

In this case of air pollutant, industries such as drugs and pharmaceuticals (20 units), cement (25 units), thermal power plants (39 units), and sugar (41 units) emit more pollutants compared to other industries. The amount of pollutant emitted into air is mentioned in the braces. The method helps to understand which industry produces the more pollution and can be closed to avoid more pollution or take immediate necessary steps to reduce the pollution. Figure 2.12 represents interpretation and explanation results obtained by LIME model. Table 2.1 gives the details of the industry pollutants in Tamil Nadu state in the year 2021. The data are obtained from open source,

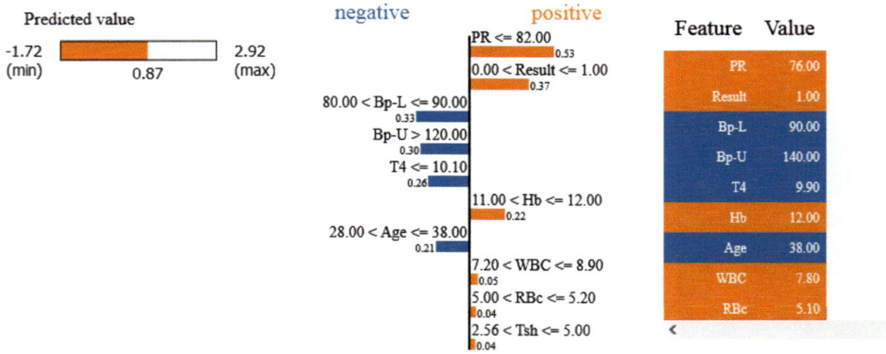


**Figure 2.10** Interpretation of LIME.

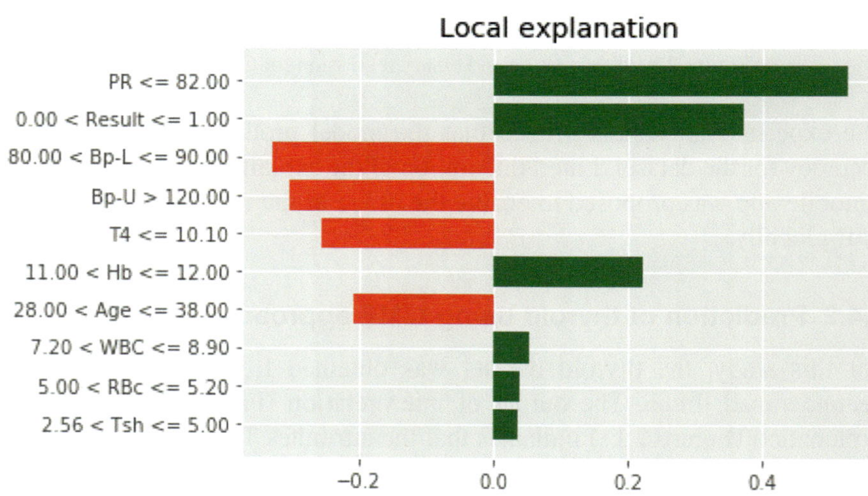


**Figure 2.11** Local explanation.

www.data.gov.in. This approach can be suggested in predicting the major pollutant and attain carbon net-zero globally. Hence, the XAI method is the best suited model for carbon net-zero.

### 2.4.4 Binary classification of breast cancer – LIME method

This case study classifies whether the cancer is malignant or benign based on the LIME method, and Figure 2.13 represents the interpretation of breast cancer prediction [19].

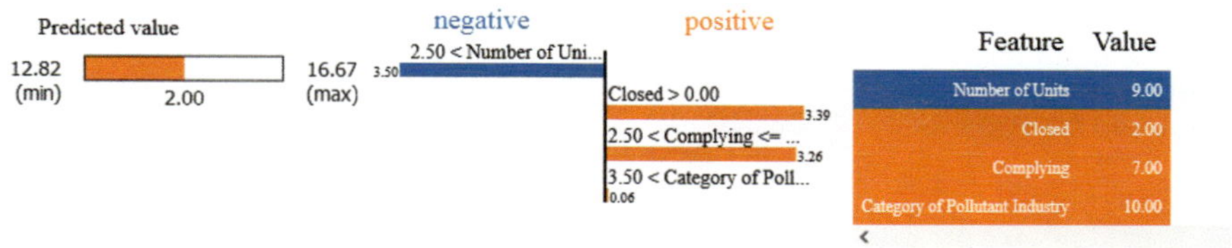


**Figure 2.12** Interpretation of air pollution using LIME.

**Table 2.1** List of pollutant industries in Tamil Nadu (2021).

| S. No. | Category of industries | Number of units | Complying | Defaulting | Closed |
|---|---|---|---|---|---|
| 1 | Aluminum smelting | 0 | 0 | NA | NA |
| 2 | Basic drugs and pharmaceuticals Manufacturing | 20 | 20 | NA | NA |
| 3 | Chlor alkali/caustic soda | 3 | 3 | NA | NA |
| 4 | Cement | 25 | 25 | NA | NA |
| 5 | Copper smelting | 1 | NA | NA | 1 |
| 6 | Dyes and dye intermediate | 1 | 1 | NA | NA |
| 7 | Fermentation (distillery) | 17 | 12 | NA | 5 |
| 8 | Fertilizer | 7 | 7 | NA | NA |
| 9 | Integrated iron and steel | 2 | 2 | NA | NA |
| 10 | Leather processing including tanneries | 9 | 7 | NA | 2 |
| 11 | Oil refinery | 3 | 3 | NA | NA |
| 12 | Pesticide formulation and manufacturing | 1 | 1 | NA | NA |
| 13 | Pulp and paper | 2 | 2 | NA | NA |
| 14 | Petrochemical | 12 | 12 | NA | NA |
| 15 | Sugar | 41 | 36 | NA | 5 |
| 16 | Thermal power plants | 39 | 39 | NA | NA |

## 2.5 Multiclassification of ECG Signals using GRAD-CAM

Yet, in another case study, Ganeshkumar [20] proposed the technique (Figure 2.14) for multiclassification using CNN and GRAD-CAM. The authors [19] trained the model on 6311 ECG records and tested the model with 280 ECG records. The model achieved a subset accuracy of 96.2%, a hamming loss of 0.037, a precision of 0.986, a recall of 0.949, and an $F1$-score of 0.967.

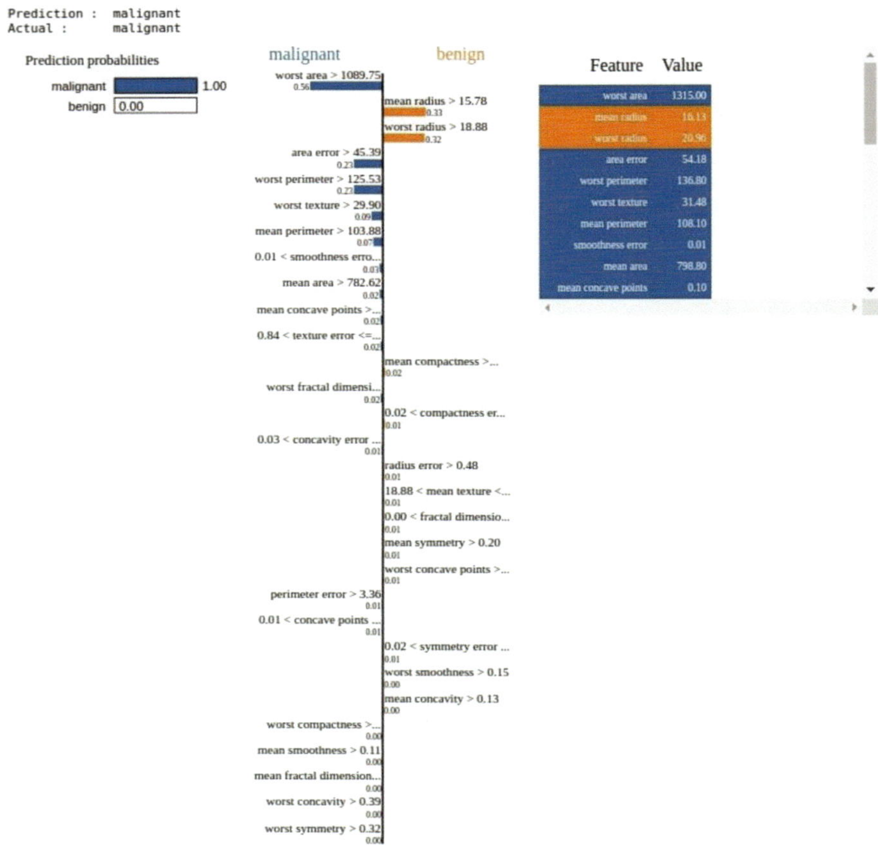


**Figure 2.13** Interpretation of the prediction of breast cancer [19].

## 2.6 Conclusion

The recent large-scale annotated clinical databases, DL models for innovation, open-source software packages are an inexpensive and rapidly increasing computing capacity and cloud storage has extensive growth in AI. The following were observed:

1. LIME outcome provides an intuition into the inner workings of ML algorithms to achieve prediction.
2. LIME algorithms help in providing interpretable output for any type of black-box algorithm.
3. Building trust on this powerful method can achieve higher accuracy and interpretability.

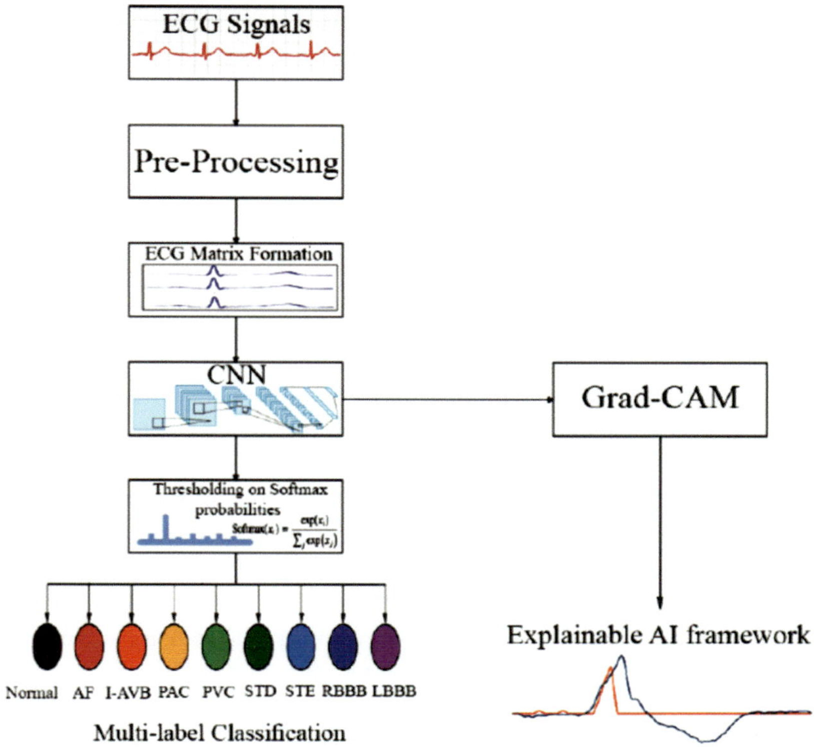


**Figure 2.14** Multiclassification of ECG using LIME [20].

## Acknowledgments

This chapter is dedicated to Prof. Iyyanki Muralikrishna, who spent his valuable and precious time for training and guiding me. I thank him for his encouragement.

## References

[1] Iyyanki M, Jayanthi P and Manickam V. (2020). Machine Learning For Health Data Analytics – A Few Case Studies Of Application Of Regression. *IGI Global. Challenges and Applications for Implementing Machine Learning in Computer Vision.* 241–270. ISBN13: 9781799801825, DOI: 10.4018/978-1-7998-0182-5.

[2] Jayanthi P and Iyyanki M. (2020). Deep Learning Techniques for Prediction, Detection, and Segmentation of Brain Tumors. *IGI Global*. Deep Neural Networks *for* Multimodal Imaging *and*

Biomedical Applications. 118–154. ISBN13: 9781799835912, DOI: 10.4018/978-1-7998-3591-2

[3] Zhang Y, Weng Y and Lund J. (2022). Applications of Explainable Artificial Intelligence in Diagnosis and Surgery. Diagnostics 2022, 12, 237.

[4] Yang G, Ye Q and Xia J. (2022). Unbox the black-box for the medical explainable AI via multi-modal and multi-centre data fusion: A mini-review, two showcases and beyond, Information Fusion. Vol 77. pp 29–52, ISSN 1566-2535, https://doi.org/10.1016/j.inffus.2021.07.016

[5] Langer M, Oster D, Speith T, Hermanns H, Kastner L, Schmidt E, Sesing A and Baum K. (2021). What do we want from Explainabile Artificial Intelligence (XAI)? – A stakeholder perspective on XAI and a conceptual model guiding interdisciplinary XAI research. Artificial Intelligence. doi: 10.1016/j.artint.2021.103473

[6] Tjoa E and Guan C. (2021) A Survey on Explainable Artificial Intelligence (XAI): Toward Medical XAI. IEEE Trans Neural Netw Learn Syst. 32(11):4793–4813. doi: 10.1109/TNNLS.2020.3027314.

[7] Lötsch J, Kringel D and Ultsch A (2022). Explainable Artificial Intelligence (XAI) in Biomedicine. Making AI Decisions Trustworthy for Physicians and Patients. Biomedinformatics 2, 1–17.https://doi.org/10.3390/biomedinformatics2010001

[8] Aghamohammadi M, Madan M, Hong J K and Watson I. (2019). Predicting Heart Attack Through Explainable Artificial Intelligence. In: Computational Science – ICCS 2019. Lecture Notes in Computer Science, vol 11537. Springer, Cham. https://doi.org/10.1007/978-3-030-22741-8_45

[9] Aggarwal R, Podder P and Khamparia A. (2022). ECG Classification and Analysis for Heart Disease Prediction Using XAI-Driven Machine Learning Algorithms. In: Khamparia, A., Gupta, D., Khanna, A., Balas, V.E. (eds) Biomedical Data Analysis and Processing Using Explainable (XAI) and Responsive Artificial Intelligence (RAI). Intelligent Systems Reference Library, vol 222. Springer, Singapore. https://doi.org/10.1007/978-981-19-1476-8_7

[10] Naik H, Goradia P, Desai V, Desai Y and Iyyanki M. (2021). Explainable Artificial Intelligence (XAI) for Population Health Management – An Appraisal. *European Journal of Electrical Engineering and Computer Science*. 5, 6 (Dec. 2021), 64–76. DOI:https://doi.org/10.24018/ejece.2021.5.6.368.

[11] Gozzi N, Malandri L, Mercorio F and Pedrocchi A. (2022). XAI for myo-controlled prosthesis: Explaining EMG data for hand gesture

classification, Knowledge-Based Systems, Vol 240. 108053, ISSN 0950-7051, https://doi.org/10.1016/j.knosys.2021.108053.

[12] Madanu R, Abbod M F, Hsiao F J, Chen W T and Shieh J S. (2022). Explainable AI (XAI) Applied in Machine Learning for Pain Modeling: A Review. Technologies 10, 74. https://doi.org/10.3390/technologies10030074

[13] Dave D, Naik H, Singhal S and Patel, P. (2020). Explainable AI meets Healthcare: A Study on Heart Disease Dataset. *ArXiv, abs/2011.03195.*

[14] Moreno-Sanchez P A. (2020). Development of an Explainable Prediction Model of Heart Failure Survival by Using Ensemble Trees. *IEEE International Conference on Big Data (Big Data)* 2020, pp. 4902–4910, doi: 10.1109/BigData50022.2020.9378460.

[15] Ahuja A S and Halperin L S. (2019). Understanding the advent of artificial intelligence in ophthalmology. J Curr Ophthalmol. vol (2): 115–117. doi: 10.1016/j.joco.2019.05.001. PMID: 31317087; PMCID: PMC6611924.

[16] Kök I, Okay F Y, Muyanl O and Özdemir S. (2022). Explainable Artificial Intelligence (XAI) for Internet of Things: A Survey. arXiv:2206.04800v1

[17] Muddamsetty S M, Jahromi M N S and Moeslund T B. (2021). Expert Level Evaluations for Explainable AI (XAI) Methods in the Medical Domain. In: Pattern Recognition. ICPR International Workshops and Challenges. ICPR 2021. Lecture Notes in Computer Science(), vol 12663. Springer, Cham. https://doi.org/10.1007/978-3-030-68796-0_3

[18] Gabbay F, Bar-Lev S, Montano O and Hadad N. (2021). A LIME-Based Explainable Machine Learning Model for Predicting the Severity Level of COVID-19 Diagnosed Patients. Appl. Sci. 2021.11, 10417. https://doi.org/10.3390/app112110417

[19] https://coderzcolumn.com/tutorials/machine-learning/how-to-use-lime-to-understand-sklearn-models-predictions

[20] Ganeshkumar M, Ravi V, Sowmya V, Gopalakrishnan E A, Soman K P. (2021). Explainable Deep Learning-Based Approach for Multilabel Classification of Electrocardiogram in *IEEE Transactions on Engineering.* https://ieeexplore.ieee.org/document/9537612

# 3

# Explainable Artificial Intelligence (XAI) in the Veterinary and Animal Sciences Field

**Amjad Islam Aqib[1], Mahreen Fatima[2], Afshan Muneer[3], Khazeena Atta[4], Muhammad Arslan[5], C-Neen Fatima Zaheer[6], Sadia Muneer[7] and Maheen Murtaza[3]**

[1]Department of Medicine, Cholistan University of Veterinary and Animal Sciences, Pakistan
[2]Faculty of Biosciences, Cholistan University of Veterinary and Animal Sciences, Pakistan
[3]Department of Zoology, Cholistan University of Veterinary and Animal Sciences, Pakistan
[4]Institute of Biochemistry and Biotechnology, University of Veterinary and Animal Sciences, Pakistan
[5]Department of Poultry Science, Cholistan University of Veterinary and Animal Sciences, Pakistan
[6]Faculty of Veterinary Science, University of Agriculture, Pakistan
[7]Institute of Microbiology, University of Agriculture, Pakistan

## Abstract

Artificial intelligence holds great promise in medical imaging and machine learning. However, artificial intelligence algorithms cannot completely explain decision-making cognitive processes. This circumstance has raised the explainability, sometimes known as the black box, in challenges of XAI in applications: an algorithm merely answers without explaining why the provided pictures were chosen. Explainable artificial intelligence (XAI) has emerged as a solution to this challenge and has grabbed the interest of many academics. In this review, we share our thoughts on current and future machine learning and possible next steps for the veterinary and animal sciences field. First, we discuss the explainable artificial intelligence in biomedical applications. Following that, we will discuss how AI-powered models may play a more sustainable role in the animal scientific environment. Lastly, we provide recommendations for XAI future perspective in animal field on how to support themselves, the dairy farmers, poultry farmers, and challenges to using XAI in veterinary and animal sciences, considering the opportunities and challenges of XAI in applications.

## 3.1 Introduction

Artificial intelligence (AI) is a field that studies computer science. This contains creating computer programs to perform things that normally need human intelligence. Algorithms for artificial intelligence can be concerned with learning, perception, problem-solving, language comprehension, and/or logical reasoning. Machines exhibit artificial intelligence, often known as mechanical intelligence, as opposed to humans and other animals, who express natural intellect. It is intended to do tasks such as speech recognition, learning, planning, and problem-solving [1]. In the last years, there has been a significant increase in the number of research articles, conferences, and symposia on explainable artificial intelligence (XAI) around the world. This has led to an abundance of domain-dependent and context-dependent methods to deal with the interpretation of machine learning (ML) models and the creation of explanations for humans. Unfortunately, this trend is not yet over; there is a wealth of knowledge in this field that is dispersed and in need of organization. The purpose of this article is to systematically review research works in the field of XAI and attempt to define some field boundaries [2].

Animal husbandry, as an agricultural process, is a difficult task within the scope of agriculture, involving multiple challenges. The use of technology in farming is critical for overcoming the challenges of animal traceability, health information, and performance recording. Furthermore, as the world's population continues to grow, there is a need to increase food production (meat) by ensuring the welfare of farm animals in order to keep up with population growth. The welfare of farm animals will ensure the availability of nutritious, high-quality food all over the world. Furthermore, the analysis and management of large datasets on employment and small- and large-scale cattle rearing, as well as technologies applicable to information delivery and communication, will aid in the protection and comprehension of the convertible agricultural system [3].

Identifying the most relevant data for animal health managers is a challenging combination of control measures based on local (such as farm characteristics, productivity objectives, etc.) and regional (such as available resources, farm location, administrative preferences, etc.) characteristics.

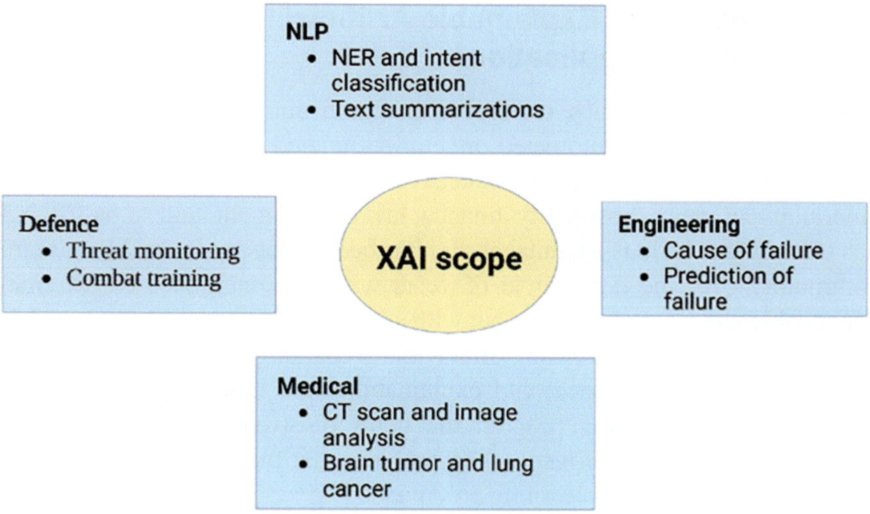


**Figure 3.1** Scope of explainable artificial intelligence in different fields NLP(natural language process) for classification and text summarization, Engineering could be used to find cause and prediction of any project , in medical and defence could be sed for CT scan brain and lungs tumor diagnosis and in threat monitoring respectively.

Mechanical modeling can be used to evaluate, compare, and prioritize a variety of options. However, most available models clearly do not coordinate human decision-making, whereas control decisions (such as unregulated diseases) are frequently made by farmers, sometimes with large-scale health and decision-making consequences (such as pathogen spread, dissemination of information and rumors, area of influence, etc.). The goal of recent research is to integrate humans and their decisions by deploying the best control and favorable strategy via AI or health economics practices [4]. However, some challenges exist for medical AI applications, such as the black-box nature of some AI models. Because these black-box models are difficult to explain, medical experts are hesitant to make explainable clinical inferences. Medical AI applications must be transparent in order to gain the trust of doctors. XAI research has recently received a lot of attention. XAI is critical for accepting and practically integrating medical AI applications. Many studies have used deep learning methods for medical applications in addition to traditional machine learning methods. Without the use of feature engineering, a deep learning algorithm can learn representations of raw data. Deep learning techniques that are commonly used include multi-layer perceptron (MLPs), deep neural networks (DNNs), convolutional neural networks (CNNs), and recurrent neural networks (RNNs) [5] (Figure 3.1).

## 3.2 Mechanism of Explainable Artificial Intelligence in Biomedical Application

ML and AI algorithms have recently been significantly improved and are now being used to develop automated or semi-automated systems in almost every domain, including construction, education, healthcare, manufacturing, travel, entertainment, news, hospitality, finance, law enforcement, and so on [6]. XAI has offered tremendous advantages and has been a hotspot in the ML research community over the last couple of years with the emergence of extremely dependable and accurate models but with a lack of interpretability and explainability. Specifically, healthcare offers more challenges which demands for model fidelity, performance, and explainability are much higher than other domains. XAI is a research program that helps to solve the so-called *black-box problem in artificial intelligence*: the problem that many computing systems developed using machine learning are opaque [7].

Scientists sometimes confuse the words interpretability and exploitability, although they have practical distinctions [8]. Despite various attempts to distinguish between these two concepts, there is no formal mathematical definition for interpretability and explainability. Explainability is defined as the ability to interact with humans in simple and intelligible ways [9]. The interpretability of model outputs, on the other hand, is mostly determined by the intuition underpinning the model's outputs. XAI aids in communicating automated options to impacted patients in a straightforward and understandable manner [10]. Healthcare is one of the high-profile areas and XAI is gaining more scientific interests in the field of biomedical sciences and healthcare. The ground mechanics and logic of ML system are linked to XAI [11]. These intelligible models may aid in gaining a deeper and more accurate understanding of human disorders. An interpretable model's underlying mechanics or internal logics may be incomprehensible to humans [12]. As a result, when it comes to ML systems, explainability does not always imply interpretability, and vice versa. As a result, explainability alone is insufficient, and the presence of interpretability is also required. For a complete knowledge of XAI, a variety of models have been supplied. In healthcare systems, interactive and interpretable ML modeling solutions that incorporate both machine learning and domain experts have been deployed [13, 14].

XAI is a field of machine learning that ensures the accessibility of complicated techniques in the field of biomedical and healthcare domains such as detection of critical illnesses by analysis of the electronic health record at early stages [15, 16], prediction of future disease by analyzing genomic data [17], and smart clinical decision supporting systems [18]. The medical data are divergent and vast, which include both structured and unstructured data and AI-based algorithms are more promising in the healthcare and biomedical domains. The mechanism of XAI implies various steps such as data acquisition, data preprocessing, configuring, simulation, assessment tuning, and recalibration. In healthcare and medical domains to make the model trustworthy, the models need to be understandable and transparent at each evaluation step [19]. XAI can help with illness knowledge and developing faith that the findings discovered by ML are not fake. Hence, XAI should have the following goals: causality, trustworthiness, informativeness, transferability, accessibility, trust, privacy awareness, fairness, and interactivity [20].

## 3.3 XAI in Diagnosis, Prevention, and Treatment

Clinical diagnosis is mostly based on signs and symptoms of the disease. It is quite difficult and challenging to diagnose a disease at an early stage based on the common signs and symptoms because of the similarity of symptoms of more than one disease. Delay in diagnosis has promising effects on the severity of symptoms leading to life-threatening disorders. Advanced and specialized processes for sickness diagnosis, prevention, management, and treatment are required to properly manage the growing patient population. Since the 1990s, machine learning has been applied in diagnostic medicine [21]. Advances in technology provided easier, faster, and reliable methods for applying machine learning in various fields of medicine, such as diabetes [22], cancer [23], respiratory diseases [24], etc. Deep learning has provided excellent results in classification and prediction. However, the parameters inside model structures lack practical meanings and are unexplainable. Explainable artificial intelligence has become a popular and emerging field in recent years [25, 26]. The fundamental goal of XAI is to persuade consumers that machine learning technologies are more transparent and can deliver reliable predictions [27]. XAI is a set of algorithms that improves on existing machine learning technologies by providing proof for predictions. In radiology, for example, a normal ML algorithm may predict that an image has cancer signs; an XAI system, on the other hand, will propose where and what that evidence is, such as a 3-cm right lower lobe nodule [28].

Lundberg et al. in 2018 where they developed an XAI-based warning system called "prescience." This system predicts hypoxemia (low oxygen levels in the blood) during surgery just 5 minutes after it occurs. Typically, real-time blood oxygen monitoring through pulse oximetry only allows anesthesiologists to take reactive actions to minimize the duration of hypoxemic episodes after their occurrence. However, the prescience system provides the physicians with a risk score and monitors vital signs that update in real time. The system also lists risk factors such as patient comorbidities and vital sign abnormalities [29, 30]. In 2022, Thimoteo *et al.* used XAI techniques in diagnosis of COVID-19 based on pathogen variables and blood tests. Two glass-box models, explainable boosting and logistic regression models, support vector and random forest machine, and two black-box models were used to diagnose the disease. Glass-box models feature importance and brought an insight into the most relevant features, while sharply additive explanations were used to explain predictions for the black-box models. All global information showed that white blood cells such as eosinophils are among the essential features to help diagnose COVID-19 [31].

Alzheimer's disease is a neurological illness that causes brain shrinkage and cell death. It is the leading cause of dementia. Thus far, no cure for Alzheimer's has been discovered. As a result, it is critical to detect it early [32]. Sudar et al. sought to detect the phases of Alzheimer's disease using photos as input in 2022 using the layer-wise relevance propagation (LRP) approach in XAI [33]. Early intervention and detection of atrial fibrillation (AF) is a cornerstone for sound treatment and prevention of mortality. Due to lack of interpretability, deep learning models (DLM) cannot be applied in clinical practice [34]. Jo *et al.* 2021 developed an explainable DLM to diagnose AF using electrocardiogram (ECG) and validated its performance through various ECG formats. The results of this study indicated that XAI can be used to the DLM using ECG and improved the transparency of the DLM for its applications in clinical practice [35]. XAI can be used for the diagnosis of various diseases such as neurological disorders [36], Parkinson's disease [37], non-communicable disease [38], obesity [39], heart rate variability and other cardiovascular disorders [40, 41], allergy [42], rheumatoid arthritis [43], hepatitis [44], etc.

Among the currently accessible technologies, XAI has been recognized as one of the most successful and effective scientific procedures for mankind. Recent research has demonstrated the significance and consequences of machine learning for image recognition in cases where traditional techniques were unable to recognize early indications of disease, particularly in the case of cancer, where XAI aids in early diagnosis and therapy. This is especially true for nations where healthcare expenses, budgets, and other similar restraints make it difficult to provide adequate treatment [45]. In light of digital health data, artificial intelligence in medicine (AIM) has contributed to healthcare [46]. However, despite their promising performance, the development of AIM technologies for actual clinical practice is relatively difficult due to factors such as inadequate data, possible bias, and the lack of equivalent mechanisms to assure efficacy and safety in the real world [47]. Some scientists contend that since physicians can rely on medications like aspirin despite not knowing the underlying process, why should they expect AI to provide explanations if its performance is good? [48]. Drugs, on the other hand, must undergo randomized clinical studies before they can be commercialized. In the event of substantial adverse effects, post-marketing surveillance directs regulatory agencies, such as the Food and Drug Administration (FDA) in the United States, to remove the product from the market. XAI increases medical professionals' trust in AIM by assisting them in determining if AIM choices reach consensus and are legitimate [49]. As a result, XAI in medicine is critical for facilitating the deployment of artificial intelligence in clinical decision support systems [48, 50].

## 3.4 XAI in Dairy Farming

Let us first define artificial intelligence (AI), which usually stands for artificial insemination in dairy circles. Software using AI may solve issues and carry out tasks that would otherwise require human intelligence. The identification of "normal" or expected shapes, colors, patterns, and so on, and the subsequent detection of deviations from these norms, are widespread and well-established applications of AI. Already, artificial intelligence (AI) in robotic milking systems chooses whether or not to milk a cow at a specific time and notifies the farmer of any changes to regular feeding habits, milk quality, and other factors. In order to maximize pasture use, some dairy producers are now adopting virtual fencing systems, which are akin to technology for canine companions. The cows have GPS-enabled collars that, when necessary, move them with beeps or a gentle electrical pulse. AI may also be used in breeding; the computer can offer breeding alternatives based on facts such as milk output, feed consumption, and other aspects. Scientists from Spain have defined an intelligent edge-IoT (Internet of Things) platform for tracking cows and plants in a dairy development environment, as well as providing the user with rich data on dairy products to ensure their quality and safety. As per scientists, AI might help the dairy industry make required market adjustments by making it more resource-efficient, ecologically friendly, visible, and safe (Figure 3.2).

Artificial intelligence is becoming more and more common in dairy farming, and it is expanding really quickly. By keeping dairy cows in good health and preserving their physiological and physical circumstances, it can primarily alter the situation for dairy farmers. This knowledge-based technology has great promise and might close the gaps in dairy production, which would help the dairy industry indirectly. AI has many benefits in dairy farming, including observing dairy cow activity, increasing milk output and farm

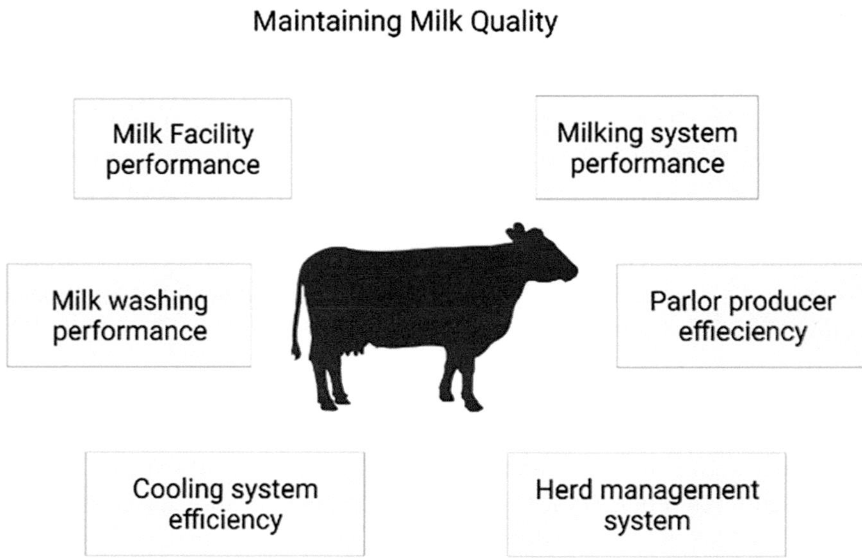


**Figure 3.2** Maintaining milk quality by XAI: XAI machines has many operational programs in livestock management such as monitoring dairy management increasing milk production, production on the farm and diagnosis diseases.

productivity, identifying mastitis in dairy cows, identifying odors on dairy farms, and creating intelligent cow pens that employ image analysis. In the end, it offers fresh optimism and wide-open possibilities for the overall quality and development of the dairy industry through a successful business strategy in dairy farming.

Opportunities include developing more precise diets, enhancing pastures used for grazing so that the supply of macronutrients and micronutrients matches animal needs, and breeding new plants. Artificial intelligence and robots used in pasture management will help match animal needs with daily supply. Better consumer knowledge of the perceived higher nutritional content of milk from grazed cows, as well as greater understanding of the benefits of grazing for animal health, welfare, and behavioral benefits, could assist in the future sustainability of demand for milk from dairy cows on pasture [51].

Future farms will use robotics, automation, and on- and off-farm sensors to better manage their herds, adhere to rules, and leave less of an environmental footprint. Artificial intelligence will transform data from sensors, robotics, and automated equipment into useful outputs that can be used by management.

The prediction of complicated events, including the timing of conception, is being improved using artificial intelligence and machine learning; as

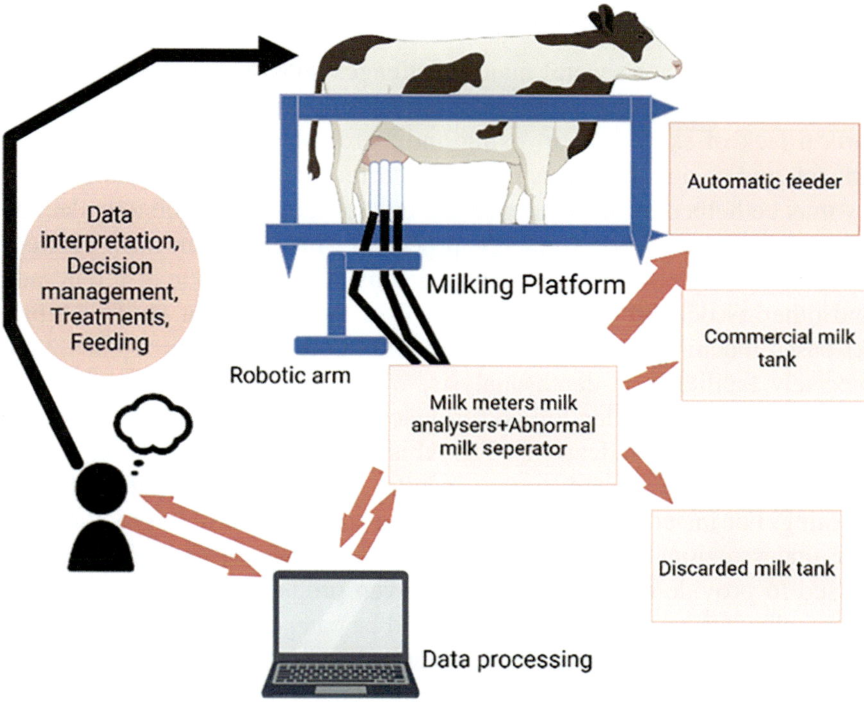


**Figure 3.3** Milking platform Automatic milking system(AMS): In addition to milk yield and composition, the frequency and intervals of milking determine the SCC and bacteriological characteristics of the milk, which are influenced by many factors. In addition, AMS equipment allows large amounts of data to be recorded about individual cows and herd performance.

feedback from sensors, robots, and automated systems is incorporated through software that learns and increases prediction or diagnosis accuracy, this field will experience rapid advancements. Information regarding the quality and digestibility of feed will be provided by sensors monitoring crop fields, silos, and other feed storage facilities. Field-specific and storage circumstances have an impact on this. Data from individual cow consumption tracked by three-dimensional imaging devices will be added to this sensor data. Mammary gland, liver, and other organs will be monitored using biodegradable, implantable sensors. The health of the udder and teats, as well as the content of the milk and important hormones, will be tracked by in-line detectors from each teat cup. Additionally, when cows go to and from milking robots, automated systems will evaluate cow BW, physical health, and changes in gait to forecast lameness. To describe changes in immunological and disease state that are reflected in perturbations in important DNA sequences throughout the genome, milk somatic cell DNA will be studied [52] (Figure 3.3).

## 3.5 XAI in Poultry Farming

Poultry farmers face several major challenges with such industry-level production, including pressure on production costs, concerns about animal welfare, a lack of skilled labor, rising antimicrobial resistance, environmental impact, and so on. Numerous problems currently faced in the poultry industry may be helped by AI. However, the bulk of farms continue to collect data manually before having computers process it. A chicken farm is predicted to be able to produce 4.1 million data points by 2050, thanks to different radars and other associated devices attached over the internet of stuffs. Utilizing AI-based machineries to gather information in real time, automatically, and precisely facilitates in-depth analysis, which may enable us to take quick action to improve production performance. AI is capable of both supervised and unsupervised data learning. The AI is trained using pre-existing fact collections that are restricted to only specific governed work under supervised learning. For instance, estimating expected body weight for a specific broiler line under regional circumstances. Enormous totals of data might be processed to provide early warning of a given product below unsubstantiated knowledge, where figures together would be categorized, and developments recognized without explicit programming using cloud resources. Big data and data mining would be the most useful tools in the hands of poultry producers to maximize the return on their investment. Only a small number of ICT organizations are concentrating on performance prediction based on records and data collected in real time, and this would assist the farmer in making decisions to optimize agricultural produce. In high-tech farms, a variety of sensors were used to measure bird weight, temperature, feed and water intake, humidity, ammonia levels, $CO_2$ levels, and many other characteristics. Computer-assisted technology and robotics have the potential to minimize human involvement with farm birds while simultaneously reducing the source of infection and increasing productivity in comparison to humans. The use of AI might lower the mistake rate to insignificant levels and work around the clock, improving agricultural efficiency and optimizing farm profit. In the near future, AI might turn conservative manufacturing agribusiness into smooth poultry farming or AI-assisted poultry farming.

In poultry buildings, innovative technology is often used, such as automated feed and water supply via automation knowledge. In recent years, research on enhancing poultry production to boost overall efficiency has continued. With the organized system designs for cage production systems, diverse automation apparatus has developed efficient pieces inside the systems. An excellent instance is the extremely automatic equipment used to gather and sort eggs for layer chickens [53].

Poultry refers to the community raising of birds such as turkeys, quails, geese, and ostriches, with chickens being the most frequent. The poultry industry's two primary functions are egg and meat production. A poultry farm used to house a few hundred birds, and all poultry farm management duties, including animal monitoring, were handled by humans. The number of poultry farms, however, will grow in tandem with the increase in demand for chicken products. Because chickens and hens are weak and prone to disease, individual bird monitoring is required so that signs of various diseases may be discovered in time to manage the disease pandemic. Obviously, if the farm is entirely controlled by humans, the number of staff needed to monitor animals on an individual bird level is far larger, resulting in higher production costs. Furthermore, the natural habitat of poultry birds is shrinking as the number of human employees increases. Furthermore, it raises concerns about the health of poultry workers. Because most poultry bird illnesses are very infectious and communicable, they also impact people. If a lethal illness emerges in poultry, the situation becomes extremely severe [53].

Monitoring environmental conditions and chicken health, egg harvesting, and stimulating bird mobility are all part of poultry production. Approaches to meeting technical demands have included the development of intelligent moveable equipment for use with chicks in poultry houses. The most notable outcomes are the Octopus Poultry Safe (OPS) robot for autonomously cleaning poultry buildings, Poultry Bot for selecting eggs, and Spoutnic for instructing hens to walk. This research and development trend is projected to continue. An expanding research focus is on the collaborations of automated chores in order to attain great efficacy in total poultry house management.

Various technologies are emerging to assist farmers in increasing their efficiency. Every discipline requires evolution to reach its pinnacle. The only issue is when it will happen. To keep up with the changing trends, AI (artificial intelligence) must be introduced into the poultry industry (Figure 3.4).

### 3.5.1 Poultry drones

Drones have the potential to be employed in the poultry sector. Despite concerns that these drones may cause flock anxiety and stress, they may be employed on free-range or yard farms where poultry birds can roam freely. Farming nondescript birds is the buzz of the town. These drones serve as nannies for these unassuming birds (large scale). Regular aviculture monitoring with drones is beneficial for flock security.

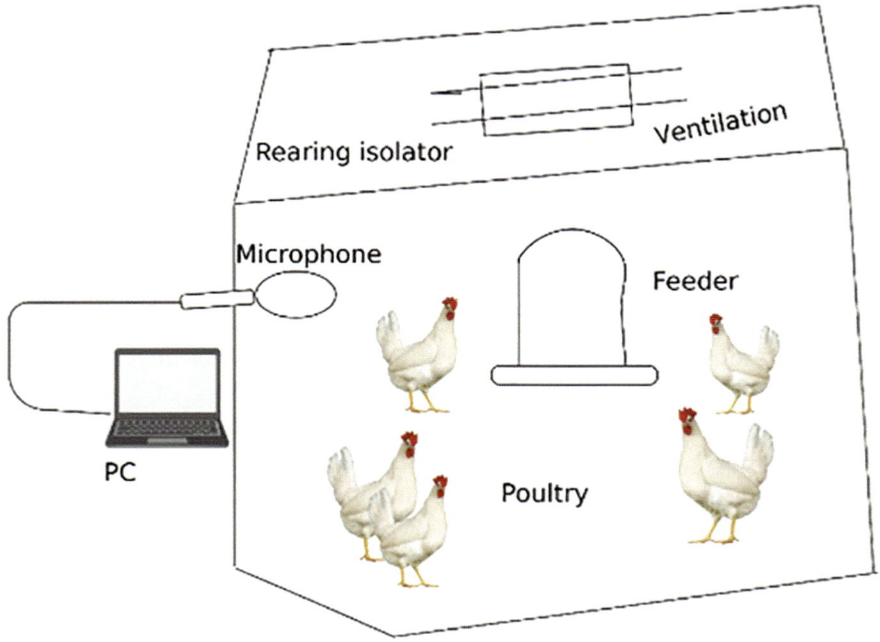


**Figure 3.4** Detecting feeding behavior through the intelligence method: A time sequence model and audio analysis can be used to detect changes in eating vocalizations based on differences between eating and normal vocalizations of poultry.

### 3.5.2 Avian illness detection models

Aside from a high fever, sick birds may exhibit symptoms such as nasal and saliva discharges. Images or views provided from more precise drones in free range and three-dimensional models in control buildings are put into specifically constructed symptom detector analyzers to detect the disease at an early stage, as the sickness is infectious and leads to decreased productivity.

It also assists farmers in preserving the lives of chicks since clogging clogs the bird's snout, resulting in death. Devices are trained to distinguish between healthy and affected birds by annotating the secretions on the beaks of chickens. Tools aid in accurately distinguishing the target form and texture of the secretion.

### 3.5.3 Models for detecting behavioral disorders

Pecking (biting anything with the beak) behavior frequently compromises the flock's health and well-being. Because death happens within 10 minutes of pecking, early diagnosis becomes critical. Devices that notify farmers about cannibalism within the period of destruction will improve the welfare and production of chickens.

Every year, current chicken production methods result in the early death and rejection of billions of chickens before they are processed for meat. This loss of life has major consequences for animal care, agricultural efficiency, and the economy. The best way to avoid these losses is to do continuously individualized and/or group-level animal evaluations. Personalized and per-herd evaluations of animals were previously regarded to be wrong and inefficient on large-scale farms, but with the introduction of artificial intelligence (AI) assisted technology, they became feasible and effective [54]. The concept of artificial intelligence and its key techniques were introduced, and then there were research and development and application from aspects such as intelligent diagnosis systems for poultry disease, intelligent decision-making platforms for poultry production, intelligent environment monitoring technology, intelligent detection technology of poultry body temperatures, intelligent listening technology for poultry sound, intelligent monitoring technology for poultry sound, intelligent monitoring technology for poultry sound, and intelligent monitoring robots [55].

**Challenges to using XAI in veterinary and animal sciences:**

Artificial intelligence is homolog to human intelligence but risks and concerns related to its use are jeopardizing the use of these cybernetics and robotics. The progression and effective installation of artificial intelligence is yet an unexplored field of computer science and technology. That is predominantly based on orthodox thoughts and estimated apprehensions at a time where advancements in veterinary businesses and medicine are urged to be fulfilled [56].

- Concerns to the extent of accuracy and precision in task performance and crisis management.
- Need of high monetary investments at commercial level installations and reduction of profits initially.
- Fear of breach in data sourcing and privacy policy's integrity at farms.
- Estimates that uniformity in animal products and their qualities will cause loss to trades and niche competition amongst veterinary businesses.
- Lack of satisfactory data about the implementation of this technology on industrial levels.

- Loss of complete and intact governmental legality concerning AI.
- Lack of trained workers or officials regarding sophisticated automation in veterinary radiology.
- Welfare and ethical issues related to the use of the technologies detecting pre-natal defects that lead to deliberate death of embryo.
- Less experimental trials on animals and robotic dealings with them also lead to many concerns.
- Additional costs on repair and maintenance, disinfection of robotics, and machinery amid epidemiology [57].

The machine learning is also leading to many projected risks as blind visionary insights that reduce the innovation in human minds. This technology is also challenging to be installed and used because AI is not capable enough to replicate all aspects of human cognitive abilities and the six senses that humans possess [58, 59]. Use of AI may also leave its marks as a mere source of human lethargy and unemployment. There is lack of complete awareness regarding the automation and cybernetics that also generates many questions in mind. These estimated logical reasoning and necessity of huge economic investments are the main challenges to the use of AI. However, these very basic reasons may be putting controversies on machine malware, data integrity, work efficiency, legality, and cost effectiveness of these technologies [60].

**Challenges of XAI in applications:**

The main purpose of machine learning (ML) is to learn the right decision system respectively, predictors that can help automate tasks, which otherwise humans will have to do. As ML is increasingly used in real-world applications, there has been a general consensus that high prediction accuracy alone may not be practically sufficient [61]. The challenge of recognizing and integrating these necessities cannot be addressed with the same discipline in isolation. Accurate patterns are typically more complicated and difficult to comprehend. In the field, this is especially significant of general trade-off power systems as a general consumer will generally demand both precision and impressive performance clarity, so that there is a high level of reliability. Only when a concept of what knowledge might be valuable and can be productively provided, at a defined perspective and to a particular stakeholder, is present does it make sense to extract usable information from black-box models. This is XAI research, which is situated at the crossroads of several fields such as ML/AI, human–computer interface (HCI) research, and branches of social sciences [62, 63].

The cornerstone for the application of XAI at medicine is the requirement because of the added value that originates from medical professionals knowing why a machine-based decision was reached. As a result, there is an increasing demand for AI methods that are not only effective but also dependable, transparent, interpretable, and explainable to a human expert. It also has significant implications for the public, politics, and government, as the defining ability of AI technology increases the credibility of medical experts [64].

Process monitoring refers to observing production processes to detect any problems. Time-series data from several hundred signals, i.e., process signals, are theoretically available immediately from the automation system in many plants. Operators analyze this process using a variety of process graphics. Process engineers and automation engineers may also be required to monitor numerous plants at the same time. Exceptional situations according to management consortium guidelines, abuse of information, inconsistencies, and non-availability can all lead to failure in human surveillance-related conditions. Not surprisingly, consistently observing such a large number of data is a psychologically demanding activity [65].

ML solutions can assist users in assessing and responding to difficult situations. Once a problem or abnormality is detected in an action or device (such as a pump or compressor), a condition is diagnosed in order to determine the source of the problem. Additional sensing, such as vibration sensors, can frequently assist localization of a problem, such as pipe-in-the-wall leaks. In fact, some events that require operator responses such as irritation or foam are relatively frequent. To better respond to or avoid such incidents, the forecasting of the event can help operators. The phrase "soft sensor" refers to data-driven technologies that provide anticipated values for physical or chemical qualities that cannot be directly or reliably measured [66]. Recognizing these challenges, the international community of explainable AI (XAI) researchers has grown significantly over the last half-decade, particularly in medical areas. The correct definition and extent of explanation are open questions that are prone to disagreement within the scientific community [67].

In general, humans remain silent in adopting, given the increased demand for moral AI, strategies that are not directly interpretable, viable, or dependable must be developed. It is common to believe that focusing just on performance will make the system more opaque. However, increases in a system's understanding might lead to the remedy of its flaws. Consideration of interpretation as an extra design motivation while creating an ML model can improve its implementation for three reasons:

1. Interpretation contributes to decision-making neutrality, i.e., detecting bias in training datasets and, as a result, detecting correct bias.
2. Interpretation facilitates consolidation delivery by revealing any competing issues that can modify prediction.
3. Interpretation can ensure that only relevant variables are used to assess production, meaning that there is a basic truth in model reasoning [68].

**XAI future perspective:**

In this section, we will discuss how XAI approach is used in the analysis of medical images and how computer vision technologies are being adapted. We divide explanation ways into three types: visual, textual, and example-based, and we divide each procedure into model-based vs. post-hawk, model-specific versus model-agnostic, and global versus local clarity frameworks [69].The most typical kind of XAI in medical photo analysis is a visual explanation, also known as significant mapping. The major maps depict the key elements of the decision-making picture. The majority of popular mapping systems employ back-propaganda-based methodologies, although some employ trouble-based or multiple example-based learning methods.

Shen et al. [68] called it rating CNN to predict the stigma of lung noodles on CT. They identified five textual descriptions of picture qualities that are typical of lung nodule malignancy and are normally evaluated by a radiologist. The challenge of locating text descriptions was linked with the critical function of determining lung nodal notoriety. While his ratings did not much outperform those of a typical CNN, the technique did include human interpretation elements of noodles. An example-based explanation is an XAI technique that provides examples of data points that are currently being analyzed. This is useful when attempting to explain why a neural network made a decision, and it is related to how humans explain the cause. For example, when a pathologist examines a patient's biopsy that shows similarities with the first patient examined by a pathologist, medical judgment can be increased by knowing the first biopsy diagnosis. We need to find a common ground for discussion in order to take a systematic approach to human-centric XAI. In broad terms, the current fidelity in XAI can be presented as the relevant social groups (e.g., AI researchers, policymakers, practitioners, etc.) who have interpretive faculty (interpretations) on field construction. Relevant terms such as clarity, interpretation, intuition, and transparency have been used interchangeably in various communities. Many people define clarity as a property of the AI system's operation or decisions that are simple for people to understand. Clarity is frequently regarded as more general than model transparency or direct interpretation models [68]. MYCIN, an expert system that recommended the diagnosis and treatment of bacterial infections in the 1970s, may already explain its reasoning for diagnostic or instructional purposes. In an essay at the Computer Science Conference on Innovative Applications of Artificial Intelligence two years later, the FSC was described as an "XAI system" for the tactical behavior of the tiny unit. A more contemporary, machine-learning-based, and often referenced XAI definition is: XAI's goal is to "build a defining model while keeping a high degree of learning performance (predictability accuracy) and enabling human customers to comprehend, trust, and govern the next generation of artificially intelligent partners." In literature, the interpretations of the term are frequently used interchangeably. One way to think about potential differences is as follows: We refer to interpretive machine learning or interpretive AI when a person can directly understand the reasoning and actions of the machine without any additional explanations. As a result, the interpretation might be regarded as a passive property of artifacts. However, if a person must be specified as a proxy in order to comprehend the system's learning and reasoning processes; for example, because the artificial neural network is extremely sophisticated, explainable AI research is discussed. Various tools have been developed and classified in computer science, which is conducting the majority of the research on XAI, to explain the internal work of AI. Some of these approaches interpret the same machine learning model prediction, while others interpret the entire model, distinguishing between "local" and "global" interpretations. Output is defined as "feature intensity" (saying that data is supported, or model prediction is opposed), "instances" (returning data examples as examples for model behavior explanation), "model internal" (returning model internal representations, such as model neurons), and "surrogate models" (returning an internally interpretive, transparent model that targets black-box estimates of the model). Some XAI approaches are applicable to any machine learning model ("explanations versus model"), while others are exclusively applicable to neural networks ("model specific explanations") [69].

## 3.6 Conclusion

XAI is an emerging field that is gaining significant attention in biomedical sciences and healthcare systems, XAI-based interactive and interpretable modeling solutions have been successfully deployed for detecting critical illnesses, predicting future diseases, and supporting smart clinical decision-making.

The application of machine learning and artificial intelligence in various fields such as veterinary and animal sciences, diagnostic medicine, and robotic milking systems. The solution-based framework developed by AI developers can be used for application model development and monitoring methods. We study AI, robotics, and machine learning, and one common area of research is Explainable AI (XAI). Given the various ways in which AI can be achieved, it is important to establish guidelines and best practices for its development.

## References

[1] Saleh, Z. (2019). Artificial Intelligence Definition, Ethics and Standards.

[2] Vilone, G., & Longo, L. (2020). *Explainable Artificial Intelligence: a Systematic Review.*

[3] Bello, R.-W., Mohamed, A. S. A., & Talib, A. (2022). *Smart animal husbandry: A review of its data, applications, techniques, challenges and opportunities.*

[4] Ezanno, P., Picault, S., Beaunée, G., Bailly, X., Muñoz, F., Duboz, R.,... Guégan, J.-F. (2021). Research perspectives on animal health in the era of artificial intelligence. *Veterinary research, 52*(1), 1–15.

[5] Zhang, Y., Weng, Y., & Lund, J. (2022). Applications of Explainable Artificial Intelligence in Diagnosis and Surgery. *Diagnostics, 12*(2), 237.

[6] Rai, A. (2020). Explainable AI: From black box to glass box. Journal of the Academy of Marketing Science, 48(1), 137–141.

[7] Gunning, D., & Aha, D. (2019). DARPA's explainable artificial intelligence (XAI) program. AI magazine, 40(2), 44–58.

[8] Lotsch, J.; Kringel, D.; Ultsch, A. Explainable artificial intelligence (XAI) in biomedicine: Making AI decisions trustworthy for physicians and patients. Biomedinformatics 2022, 2, 1–17. [CrossRef]

[9] Linardatos, P.; Papastefanopoulos, V.; Kotasiantis, S. Explainable AI: A review of machine learning interpretability methods. Entropy 2021, 23, 18. [CrossRef]

[10] Lipton, Z.C. The mythos of model interpretability. Queue 2018, 16, 31–57. [CrossRef]

[11] Doshi-Velez, F.; Kim, B. Towards a rigorous science of interpretable machine learning. arXiv 2017, arXiv:1702.08608.

[12] Gilpin, L.H.; Bau, D.; Yuan, B.Z.; Bajwa, A.; Specter, M.; Kagal, L. Explaining explanations: An overview of interpretability of machine learning. In Proceedings of the 2018 IEEE 5th International Conference on Data Science and Advanced Analytics (DSAA), Turin, Italy, 1–3 October 2018; pp. 80–89.

[13] Datta, A.; Flynn, N.R.; Barnette, D.A.; Woeltje, K.F.; Miller, J.P.; Swamidass, S.J. Machine learning liver-injuring drug interactions with non-steroidal anti-inflammatory drugs (NSAIDs) from a retrospective electronic health record (EHR) cohort. PLoS Comput. Biol. 2021, 17, E1009053. [CrossRef] [PubMed]

[14] Shamshirband, S.; Fathi, M.; Dehzangi, A.; Chronopoulos, A.T.; Alinejad-Rokny, H. A review on deep learning approaches in healthcare systems: Taxonomies, challenges, and open issues. J. Biomed. Infomat. 2021, 113, E103627. [CrossRef] [PubMed]

[15] J. Amann, A. Blasimme, E. Blasimme, D. Vayena, D. Frey, and V. I. Madai, "Explainability for artificial intelligence in healthcare: a multidisciplinary perspective," BMC Medical Informatics and Decision Making, vol. 20, no. 1, p. 310, 2020.

[16] A. Holzinger, "Explainable AI and multi-modal causability in medicine," I-Com, vol. 19, no. 3, pp. 171–179, 2021.

[17] S. J. Schrodi, S. Mukherjee, Y. Shan *et al.*, "Genetic-based prediction of disease traits: prediction is very difficult, especially about the futureaˆ€," Frontiers in Genetics, vol. 5, 2014.

[18] S. M. Lauritsen, M. Kristensen, M. V. Olsen *et al.*, "Explainable artificial intelligence model to predict acute critical illness from electronic health records," Nature Communications, vol. 11, no. 1, p. 3852, 2020

[19] A. Lakhan, M. A. Mohammed, J. Nedoma et al., "Federatedlearning based privacy preservation and fraud-enabled blockchain IoMT system for healthcare," IEEE Journal of Biomedical and Health Informatics, p. 1, 2022.

[20] Lötsch, J., Kringel, D., & Ultsch, A. (2021). Explainable artificial intelligence (XAI) in biomedicine: Making AI decisions trustworthy for physicians and patients. BioMedInformatics, 2(1), 1-17.

[21] Singh, P., Singh, S. P., & Singh, D. S. (2019). An introduction and review on machine learning applications in medicine and healthcare. In 2019 IEEE conference on information and communication technologyy (pp. 1–6). https://doi.org/10.1109/CICT48419.2019. 9066250.

[22] Zou, Q., Qu, K., Luo, Y., Yin, D., Ju, Y., & Tang, H. (2018). Predicting diabetes mellitus with machine learning techniques. Frontiers in Genetics. https://doi.org/10.3389/fgene.2018.00515.

[23] Liu, Y., Gadepalli, K., Norouzi, M., Dahl, G. E., Kohlberger, T., Boyko, A., Venugopalan, S., Timofeev, A., Nelson, P. Q., Corrado, G.S., Hipp, J. D., Peng, L., & Stumpe, M. C. (2017). Detecting cancer metastases on gigapixel pathology images. MICCAI Tutorial (2017) arXiv:1703.02442v2.

[24] Amaral, J. L. M., Lopes, A. J., Jansen, J. M., Faria, A. C. D., & Melo, P. L. (2012). Machine learning algorithms and forced oscillation measurements applied to the automatic identification of chronic obstructive pulmonary disease. Computer Methods and Programs in Biomedicine, 105(3), 183–193. https://doi.org/10.1016/j.cmpb. 2011.09.009.

[25] A. Adadi and M. Berrada, "Peeking inside the black-box: A survey on explainable artificial intelligence (XAI)," IEEE Access, vol. 6, pp. 52138–52160, 2018.

[26] E. Tjoa and C. Guan, "A survey on explainable artificial intelligence (XAI): Towards medical XAI," 2019, arXiv:1907.07374. [Online]. Available: http://arxiv.org/abs/1907.07374S

[27] A. B. Tickle, R. Andrews, M. Golea, and J. Diederich, "The truth will come to light: Directions and challenges in extracting the knowledge embedded within trained artificial neural networks," IEEE Trans. Neural Netw., vol. 9, no. 6, pp. 1057–1068, Nov. 1998.

[28] L. H. Gilpin, D. Bau, B. Z. Yuan, A. Bajwa, M. Specter, and L. Kagal, "Explaining explanations: An overview of interpretability of machine learning," in Proc. IEEE 5th Int. Conf. Data Sci. Adv. Analytics (DSAA), Oct. 2018, pp. 80–89.

[29] Gordon L, Grantcharov T, Rudzicz F. Explainable Artificial Intelligence for Safe Intraoperative Decision Support. JAMA Surg. 2019;154(11):1064–1065. doi:10.1001/jamasurg.2019.2821.

[30] Lundberg SM, Nair B, Vavilala MS, *et al.* Explainable machine-learning predictions for the prevention of hypoxaemia during surgery. Nat Biomed Eng. 2018;2(10):749–760. doi:10.1038/ s41551-018-0304-0

[31] Thimoteo, L. M., Vellasco, M. M., Amaral, J., Figueiredo, K., Yokoyama, C. L., & Marques, E. (2022). Explainable artificial intelligence for COVID-19 diagnosis through blood test variables. Journal of Control, Automation and Electrical Systems, 33(2), 625–644.

[32] Sudar, K. M., Nagaraj, P., Nithisaa, S., Aishwarya, R., Aakash, M., & Lakshmi, S. I. (2022, April). Alzheimer's Disease Analysis using Explainable Artificial Intelligence (XAI). In 2022 International Conference on Sustainable Computing and Data Communication Systems (ICSCDS) (pp. 419–423). IEEE.

[33] Jo, Y. Y., Cho, Y., Lee, S. Y., Kwon, J. M., Kim, K. H., Jeon, K. H., ... & Oh, B. H. (2021). Explainable artificial intelligence to detect atrial fibrillation using electrocardiogram. International Journal of Cardiology, 328, 104–110.

[34] Shahtalebi, S., Atashzar, S. F., Patel, R. V., Jog, M. S., & Mohammadi, A. (2021). A deep explainable artificial intelligent framework for neurological disorders discrimination. Scientific reports, 11(1), 1–18.

[35] Cavaliere, F., Della Cioppa, A., Marcelli, A., Parziale, A., & Senatore, R. (2020, July). Parkinson's disease diagnosis: towards grammar-based explainable artificial intelligence. In 2020 IEEE symposium on computers and communications (ISCC) (pp. 1–6). IEEE.

[36] Davagdorj, K., Bae, J. W., Pham, V. H., Theera-Umpon, N., & Ryu, K. H. (2021). Explainable artificial intelligence based framework for non-communicable diseases prediction. IEEE Access, 9, 123672–123688.

[37] Anguita-Ruiz, A., Segura-Delgado, A., Alcalá, R., Aguilera, C. M., & Alcalá-Fdez, J. (2020). eXplainable Artificial Intelligence (XAI) for the identification of biologically relevant gene expression patterns in longitudinal human studies, insights from obesity research. PLoS computational biology, 16(4), e1007792.

[38] Sanjana, K., Sowmya, V., Gopalakrishnan, E. A., & Soman, K. P. (2020). Explainable artificial intelligence for heart rate variability in ECG signal. Healthcare Technology Letters, 7(6), 146.

[39] Westerlund, A. M., Hawe, J. S., Heinig, M., & Schunkert, H. (2021). Risk prediction of cardiovascular events by exploration of molecular data with explainable artificial intelligence. International Journal of Molecular Sciences, 22(19), 10291.

[40] Chaves, J. M. Z., Chaudhari, A. S., Wentland, A. L., Desai, A. D., Banerjee, I., Boutin, R. D., ... & Patel, B. (2021). Opportunistic assessment of ischemic heart disease risk using abdominopelvic computed tomography and medical record data: a multimodal explainable artificial intelligence approach. medRxiv.

[41] Kavya, R., Christopher, J., Panda, S., & Lazarus, Y. B. (2021). Machine learning and XAI approaches for allergy diagnosis. Biomedical Signal Processing and Control, 69, 102681.

[42] San Koo, B., Eun, S., Shin, K., Yoon, H., Hong, C., Kim, D. H., ... & Oh, J. S. (2021). Explainable artificial intelligence for predicting remission in patients with rheumatoid arthritis treated with biologics.

[43] Peng, J., Zou, K., Zhou, M., Teng, Y., Zhu, X., Zhang, F., & Xu, J. (2021). An explainable artificial intelligence framework for the deterioration risk prediction of hepatitis patients. Journal of Medical Systems, 45(5), 1-9.

[44] Wani, S. U. D., Khan, N. A., Thakur, G., Gautam, S. P., Ali, M., Alam, P., ... & Shakeel, F. (2022, March). Utilization of artificial intelligence in disease prevention: diagnosis, treatment, and implications for the healthcare workforce. In Healthcare (Vol. 10, No. 4, p. 608). MDPI.

[45] Rajkomar A, Oren E, Chen K, *et al.* Scalable and accurate deep learning with electronic health records. NPJ Digit Med 2018; 1 (1): 1–10.

[46] Jensen PB, Jensen LJ, Brunak S. Mining electronic health records: towards better research applications and clinical care. Nat Rev Genet 2012; 13 (6): 395–405.

[47] Wang F, Kaushal R, Khullar D. Should health care demand interpretable artificial intelligence or accept 'black box' medicine. Ann Intern Med 2020; 172 (1): 59.

[48] Nundy S, Montgomery T, Wachter RM. Promoting trust between patients and physicians in the era of artificial intelligence. JAMA 2019; 322 (6): 497–8.

[49] Holzinger A, Langs G, Denk H, Zatloukal K, Mu¨ller H. Causability and explainability of artificial intelligence in medicine. Wiley Interdiscip Rev: Data Min Knowl Discov 2019; 9 (4): e1312.

[50] Vellido A. The importance of interpretability and visualization in machine learning for applications in medicine and health care. Neural Comput Appl 2019. doi: 10.1007/s00521-019-04051-w.

[51] Wilkinson, J. M., Lee, M. R., Rivero, M. J., & Chamberlain, A. T. (2020). Some challenges and opportunities for grazing dairy cows on temperate pastures. *Grass and Forage Science, 75*(1), 1-17.

[52] Britt, J., Cushman, R., Dechow, C., Dobson, H., Humblot, P., Hutjens, M., … Stevenson, J. (2018). Invited review: Learning from the future—A vision for dairy farms and cows in 2067. *Journal of dairy science, 101*(5), 3722–3741.

[53] Ren, G., Lin, T., Ying, Y., Chowdhary, G., & Ting, K. (2020). Agricultural robotics research applicable to poultry production: A review. *Computers and Electronics in Agriculture, 169*, 105216

[54] Neethirajan, S. (2022). Automated tracking systems for the assessment of farmed poultry. *Animals, 12*(3), 232.

[55] Lin, J., Zhu, W., Sun, K., Yin, R., & Li, H. (2018). Application of artificial intelligence technology in poultry production. *China Poultry, 40*(9), 61–63.

[56] Collin, C., Lyne, P., & Grange, J. (1995). Microbiological methods. Butter Worth: Oxford.

[57] Bao, J., & Xie, Q. (2022). Artificial intelligence in animal farming: A systematic literature review. *Journal of Cleaner Production, 331*, 129956. doi: 10.1016/j.jclepro.2021.129956

[58] Basran, P. S., & Appleby, R. B. (2022). The unmet potential of artificial intelligence in veterinary medicine. *American Journal of Veterinary Research, 83*(5), 38–392.

[59] Bao, J., & Xie, Q. (2022). Artificial intelligence in animal farming: A systematic literature review. *Journal of Cleaner Production, 331*, 129956. doi: 10.1016/j.jclepro.2021.129956

[60] Khurshid Wani, A., Akhtar, N., Singh, R., Prakash, A., Raza, S. H. A., Cavalu, S., … Hashem, N. (2022). Genome centric engineering using ZFNs, TALENs and CRISPR-Cas9 systems for trait improvement and disease control in Animals. *Veterinary Research Communications*. doi: 10.1007/s11259-022-09967-8. Samek, W., Montavon, G., Lapuschkin, S., Anders, C. J., & Müller, K.-R. (2021). Explaining deep neural networks and beyond: A review of methods and applications. *Proceedings of the IEEE, 109*(3), 247–278.

[61] Holzinger, A., Carrington, A., & Müller, H. (2020). Measuring the quality of explanations: the system causability scale (SCS). *KI-Künstliche Intelligenz, 34*(2), 193–198.

[62] Machlev, R., Heistrene, L., Perl, M., Levy, K., Belikov, J., Mannor, S., & Levron, Y. (2022). Explainable Artificial Intelligence (XAI) techniques for energy and power systems: Review, challenges and opportunities. *Energy and AI*, 100169.

[63] Antoniadi, A. M., Du, Y., Guendouz, Y., Wei, L., Mazo, C., Becker, B. A., & Mooney, C. (2021). Current challenges and future opportunities for XAI in machine learning-based clinical decision support systems: a systematic review. *Applied Sciences, 11*(11), 5088.

[64] Kotriwala, A., Klöpper, B., Dix, M., Gopalakrishnan, G., Ziobro, D., & Potschka, A. (2021). *XAI for Operations in the Process Industry-Applications, Theses, and Research Directions.* Paper presented at the AAAI Spring Symposium: Combining Machine Learning with Knowledge Engineering.

[65] Tjoa, E., & Guan, C. (2020). A survey on explainable artificial intelligence (xai): Toward medical xai. *IEEE transactions on neural networks and learning systems, 32*(11), 4793–4813.

[66] Arrieta, A. B., Díaz-Rodríguez, N., Del Ser, J., Bennetot, A., Tabik, S., Barbado, A., Benjamins, R. (2020). Explainable Artificial Intelligence (XAI): Concepts, taxonomies, opportunities and challenges toward responsible AI. *Information fusion, 58*, 82–115.

[67] Olden, J. D., Joy, M. K., & Death, R. G. (2004). An accurate comparison of methods for quantifying variable importance in artificial neural networks using simulated data. *Ecological modeling, 178*(3–4), 389–397.

[68] Shen, S., Han, S. X., Aberle, D. R., Bui, A. A., & Hsu, W. (2019). An interpretable deep hierarchical semantic convolutional neural network for lung nodule malignancy classification. *Expert systems with applications, 128*, 84–95.

[69] Ehsan, U., Wintersberger, P., Liao, Q. V., Mara, M., Streit, M., Wachter, S., Riedl, M. O. (2021). *Operationalizing human-centered perspectives in explainable AI.* Paper presented at the Extended Abstracts of the 2021 CHI Conference on Human Factors in Computing Systems.

# 4

# Interpretable Analysis of the Potential Impact of Various Versions of Corona Virus: A Case Study

**Pawan Whig and Ashima Bhatnagar Bhatia**

Vivekananda Institute of Professional Studies -TC, India

## Abstract

It has become clear that kind of the Omicron virus contains a number of mutations, some of which are highly dangerous. Initial research suggests that variation has a higher risk of reinfection, unlike another virus. The prevalence of these occurrences with this variance appears to be increasing throughout South Africa's peripheral regions. The Twitter API, tweeps, and the Python module were used to create The Omicron Rising. The database will be updated often, and the same is done to keep up with the COVID-19 virus's most recent advances. Additionally, it has been noted that many comments about fresh Omicron occurrences found throughout the globe that certain approaches classify as positive are really sarcastic. Whether or not they express themselves in "positive" terms, their true intent is negative. Among those who have specified a nation, India seems to have the most tweets. Naturally, the study of the nation is biased toward residents of that nation. Even said, it makes sense that India would have the most tweets, given that six examples of the Omicron type have just been found there. The tweets coming from India may be a result of worry about a potential Omicron catastrophe, similar to what happened with the Delta mutation in India recently. In this book chapter, findings from this research study are highly fascinating and will be very useful for identifying the user's sentiment about the new variant.

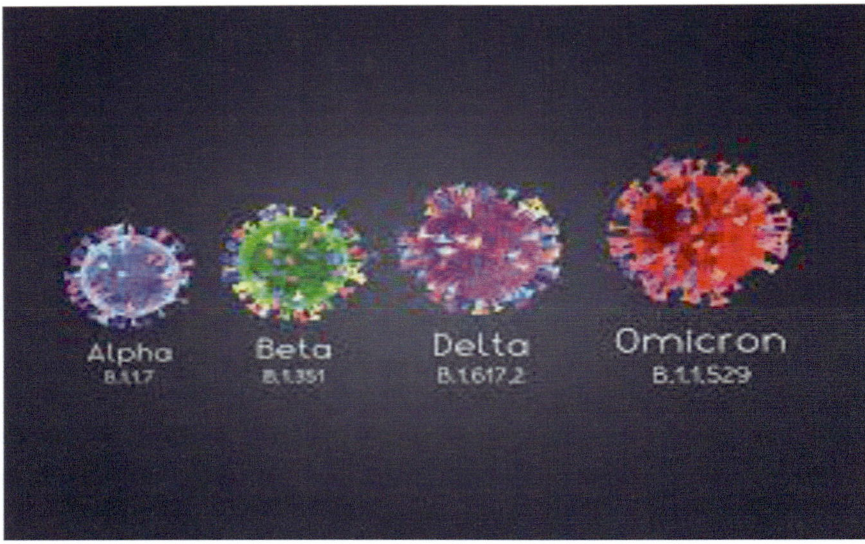


**Figure 4.1** Different versions of corona viruses.

## 4.1 Introduction

The name of the most current COVID-19 variant, Omicron, was inspired by the 15th Greek letter and was first found in South Africa [1]. The World Health Assembly had previously used 12 letters of the Greek alphabet before a new version first appeared in South Africa early in the week. Instead of Nu or Xi, the two letters that came before it, WHO chose Omicron for this one [2]. It incorporates several modifications, and early evidence indicates a higher risk of reinfection, according to the WHO [3]. The variation is thought to increase the virus's ability to spread and withstand certain, but not all, forms of vaccine protection. The WHO received a new report from South Africa on November 24. Israel, Hong Kong, Botswana, Belgium, and Belgium have all verified the virus's existence [4].

There are already five "variants of concern," as shown in Figure 4.1 each with its own Greek letter, according to a WHO tracking webpage. For instance, the variant from India is referred to as Delta, which is the fourth letter of the Greek alphabet [5, 6]. Omicron comes after other phonics variants including Alpha, which was discovered in the UK, Beta, which was found in South Africa, Gamma, which was found in Brazil, and Delta, which was discovered in India [7–10].

If additional control metrics are not implemented, the Omicron version can cause a wave of transmission in England that will result in higher levels

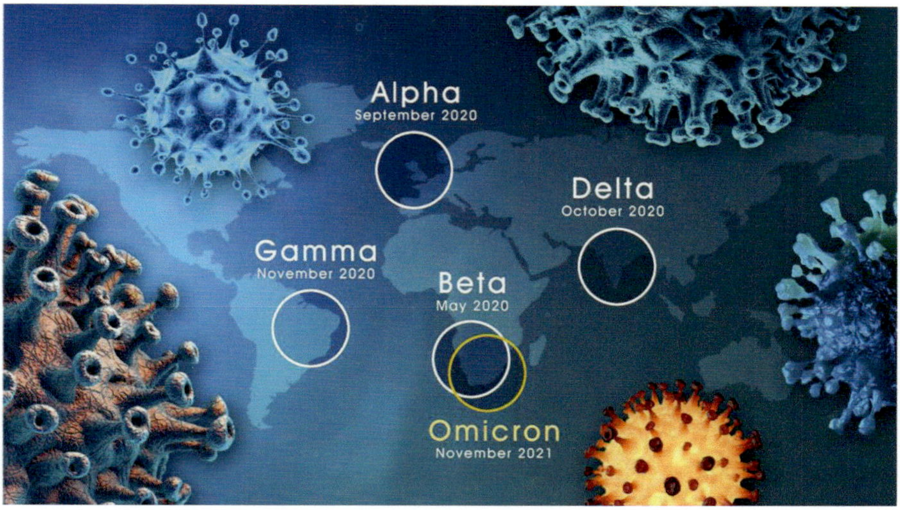


**Figure 4.2** Modification in SARS-CoV-2.

of cases and hospitalizations than any of those seen in January 2021, according to new modeling first from the London School of Hygiene and Tropical Medicine (LSHTM) [11–14].

The work is provided in a pre-print publication and has not yet undergone peer review. To explore potential avenues for Omicron's immunological escape, the researchers examined the most recent experimental findings on the antibody-evading capabilities of the Omicron variant [15–17].

The researchers selected the rate of disease transmission throughout the introduction era of Omicron to coincide with the growth of observed S gene target failure data in England given the evolving knowledge on immune evasion. The dynamics of SARS-CoV-2 infection in England over the first half of 2022 have been predicted using these scenarios [18, 19].

In this case, early 2022 implementation of control laws with a level of severity comparable to Step 2 of the roadmap, which included limiting indoor lodging, closing some concert venues, and attempting to limit gathering sizes, would have been sufficient to significantly control the wave, resulting in 53,000 hospitalizations and 7600 fatalities [20].

The lowest component (high immune escape and reduced refill efficacy) forecasts an infection wave that would cause 492,000 (418,000–537,000) hospital admissions and 74,800 (63,500–82,900) fatalities, approximately twice as many as the peak observed in January 2021 [21–24].

The most difficult adjustments in this variety are its many modifications as shown in Figure 4.2. According to the preliminary research, this variation

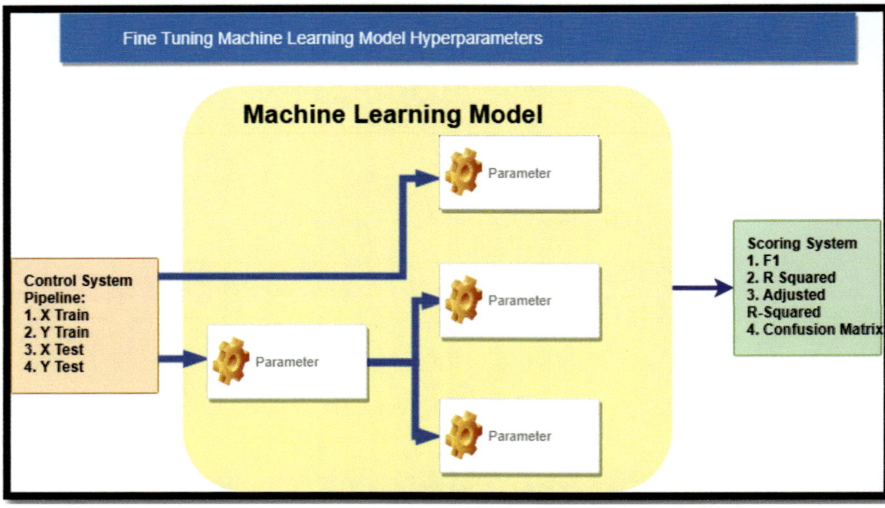


**Figure 4.3** Flowchart of the machine learning model.

has a higher risk of reinfection than other VOCs. In nearly every province of South Africa, this mutation is occurring more often.

This variation is recognized by current SARS-CoV-2 PCR assays [25–27]. Numerous laboratories have asserted that one of the three gene expressions is not picked up in commonly performed integrity checks and that this test may have been utilized as a marker for this variation pending sequencing confirmation. This variation has been identified more quickly than in past outbreaks, suggesting a higher incidence [28, 29]. The following research study examines the sentiment classification for current tweets on the new Omicron variant of COVID-19. The objective is to determine by examining tweets how people feel about the new variety [30].

## 4.2 Modeling using Machine Learning

Without having to go into the resources, anyone may construct and develop machine learning models using the Python platform. Py frameworks are code files from the past that can be imported into any source code by using the import function in Python [31]. This encourages your code to be reused. The Py frameworks may be characterized as a collection of libraries designed to make building models (such as those for machine learning) straightforward even for those who are unfamiliar with the underlying techniques. On the other side, an ML developer has to be aware of how processes work in order to know what results to anticipate and validate as shown in the flowchart in Figure 4.3.

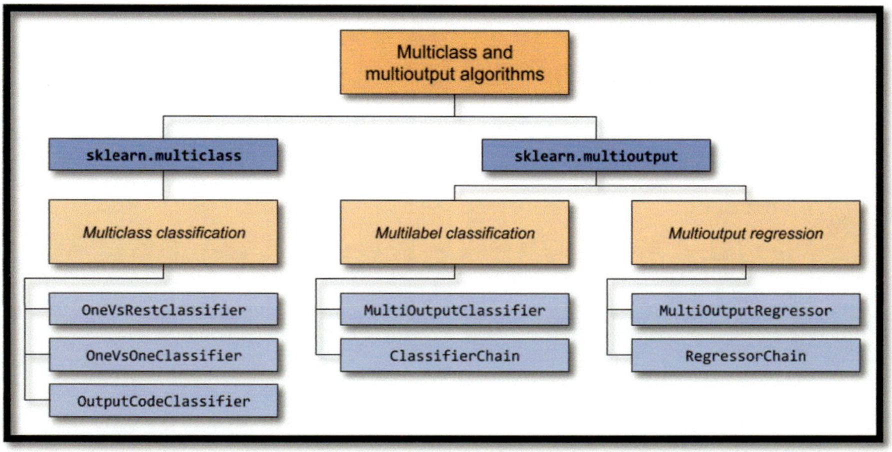


**Figure 4.4** Multiclass classification.

### 4.2.1 Multiclass classification

Problems with classification include giving input instances a class label.

Tasks with only two classifications are known as binary classification tasks. For each case, one choice is made, either to put it in one class or another. A solitary likelihood of the instance belonging to one session is forecast by a probability model, known as a binomial probability distribution, where the opposite is the likelihood for the additional class [32].

Having more than two classes might be difficult. It is possible to apply strategies created for two classes to numerous classes, and in certain cases, this is simple and multiclass classification is as shown in Figure 4.4.

Assign one of many class labels to a sample input that has been provided.

The issue may also be naturally divided into several binary classification jobs.

**Different ways of multi class classification:**
The classes, for instance, can be divided into several single vs. rest forecast issues. Then, a classical may be fitted for each subproblem, and, generally, each model uses the same kind of technique. The model that replies more powerfully than the additional mock-ups can be used to allocate a forecast when one is needed for a new example. This strategy is known as a one-vs-all (OvA) or one-vs-rest (OvR) method [33].

OvR: A method for breaking down a multiclass classification into a single binary classification issue for each class as shown in Figure 4.5.

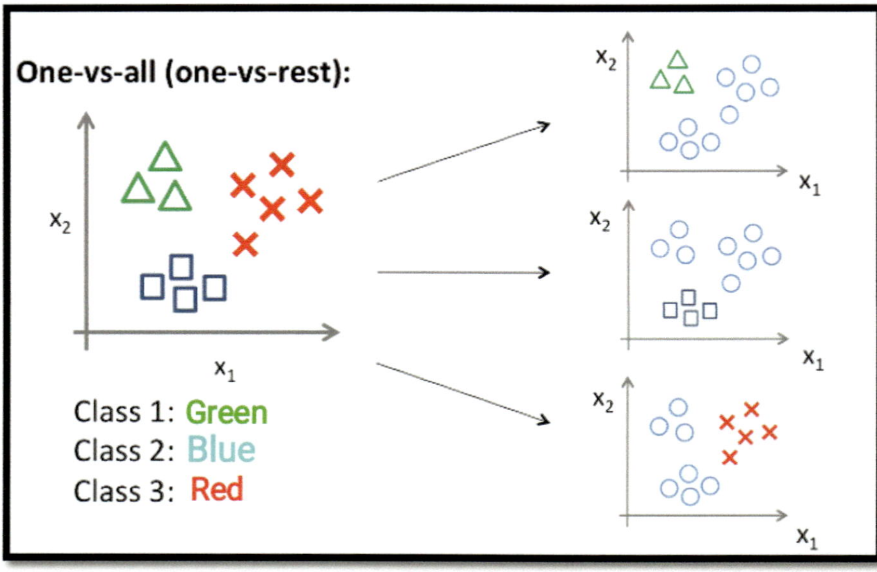


**Figure 4.5** One vs all model.

A model fit on each pair of classes can be used to the multiclass classification issue. Once more, the model with the strongest response may be used to make a forecast for a fresh case. This is known as one-vs-one (OvO).

OvR: A strategy for breaking down a multiclass organization into a single binary organization issue for each pair of lessons. It is possible to expand this method of splitting up a multiclass classification issue into many binary classification tasks. Each class can be translated into a distinct binary string of any length. Thereafter, one classifier may be fitted to predict each bit in the bit string, enabling the usage of any number of classifiers [34].

The class label with the closest match can then be assigned to the bit string. The extra bits function as error-correcting codes, sometimes outperforming the OvR and OvO approaches in terms of performance. Error-correcting output codes, or ECOC, is the name of this method.

Similar to an ensemble, many models are used in each of these scenarios. This approach involves using a champion income formula instead of an election or biased total to aggregate predictions, similar to an ensemble method. However, it differs from most traditional ensemble learning approaches in its implementation.

Contrary to ensemble learning, these strategies are made to investigate the prediction problem's natural breakdown and make use of binary classification issues that could be difficult to scale to several classes.

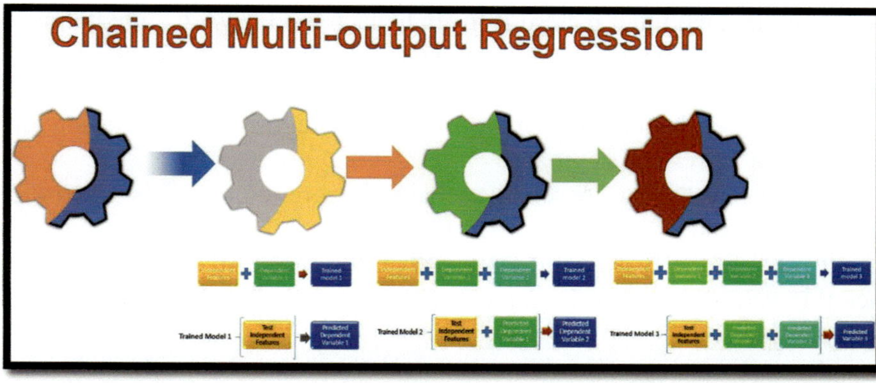


**Figure 4.6** Chained multi-output regression.

While ensemble learning is often solely concerned with improving the prediction performance of contributing models, it is not concerned with enabling new capabilities. The contributing models cannot, by definition, be utilized to solve the prediction issue independently when using methods like OvR, OvR, and ECOC.

### 4.2.2 Multi-output regression models with multiple models

Regression issues entail forecasting a numerical value from an example provided as input.

Usually, just one output value is anticipated. But there are regression issues where each input sample requires the prediction of numerous numerical values. Using one input, predict two or more numerical outcomes using multiple-output regression as shown in chained multi-output regression in Figure 4.6.

Although multi-output regression issues are another example of problems that may naturally be separated into subproblems, replicas can be created to forecast all board standards at one occasion.

The majority of regression predictive modeling approaches were created to predict a single value, similar to binary classification in the preceding section. Multiple value predictions might be challenging and need changing of the method. Some methods cannot really be adjusted for different values. To forecast each target value in a multi-output regression issue, one method is to create a distinct regression model. Typically, each model uses the same kind of algorithm. For instance, training three models—one for each goal—would be necessary for a multi-output regression with three target values.

The identical input pattern is given to each model when a prediction is needed, and each model's unique target is then forecasted. Together, these predictions make up the vector output of the approach. One reversion model is applied to each goal in a multi-production regression issue using the multi-output regression approach.

The creation of a consecutive chain of regression models is another comparable strategy. The key distinction is that although the first model's output predicts the first output target value, the second model in the chain uses this value as part of its input to forecast the second production goal value, and so on.

As a result, the cable adds a linear relationship between the deterioration replicas, enabling subsequent models in the chain to depend on earlier models in the chain for their outputs.

### 4.2.3 Different expert models

We have looked at breaking down challenges into smaller jobs based on the structure of the projected data thus far.

On the basis of the incoming data, certain issues can also be organically subdivided into smaller ones. This strength is as straightforward as splitting the contribution eye interplanetary into sections, or it could be complex, as creating separate models for the foreground and background of a picture.

A blend of experts is a more broad strategy for this from the science of neural networks (MoE).

The process begins by breaking the learning task down into smaller tasks. For each smaller job, an expert model is then developed. Finally, a gating perfect is used to determine or learn which skill to utilize for each instance and the puddle.

The approach is distinct due to two features of MoE. The first involves explicitly dividing up the input feature space, while the second involves using a gating scheme perfect that figures out which expert to believe in each circumstance, such as each input instance.

A skill can still be utilized to produce a prediction on something unrelated to its area of knowledge even if it may not be suited to a particular input.

### 4.2.4 Hybrid models

Hybrid models are a different kind of machine learning that uses many models and is roughly connected to ensemble learning.

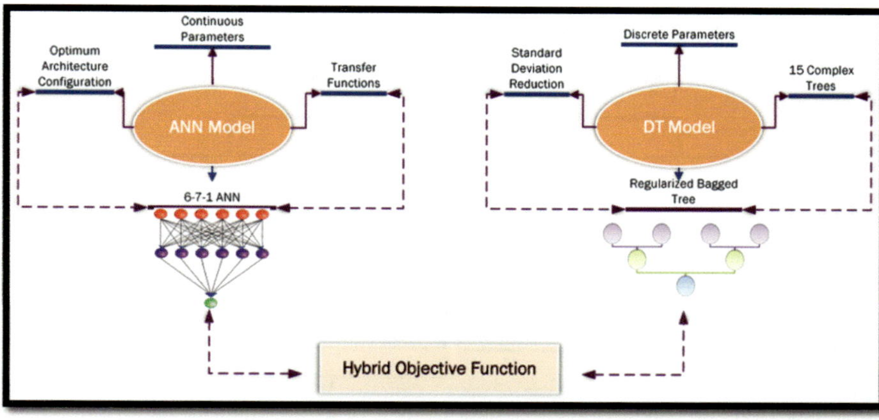


**Figure 4.7** Hybrid models.

Models that explicitly mix two or more models are known as hybrid models. As a result, it may be difficult to define exactly what a hybrid model is and what is not.

Hybrid model: A method that in some manner mixes two or more distinct machine learning models.

Two ML representations, an NN and an SVM, are used in this example. The shown forecast in Figure 4.7 is made by simply layering the models linearly on top of each other.

## 4.3 Sentimentality Analysis

The method of identifying positive or bad sentiment in text is recognized as sentiment analysis. Trades regularly employ it to analyze community media data for sentiment, evaluate product repute, and comprehend clientele.

One of the most contentious and active research areas in computer vision and natural language processing is sentiment analysis (NLP). The content, tone, context, and intent of people's writing may give businesses important information about their current and potential customers as well as their competition.

Making complicated judgments about the enterprise's scope, scalability, design, and ultimate objective is necessary while creating a corporate sentiment lexicon utilizing the best frameworks currently available.

Since sentiment analysis is a young field, the market has not yet been dominated by a particular solution or method. Even the most versatile and mature open-source NLP solutions are not the easiest to use or administer,

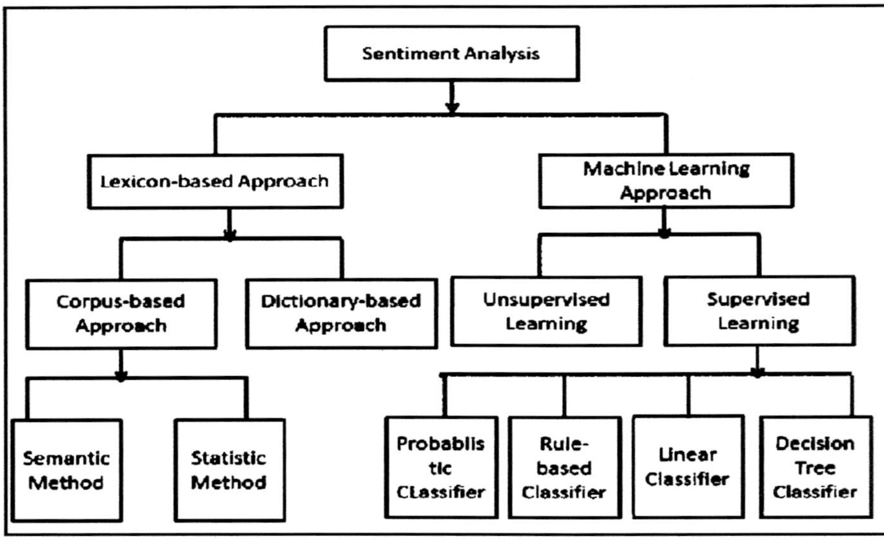


**Figure 4.8** Various sentiment analysis techniques.

and some of the most alluring alternative packages have a real interest in sentiment analysis.

A vocabulary and regulatory sentiment analyzer tuned to social networking attitudes is called VADER (valence aware dictionary and sentiment reasoner). All of it is open source. Several tools for linguistic input manipulation and analysis are included in an NLTK package. One of its sophisticated features is text classifiers, which may be used for different classifications, such as sentiment analysis.

### 4.3.1 Sentiment analysis techniques

Sentiment analysis is primarily concerned with a text's polarity, but it also extends beyond polarity to identify certain moods and emotions, urgency, and even intents. Various sentiment analysis techniques are shown in Figure 4.8.

You may construct and customize your categories to match your sentiment analysis needs based on how you wish to interpret consumer comments and inquiries. Following are a few of the most well-liked varieties of sentiment analysis in the interim.

Sentiment analysis by grade:

If your company places a premium on polarity precision, you can think about extending your polarity categories to cover various intensities of positive and negative:

Very positive

Positive

Neutral/negative

Very unfavorable

This is typically known as graded or fine-grained sentiment analysis and might be used, for instance, to evaluate 5-star reviews:

Five stars for Very positive

Very poor = 1 star

Sentiment analysis is a technique that makes use of algorithms to classify numerous connected text samples into broad positive and negative groupings. These techniques may be used with NLTK to get insights from textual data utilizing anti-oppression machine learning techniques.

### 4.3.2 Sentiment analysis across languages

Sentiment analysis across languages may be challenging. It takes a lot of time and energy to prepare. The majority of these tools – such as sentiment lexicons – are accessible online, while others – such as translated corpora or noise detection algorithms – require coding knowledge to utilize as shown in Figure 4.9.

As an alternative, you might use a language classifier to detect language in texts automatically and then train a unique sentiment analysis model to categorize texts in the language of your choice.

## 4.4 Case Study Discussion

Machine learning techniques are required to enable a sentiment analysis model to be trained so that it can learn data patterns from specialized sentiment analysis datasets. The sentiment analysis model is powered by artificial intelligence, and after being trained on these datasets, it is aware of how to respond to comparable fresh data. As shown in Figure 4.10, you need a model that has been trained on datasets that have been gathered and tagged from the hotel industry if your business is in that sector. And this is true for all business sectors.

Such datasets must cover a very broad range of business scenarios and sentiment analysis applications. Business intelligence may greatly benefit

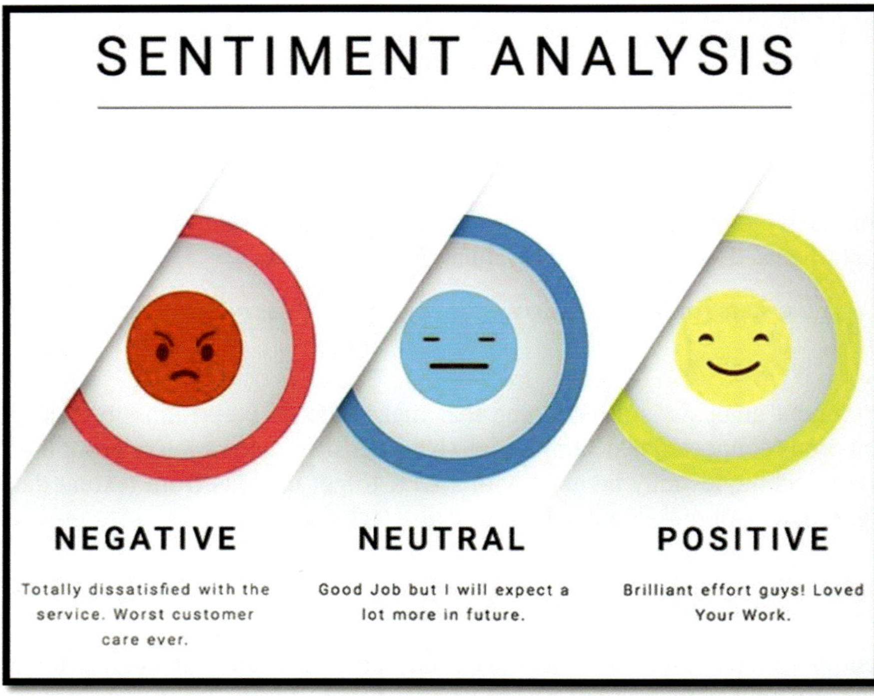


**Figure 4.9** Sentiment analysis representation.

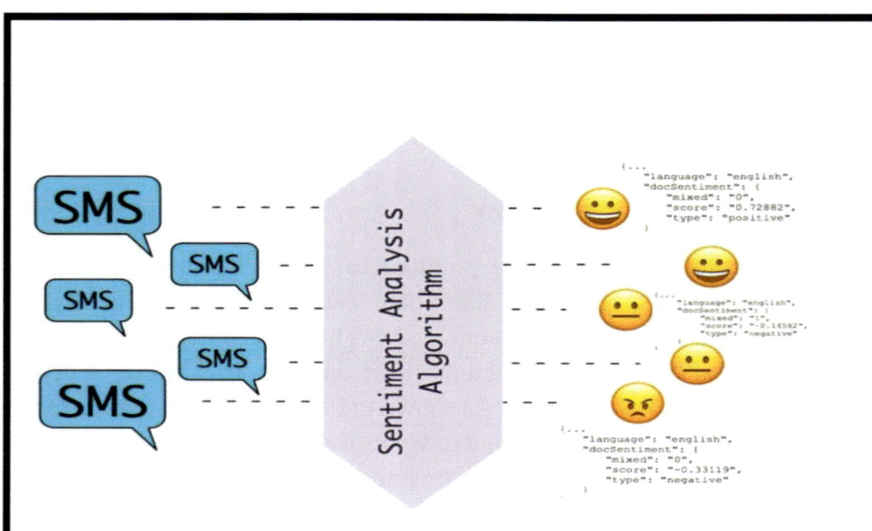


**Figure 4.10** Sentiment analysis case study.

from a well-trained sentiment model that can effectively interpret sentiment from both text and videos using video content analysis. It may assist you in gaining client data from social media sites like YouTube, TikTok, Facebook, and more in addition to reviews and surveys.

A dataset is a grouping or set of data. This collection is often displayed in a tabular format. Each column provides information about a distinct variable. In accordance with the stated question, each row represents a certain component of the dataset. The management of data includes this. For unknown quantities like the height, weight, temperature, volume, etc., of an object or random integer values, datasets represent values for each variable. This set of values is referred to as a datum. Each row's worth of data in the data collection corresponds to one or more members.

The shape of the dataset used for the analysis is obtained using the following command:

```
print(f"data shape: {tweets_df.shape}")

data shape: (3168, 16)
```

It is found that there are 3186 entries of tweets in a given dataset with 16 attributes. The attributes and datatype used will be further obtained by using the following command:

```
<class 'pandas.core.frame.DataFrame'>

RangeIndex: 3168 entries, 0 to 3167

Data columns (total 16 columns):
```

| # Column | Non-Null Count | Dtype |
|---|---|---|
| 0 id | 3168 non-null | int64 |
| 1 user_name | 3168 non-null | object |
| 2 user_location | 2296 non-null | object |
| 3 user_description | 2953 non-null | object |
| 4 user_created | 3168 non-null | object |
| 5 user_followers | 3168 non-null | int64 |
| 6 user_friends | 3168 non-null | int64 |
| 7 user_favourites | 3168 non-null | int64 |

| | | |
|---|---|---|
| 8 user_verified | 3168 non-null | bool |
| 9 date | 3168 non-null | object |
| 10 text | 3168 non-null | object |
| 11 hashtags | 2479 non-null | object |
| 12 source | 3168 non-null | object |
| 13 retweets | 3168 non-null | int64 |
| 14 favorites | 3168 non-null | int64 |
| 15 is_retweet | 3168 non-null | bool |

There are 15,168 tweets, with null values for the columns user_description, user_location, and hashtags. Missing user_description: some users do not have any description.

- Missing user_location: some users did not specify the location.
- Missing hashtags: some posts do not have any hashtag.

The frequency of tweets by date, time, and country are shown in Figures 4.11–4.13.

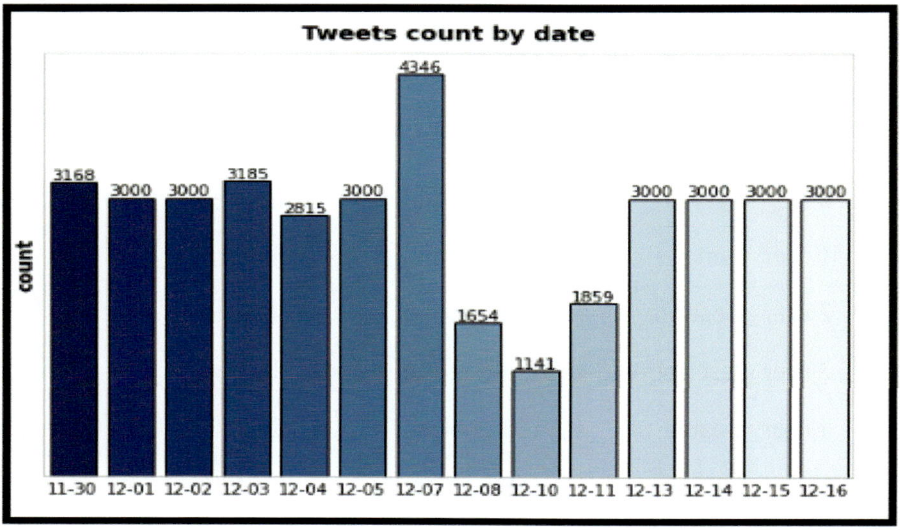


**Figure 4.11** Number of tweet counts by dates.

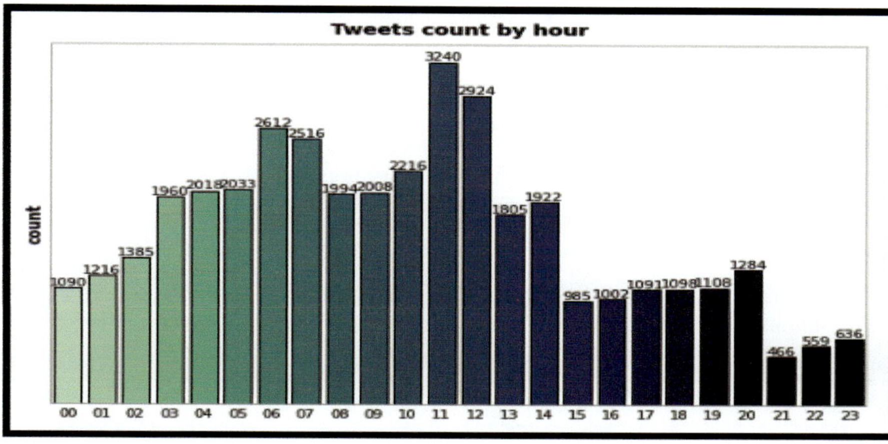


**Figure 4.12** Frequency of tweets by hour.

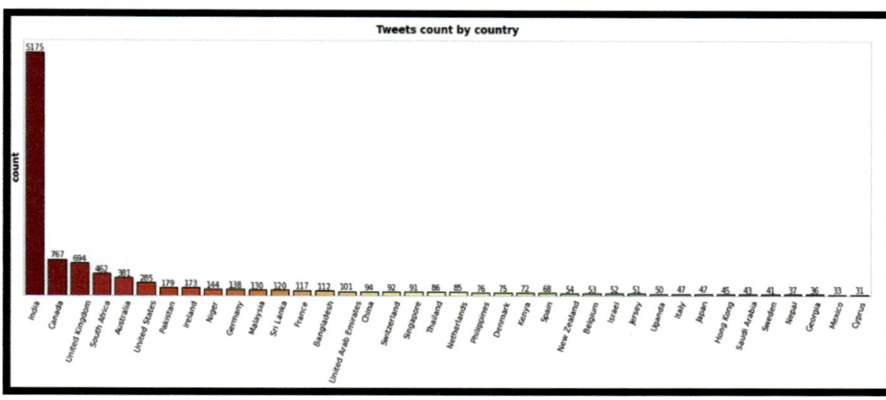


**Figure 4.13** Frequency of tweets by country.

It looks like most of the tweets have been labeled as neutral, with very few positive and negative labeled tweets. Next, we will remove external entities such as hashtags, emojis, and links to clean the tweets' text. The summary of mean, standard deviation, and quartile analysis is given by describing command, and the result obtained is shown in Table 4.1. The general positive and negative tweets using word cloud is shown in Figures 4.14 and 4.15.

Judging by the word cloud, it looks like NLTK and Vader identified as unfavorable the sentences with solid emotional words like "fear," "panic," and insults.

In the case of Textblob and flair, we cannot find any inspirational words.

**Table 4.1** Statistical analysis of data.

| | id | user_followers | user_friends | user_favourites | retweets | favorites |
|---|---|---|---|---|---|---|
| count | 3.168000e+03 | 3.168000e+03 | 3168.000000 | 3168.000000 | 3168.000000 | 3168.000000 |
| mean | 1.465672e+18 | 1.796887e+05 | 1594.637311 | 14687.523043 | 1.034722 | 4.494634 |
| std | 1.387069e+13 | 1.184551e+06 | 7425.926997 | 46019.753960 | 7.352511 | 42.359446 |
| min | 1.465648e+18 | 0.000000e+00 | 0.000000 | 0.000000 | 0.000000 | 0.000000 |
| 25% | 1.465660e+18 | 1.287500e+02 | 134.000000 | 232.750000 | 0.000000 | 0.000000 |
| 50% | 1.465673e+18 | 8.010000e+02 | 465.000000 | 2083.00000 | 0.000000 | 0.000000 |
| 75% | 4.165684e+18 | 4.610250e+03 | 1453.750000 | 10223.000000 | 0.000000 | 2.000000 |
| max | 1.465684e+18 | 1.638385e+07 | 280120.000000 | 979546.000000 | 296.000000 | 1919.000000 |

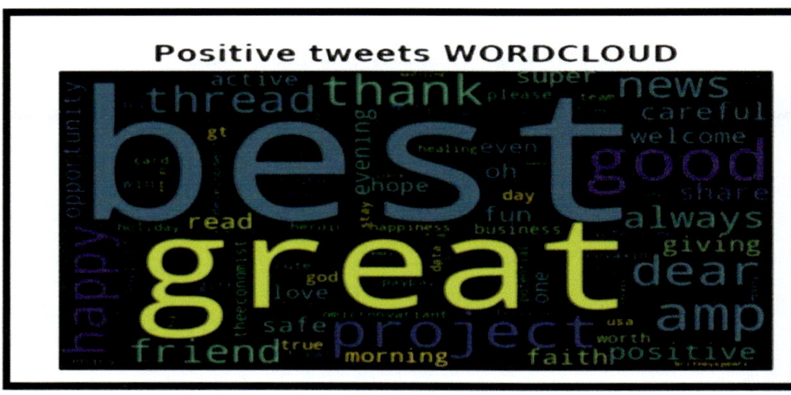


**Figure 4.14** Positive tweet analysis using word cloud.

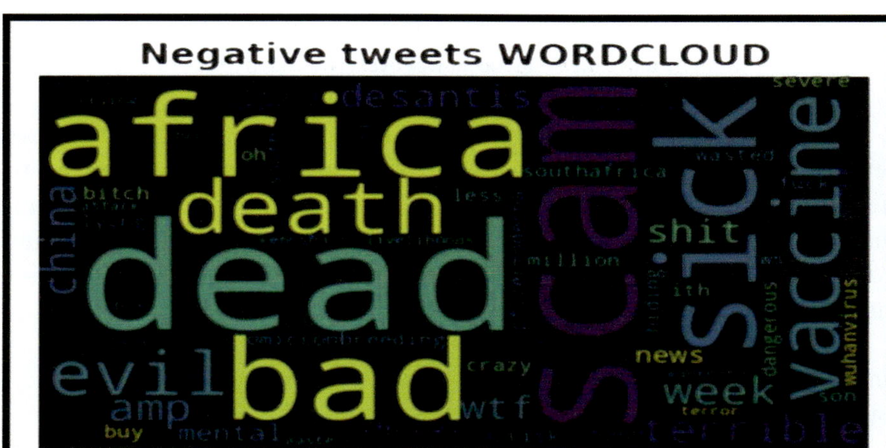


**Figure 4.15** Negative tweet analysis using world cloud.

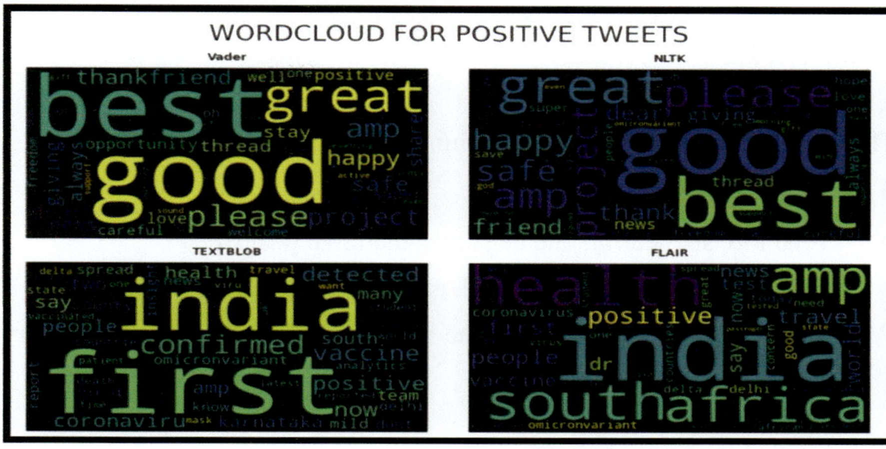


**Figure 4.16** Comparison of positive tweets using various classifiers.

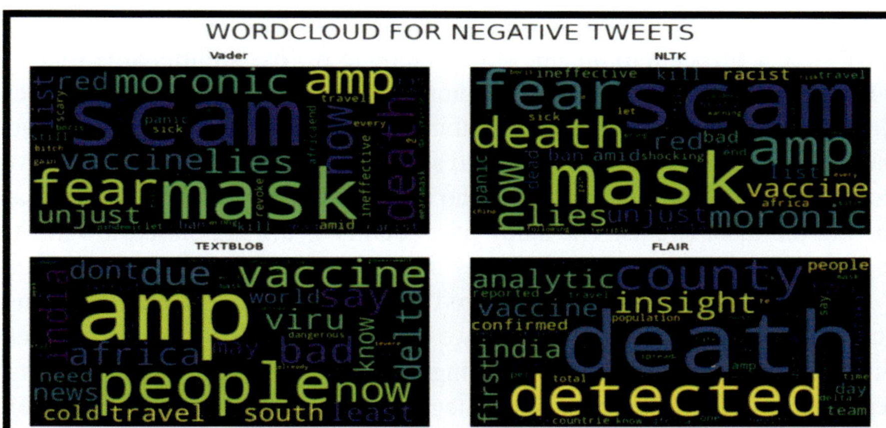


**Figure 4.17** Comparison of negative tweets using various classifiers.

**Favorite and re-tweeted tweets:**

From the above comparison shown in Figures 4.16 and 4.17, it is found that sentiment chosen by a different algorithm using favorite tweets are given as follows:

- Vader and NLTK: all neutral.
- Textblob: five neutral, one negative, and four positives.
- Flair: six negative and four neutral.

We could say that Flair performed the best here since all these tweets carry negative news.

**Also, for the re-tweeted tweets:**
The sentiments chosen by the algorithms are as follows:

- Vader and NLTK: all neutral.
- Textblob: six neutral, one negative, and three positive.
- Flair: six negative, three neutral, and one positive.

We could say that Flair performed the best here since all these tweets carry negative news.

## 4.5 Model Interpretation

### 4.5.1 Results and discussion

The word clouds produced by algorithms, which include both good and negative tweets, all seem to include strong emotive words. Additionally, we discovered in the case study that many comments on recent Omicron occurrences discovered globally that some algorithms labeled as favorable are really sarcastic. Despite the fact that they could seem to be helpful, they actually have negative intentions. Among those who have picked a nation, India ranks as having the most tweets. The study of a country is always biased toward its citizens. As was already said above, the obtained data were cleansed and extremely simple to alter and analyzed in the way that we preferred. Using straightforward manual techniques, we simply hard coded the data and then divided it into three categories, ranging from 0 to 3, based on the main patterns we noticed in the data. The categories of fear, sorrow, anger, and joy were represented by the numbers 0, 1, 2, and 3, respectively.

**Current attitude of COVID-19 cases:**
It was crucial that we contrast the general feelings between the live tweets and the previous tweets in order to assess the performance of our live Twitter emotional analysis with that of old COVID-19 tweets. There are numerous ways to scrape older COVID-19 tweets.

We may import an API called GetOldTweet3, and then move on to cleaning and analysis of the data, or just utilize the cleaned, preprocessed data from github.com while we proceed with the data analysis. Both approaches are acceptable, but because the latter is more time-effective for this task, we decided to adopt it. As a starting point for basic generalization, we chose to limit our research to just India from March 2020 to June 2020, which were pivotal dates in the global COVID-19 phase. Since the initial wave of the COVID-19 epidemic hit the world at this time, the analysis will be very indicative of the attitudes of the time. Approximately 3090 tweets on topics relevant to COVID-19, such as "Coronavirus," "Covid19," "lock down," "pandemic," etc., were located in a repository that contains cleansed data of tweets from the time period of March 2020 to June 2020.

The words "glad," "great," "excellent," "please," and "friend" were all identified by NLTK and Vader as positive phrases. Textblob and flair could not be given an expressive name. The words "fear," "death," and "scam" were among the emotional solid keywords that NLTK and Vader classified as negative in the word cloud. In the cases of Textblob and flair, there are less expressive words to be found. Furthermore, after a critical evaluation of some tweets classified as positive or negative by the four algorithms, we were able to confirm that tweets selected by Vader and NLTK have significantly more comments than those selected by Textblob and Flair, which are longer and probably have a deeper emotional meaning, not just defined by some emotional buzzwords. Flair classified more than 7/10 of the top 10 favorite and retweeted tweets as negative, in contrast to other algorithms.

## 4.6 Conclusion and Future Scope

Naturally, the study of the nation is biased toward the residents of that nation. Even said, it makes sense that India would have the most tweets, given that two Omicron examples were just found there. Concern regarding a potential Omicron crisis, similar to what happened with the Delta variant in India recently, may be the cause of the tweets coming from India. Depending on the dataset scraper's GMT, there is a tweet peak between 11:00 a.m. and 12:00 a.m. For academics in the same field, this research paper is quite helpful.

## Acknowledgements

I am highly grateful to the management of Vivekananda Institute of Professional Studies who give me an opportunity to write this book chapter well on time.

## References

[1] M. Jamshidi *et al.*, "Artificial Intelligence and COVID-19: Deep Learning Approaches for Diagnosis and Treatment," *IEEE Access*, vol. 8, pp. 109581–109595, 2020, doi: 10.1109/ACCESS.2020.3001973.

[2] P. Whig, R. R. Nadikattu, and A. Velu, "COVID-19 pandemic analysis using application of AI," *Healthcare Monitoring and Data Analysis Using IoT: Technologies and Applications*, p. 1, 2022.

[3] M. Anand, A. Velu, and P. Whig, "Prediction of Loan Behaviour with Machine Learning Models for Secure Banking," *Journal of Computer Science and Engineering (JCSE)*, vol. 3, no. 1, pp. 1–13, 2022.

[4] Y. Alkali, I. Routray, and P. Whig, "Study of various methods for reliable, efficient and Secured IoT using Artificial Intelligence," *Available at SSRN 4020364*, 2022.

[5] N. George, K. Muiz, P. Whig, and A. Velu, "Framework of Perceptive Artificial Intelligence using Natural Language Processing (PAIN)," *Artificial & Computational Intelligence/Published Online: July*, 2021.

[6] V. Parihar and S. Yadav, "Comparison Estimation of Effective Consumer Future Preferences with the Application Oof AI".

[7] P. Whig and A. Rupani, "Novel Economical Social Distancing Smart Device for COVID19," *International Journal of Electrical Engineering and Technology*, vol. 2, 2020.

[8] Y. Khera, P. Whig, and A. Velu, "efficient effective and secured electronic billing system using AI," *Vivekananda Journal of Research*, vol. 10, pp. 53–60, 2021.

[9] A. Velu and P. Whig, "Protect Personal Privacy And Wasting Time Using Nlp: A Comparative Approach Using Ai," *Vivekananda Journal of Research*, vol. 10, pp. 42–52, 2021.

[10] P. Whig and S. N. Ahmad, "Methodology for Calibrating Photocatalytic Sensor Output," *International Journal of Sustainable Development in Computing Science*, vol. 1, no. 1, pp. 1–10, 2019.

[11] R. R. Nadikattu, R. Bhandari, and P. Whig, "Improved Pattern of Adaptive Rood-Pattern Search Algorithm for Motion Estimation in Video Compression," in *Innovations in Cyber Physical Systems*, Springer, Singapore, 2021, pp. 441–448.

[12] A. Rupani and G. Sujediya, "A Review of FPGA implementation of Internet of Things," *International Journal of Innovative Research in Computer and Communication Engineering*, vol. 4, no. 9, 2016.

[13] C. M. Ruchin and P. Whig, "Design and Simulation of Dynamic UART Using Scan Path Technique (USPT)", International Journal of Electrical, Electronics & Computer Science Engineering," 2015.

[14] P. Shrivastav, P. Whig, and K. Gupta, "Bandwidth Enhancement by Slotted Stacked Arrangement and its Comparative Analysis with Conventional Single and Stacked Patch Antenna".

[15] V. Bhatia and R. Gupta, "Design of a GSM based electronic voting machine with voter tracking," *BVICA M's International Journal of Information Technology*, vol. 7, no. 1, p. 799, 2015.

[16] P. Whig, "IoT Based Novel Smart Blind Guidance System," *Journal of Computer Science and Engineering (JCSE)*, vol. 2, no. 2, pp. 80–88, 2021.

[17] A. Velu and P. Whig, "Studying the Impact of the COVID Vaccination on the World Using Data Analytics".

[18] Dr. P. W. Purva Agarwal1, "A Review-Quaternary Signed Digit Number System byReversible Logic Gate," *International Journal on Recent and Innovation Trends in Computing and Communication*, vol. 4, no. 3, 2016.

[19] R. R. Nadikattu, S. M. Mohammad, and P. Whig, "Novel economical social distancing smart device for covid-19," *International Journal of Electrical Engineering and Technology (IJEET)*, 2020.

[20] S. Chouhan, S. Chaudhary, T. Upadhay, A. Rupani, and P. Whig, "Comparative Study of Various Gates Based in Different Technologies," *Int Rob Auto J*, vol. 3, no. 2, p. 00046, 2017.

[21] P. Whig and S. N. Ahmad, "Controlling the Output Error for Photo Catalytic Sensor (PCS) Using Fuzzy Logic," *Journal of earth science and climate change*, vol. 8, no. 4, pp. 1–6, 2017.

[22] 1 S N Ahmad Pawan Whig 2 Anupam Priyam3, "Simulation & performance analysis of various R2R D/A converter using various topologies," *International Robotics & Automation Journal*, vol. 4, no. 2, pp. 128–131, 2018.

[23] P. Agarwal and P. Whig, "Low Delay Based 4 Bit QSD Adder/Subtraction Number System by Reversible Logic Gate," in *2016 8th International Conference on Computational Intelligence and Communication Networks (CICN)*, 2016, pp. 580–584.

[24] A. Rupani, P. Whig, G. Sujediya, and P. Vyas, "A robust technique for image processing based on interfacing of Raspberry-Pi and FPGA using IoT," in *2017 International Conference on Computer, Communications and Electronics (Comptelix)*, 2017, pp. 350–353.

[25] A. Rupani, D. Saini, G. Sujediya, and P. Whig, "A Review of Technology Paradigm for IOT on FPGA," *IJARCCE-International Journal of Advanced Research in Computer and Communication Engineering*, vol. 5, no. 9, 2016.

[26] J. B. Chacko and P. Whig, "Low Delay Based Full Adder/Subtractor by MIG and COG Reversible Logic Gate," in *2016 8th International*

*Conference on Computational Intelligence and Communication Networks (CICN)*, 2016, pp. 585–589.

[27] P. Whig, S. N. Ahmad, and S. Kumar, "Simulation and performance analysis of Multiple PCS sensors system," *Electronics (Basel)*, vol. 20, no. 2, pp. 85–89, 2016.

[28] V. Bhatia, P. Whig, and S. N. Ahmad, "Smart PCS Based System for Oxygen Content Measurement," 2015.

[29] A. Sharma, A. Kumar, and P. Whig, "On the performance of CDTA based novel analog inverse low pass filter using 0.35 μm CMOS parameter," *International Journal of Science, Technology & Management*, vol. 4, no. 1, pp. 594–601, 2015.

[30] P. Whig and S. N. Ahmad, "Novel FGMOS based PCS device for low power applications," *Photonic Sensors*, vol. 5, no. 2, pp. 123–127, 2015.

[31] T. Verma, P. Gupta, and P. Whig, "Sensor Controlled Sanitizer Door Knob with Scan Technique," in *Emerging ICT for Bridging the Future-Proceedings of the 49th Annual Convention of the Computer Society of India CSI Volume 2*, 2015, pp. 261–266.

[32] P. Whig and S. N. Ahmad, "Development of economical ASIC for PCS for water quality monitoring," *Journal of Circuits, Systems and Computers*, vol. 23, no. 06, p. 1450079, 2014.

[33] P. Whig and S. N. Ahmad, "A CMOS integrated CC-ISFET device for water quality monitoring," *International Journal of Computer Science Issues*, vol. 9, no. 4, pp. 1694–1814, 2012.

[34] P. Whig and S. N. Ahmad, "DVCC based readout circuitry for water quality monitoring system," *International Journal of Computer Applications*, vol. 49, no. 22, pp. 1–7, 2012.

# 5

# XAI in Biomedical Applications

**K. K. Kırboğa[1,2] and E. U. Küçüksille[3]**

[1]Bilecik Seyh Edebali University, Faculty of Engineering Bioengineering Department, Turkey
[2] Informatics Institute, Istanbul Technical University, Maslak, Istanbul, 34469, Turkey
[3]Informatics Institute, Istanbul Technical University, Maslak, Istanbul, 34469, Turkey
Email: kubra.kirboga@bilecik.edu.tr; ecirkucuksille@sdu.edu.tr

## Abstract

When the correct diagnosis or selection of therapy is made by algorithms by a machine, decisions for doctors, patients, and experts can become non-transparent, leading to the breakdown of relationships. Asking the machine to explain its algorithms is essentially a detailed understanding of the mathematical and statistical details. At this stage, the combined work of state informatics and statistics specialists and doctors and medical specialists emerges. This book chapter focuses on how and with what studies explainable AIs (XAIs) explain the decisions they make in the biomedical environment to experts.

## 5.1 Introduction

As an essential research question, "explanation" and "explanation criteria" are active topics in many computer science fields. According to a survey conducted by Miller in 2019, practical explanations can be created based on three main findings [1].

The three main findings are as follows:

(I) The first phenomenon states that people tend to understand events happening and not happening.

(II) The second fact is that the user is not overwhelmed with too much information. In the decision or recommendation phase, the user focuses on one or two possible causes instead of focusing on all possible causes.

(III) The last phenomenon uses a mental model while explaining. It is about having a social and interactive conversation while conveying information.

These three facts demonstrate the connections between the explainability of artificial intelligence and social science disputes. XAI (Explainable artificial intelligence) has recently concentrated on these occurrences and created a new concept of explainability. Different methodologies are used in biomedical investigations that use XAI in computer science. It will be feasible to develop an interpretable model in biomedicine, establish its competitive accuracy levels compared to the black-box model, and comprehend how accurately the model imitates its estimator, thanks to the explanations. The following sections will discuss the sub-approaches and types of motivation and reasoning that these systems represent.

Machine learning (ML) systems are used even when the molecular processes involved in diseases are partially known. The ML algorithm uses selected training and test data to perform specific tasks. In this way, it can generalize to unknown situations. In this process, confidence and performance are measured. Skill-based machine learning serves better for similar data. The concert will be lower for data with a different structure. However, since the scientific data are not given clearly in the biomedical field, skill-based methods are used more because the datasets are generally similar. The analysis of these algorithms can be realized by understanding the mathematical model [2].

## 5.2 Main Text

### 5.2.1 Main biomedical goals of XAI

The use of XAI in biomedical studies can serve many different purposes. In the process of explaining deep learning algorithms, the visualization of the various factors that contribute to each decision is often used [3]. One of the preferred methods for this purpose is heat maps Figure 5.1. Heat maps visually describe the contributors who were instrumental in the disclosure process. It can be emphasized with such methods that inputs are related to the output obtained [3–5]. Interpretability methods, which are the reason for the emergence of XAI, have recently increased interest in the field. Certain

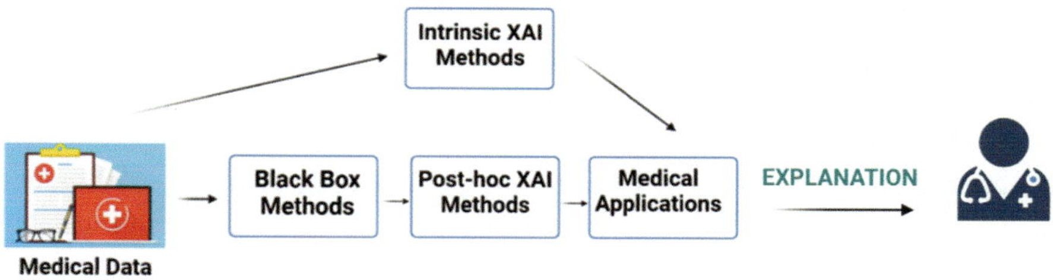


**Figure 5.1** XAI methods and use in the biomedical field.

properties of XAI have been defined to increase explainability and interpretability in the biomedical field: (i) trustworthiness, (ii) transparency, (iii) comprehensibility, (iv) accessibility, (v) transferability, (vi) fairness, (vii) trust, (viii) interaction, and (ix) privacy awareness. The importance and use of these properties in the biomedical field will be detailed in the next chapter.

#### 5.2.1.1 Trustworthiness

Trustworthiness in classification studies is based on knowing the characteristics and causes of the AI output. Using ML methods, it can be determined which clinical diagnoses can be used in a particular case. In the clinic, if a fate is to be defined due to this decision, the reliability of ML becomes very important. For the interaction between patient–physician and the method to be strong, the reliability of AI-assisted decision-making can be transformed into the context of XAI. At this stage, investigating the characteristics and causes of AI output also means restoring the trust between the patient–physician and method trio. If there is no confidence in the AI-based process in a clinical diagnosis, it is unlikely that any of the trios will rely on the recommended way [6]. In such tasks, a solution can be found with the LIME (Local Interpretable Model-agnostic Explanations) method. This method makes transparent assignments to case-related clusters based on the random forest model [7]. Some studies claim the opposite. Therefore, there is a method that needs to be developed. As a result, the relationship of machine-generated outputs to inputs in biomedical research should be clearly defined and aimed at capturing more of the main objectives.

#### 5.2.1.2 Transparency

The principle of transparency includes the transition from the black box to the white box, intelligibility, and explanations. In this way, how the AI model works can be determined mathematically, statistically, and algorithmically [8]. While statisticians, mathematicians, and computer scientists are understandable, these phrases may not make much sense to doctors and biologists. The principle of transparency can be explained through various banking or financial transaction formulas. However, the principle of transparency in the biomedical field can be interpreted through the explainability of the models. The importance of the explainability of artificial intelligence in health emerges in the decision-making process in many situations that affect our life and death. This principle is adopted through the transparency of the software and models in estimation software of disease rates with a large spread, such as cancer. Transparency, which expresses the features of disease detection software, is related to how much this system is reflected in theory. The explanations on how AI works in the prediction of diseases and the inclusion of the model are related to the principle of transparency.

#### 5.2.1.3 Comprehensibility

It is a principle based on interpreting the terms, formulations, and methods used in the decision-making of biomedical tasks and the outputs from inputs within the framework of causality and logic. This is the whole meaning of the explainability of AI, and all approaches and risks should be considered in this principle [8]. The concept of intelligibility is the essential condition for making an explanation. For output to be explained by the user, it must be understood. Here it must be considered whether the user is a patient, a doctor, a statistician, or a computer scientist. However, to communicate clearly to patients in biomedical decisions, it is necessary to have an easily understandable output that makes the decisions transparent. Many conditions are considered, such as whether doctors or clinicians can make the output understandable, given a coherent explanation to the patient. In this context, the intelligibility of XAI varies according to special interests, goals, needs, and expectations in biomedical processes, but it has an important key role in their definition.

#### 5.2.1.4 Accessibility

The principle of accessibility in the continuous self-improving AI process can be defined as improving and developing algorithms by end-users. No artificial intelligence or programming knowledge is required to be involved in the improvement and development process. For this reason, it provides excellent convenience for end-users to reach an understandable and transparent output by using hierarchical or non-hierarchical rules. The breast cancer cohort study used several non-hierarchical guidelines predicting the development of persistent pain [9]. The accessibility system allows the comparison and evaluation of AI models using interpretable information to assist the user in decision-making. It plays a crucial role in making comparisons and measuring the consistency of cases that are related or thought to be related in terms of predictive criteria.

#### 5.2.1.5 Transferability

Because biomedical tasks create a synergetic link with health, understand how an AI model works and transfer that solution to another application or study. When moved, another perspective can be presented to the underlying timeline of the problem. Therefore, transferability was cited as the second most common reason for using XAI [10]. An example is a study in the breast cancer cohort on transferability, which is an essential principle in getting to the root of the problems. Comprehensive psychological questionnaires were conducted to estimate the persistence of pain. ML was used to find the expected results and the pain context of the survey results. A shorter and more understandable questionnaire was created by taking approximately 10% of the original questionnaire. This situation created a more useful survey result for both patients and clinicians [9]. Filtering big data and using transferability in interrelated biomedical processes can be great gifts that AI-based methods offer us.

### 5.2.2 Use of XAI in Biomedical Studies

#### 5.2.2.1 Diagnosis and surgery

The progress and success of artificial intelligence in medicine have effectively supported the medical decision-making process of doctors. Diagnosis of diseases [11], surgical interventions [12], and AI are used in many medical applications. As mentioned, there are some challenges, including the black-box nature of AI. These difficulties cause poor explainability of the models and low reliability of clinical inferences. AI applications need to be more transparent to increase trust in doctors and medical workers. Therefore, integrating XAI studies into biomedicine and medicine is very important.

There are many studies researched on the diagnosis. In the ML algorithm applied for allergy diagnosis, the algorithm giving the best performance value was selected by using the *k*-fold cross-validation method. If it is based on XAI, a random forest is created, and every path in the trees contains medical data. In addition, this study is embedded in the mobile application [13]. It has been shown that by applying clustering and size reduction in an XAI framework for breast cancer, important clinical features for oncologic treatments can be summarized [14]. Yet another successful study proposes a classifier for spinal posture independent of an explainable pathological condition.

This study used Support Vector Machine (SVM) and Random Forest (RF) as ML classifiers, and LIME explained the predictions [15]. In a proposed RF model for diagnosing Alzheimer's disease (AD), Shapley Additive explanation (SHAP) was applied to select critical features in the classifier. The SHAP method explains the effects of features on the model to explain patient diagnosis and prediction of disease progression [16].

Peng et al. proposed an XAI model to assist physicians with the prognosis of hepatitis patients. They compared logistic regression (LR) and decision tree (DT) XAI methods and SVM, XGBoost, and RF models [17]. In another successful ML study, CNN-based models were proposed for chronic wound classification, and LIME was applied for its explanation. As an interesting case, they used the transfer learning technique in the CNN model. Precision, mean recall, and mean $F1$ score were 95%, 94%, and 94%, respectively. Wound images and heat maps produced with LIME and the model can greatly benefit clinicians [18]. A graph-based neural network that can extract facts from electronic medical records (EMR) has been proposed to diagnose a significant health problem of lymphedema. When this model is evaluated on accurate Chinese electronic medical records, it is seen that it exhibits an approach that can be interpreted and gives correct results in reasoning [19, 20]. The use of XAI in surgery, like diagnosis, has recently been the focus of attention. Yoo et al. presented a multi-class XGBoost model for laser surgery. The datasets achieved 78.9% accuracy. In this method, SHAP is also used to provide a clinical understanding of the methods [21]. This method has been one of the ML methods that can be used to select the laser surgery option. Another study is on surgical education. In this study, an SVM model was created with surgical data, and an accuracy of 92%, a specificity of 82%, and a sensitivity of 100% were obtained. In addition, they explained the learnable metrics extensively with the XAI method [22]. To classify surgical skill levels, which is a specific study, a fully convolutional neural (FCN) network has been created, and an interpretable medical application is presented. This classification uses the CAM technique to provide feedback; a visual post-hoc XAI detects features that affect classification decisions. In this way, behaviors were investigated according to skill level [23].

#### 5.2.2.2 Medical image analysis

DL and ML methods, especially medical imaging analysis, have advanced. This chapter focuses on XAI techniques in medical imaging and biomedicine studies. It also focuses on future opportunities for XAI in medical imaging. Various XAI criteria are used to classify DL-based medical imaging [24].

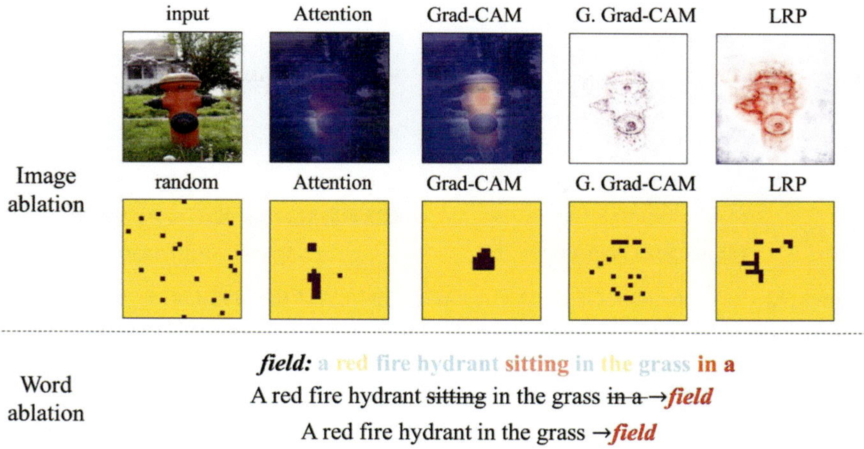


**Figure 5.2** The experiment with image ablation (upper) and word ablation (below). The first row of image ablation displays visual explanations of the word hydrant, while the second row displays masked regions with high relevance scores [25].

To analyze the predictions of the caption models, used layer-by-layer conformity propagation (LRP) and gradient-based annotated methods to caption models, which include attention mechanisms. In this study, the interpretability of the heat maps was provided by methods such as LRP, Grad-CAM, and guided Grad-CAM. As a result of the research, the observed features of the explanations and the object hallucination problem in the caption models were reduced, and an LRP inference with high sentence fluency was presented [25]. From Figure 5.2, it is seen that the words explained correspond to the image content. It has been quantitatively analyzed whether the inputs will be used as evidence by the model. An ablation experiment was designed for both image annotations and linguistic annotations.

Using LRP and gradient-based explanation methods, this study shows that quantitative and qualitative experiments and the explanation methods they use provide more information than attention, solve the contributions of visual and linguistic information in detail, and help investigate the causes of hallucination problems Figure 5.3. In another study, scans on the interpretability of computer algorithms were made and categorized. Various interpretable algorithms and different perspectives are presented to clinicians and practitioners. There are complex patterns and dimensions in interpretability research in different categories. Many additional considerations are hoped for, such as clinicians being more cautious, identifying bias regarding its interpretability, and advancing medical education with data-based mathematical-based methods. As seen in Figure 5.4, well-established processes and

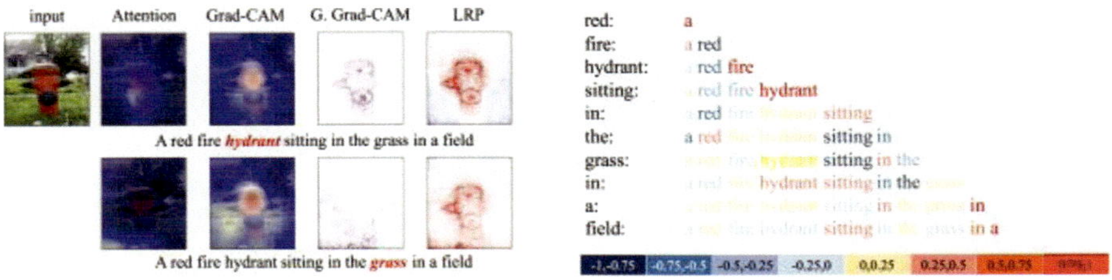


(a) image explanations (b) linguistic explanations of LRP

**Figure 5.3** (a) Attention, Grad-CAM, guided Grad-CAM (G.Grad-CAM), and LRP image explanations of the words hydrant (first row) and grass (second row). (b) For each word in the expected caption, the linguistic explanations of LRP. Blue and red colors, respectively, indicate negative and positive relevance scores [25].

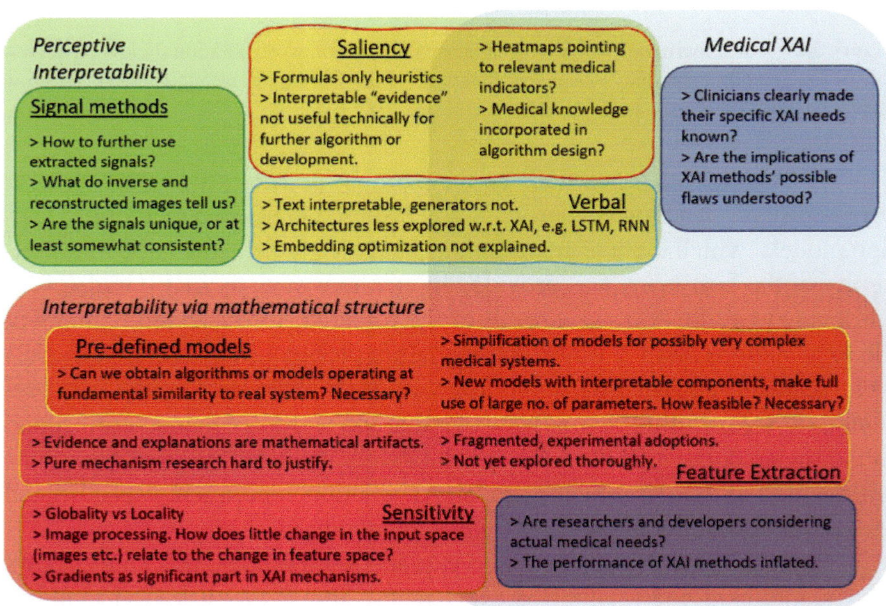


**Figure 5.4** In a Venn diagram, an overview of challenges and future potential is presented [26].

advanced ML algorithms in medical applications have been observed. Since medical ML is a young field, it is prone to development and specialization. As the studies progress, many practical methods will continue to be added, and their contribution to medical practice will become more apparent. To make conscious and more consistent interpretations, it should be studied systematically to obtain many unexplored opportunities. Thanks to mathematical techniques, interpretability is developing, and the interpretability of algorithms

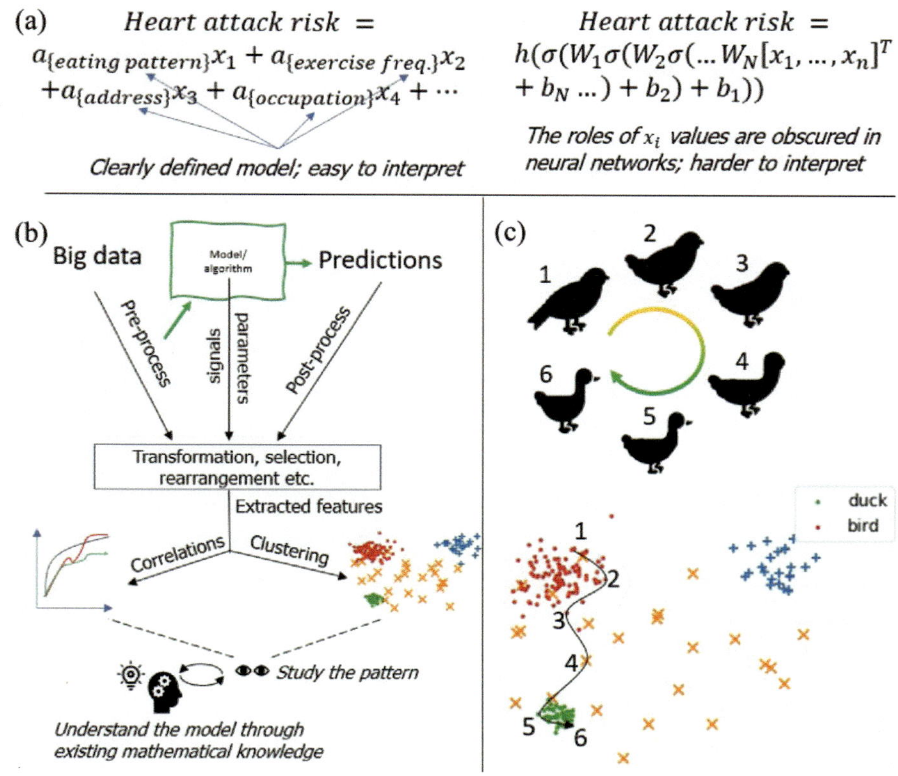


**Figure 5.5** An overview of the interpretability of mathematical structures. (a) Easy-to-understand modeling, such as linear models, helps improve interpretability. (b) Feature extraction. In comprehensions that require mathematical knowledge, the data and parameters in the model are transformed and selectively selected. (c) Sensitivity. It serves to explain how different data are represented differently. In the figure, the transformation of bird to duck can be traced using clustering [26].

is improving in richer ways. Figure 5.5 also provides an overview of the usability and interpretability of these algorithms in medical applications [26].

Many different mathematical methods are used to determine the working mechanisms of ML and NN algorithms. NN stores the information of deep and shallow layers. The concept activation vector (CAV) shows a similar trend. As shown in Figure 5.6, many different methods can be used regarding clustering and subspace of image analysis.

#### 5.2.2.3 Biological process

The proposed ML approaches for modeling ohmic data are based on black-box algorithms. More interpretable models are demanded to elucidate

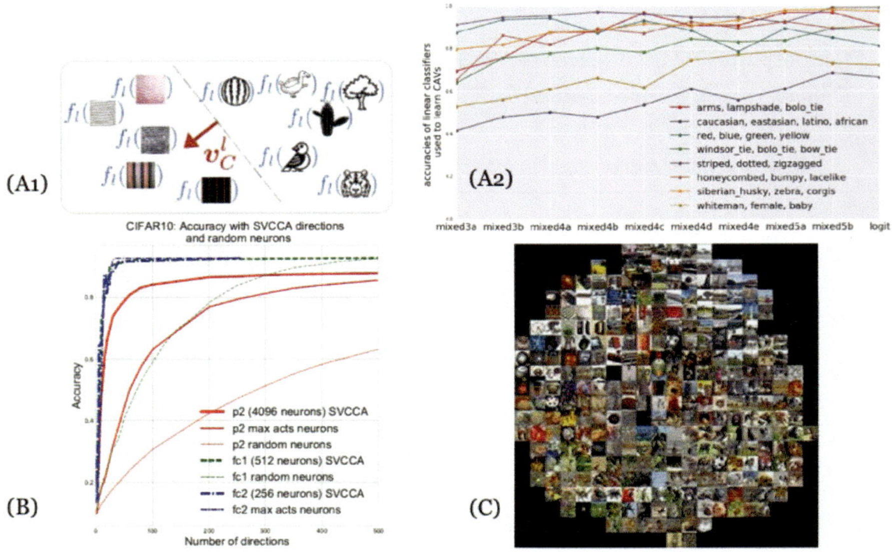


**Figure 5.6** (a1) With the TCAV [27] method, a hyperplane CAV that separates the target concepts from each other can be found. (a2) The CAV accuracies applied to different layers and the content of the concepts involved in deep and shallow layers are shown. (b) SVCCA [28] finds the concept of the subspace most meaningful and contains the most information. (c) t-SNE organizes dog images in a meaningful way [26].

explanatory aspects such as model accuracy and predictive ability. The XAI revolution offers methods quite suitable for illustrative purposes. In this way, more explanatory biologically more robust models can be obtained. Gene models were validated, and biologically relevant gene–gene relationships were examined in a study involving the rule-based XAI strategy from human gene expression data.

Regulatory mechanisms among thousands of genes control biological processes in humans. To understand the mechanism of genes interacting with each other in a four-dimensional space, gene–gene temporal interactions need to be analyzed. More biologically meaningful results have become necessary as AI approaches to this problem. Many of these methods can be applied to gene expression data. New therapeutic targets may emerge, and complex processes can be significantly expanded, thanks to the new pipeline applied to data from obesity research.

Figure 5.7 shows the critical importance of confirming the study results with obesity data and distinguishing between real and fake. Work supported by acceptable rules and metrics (support = 90% and confidence = 85%) [29].

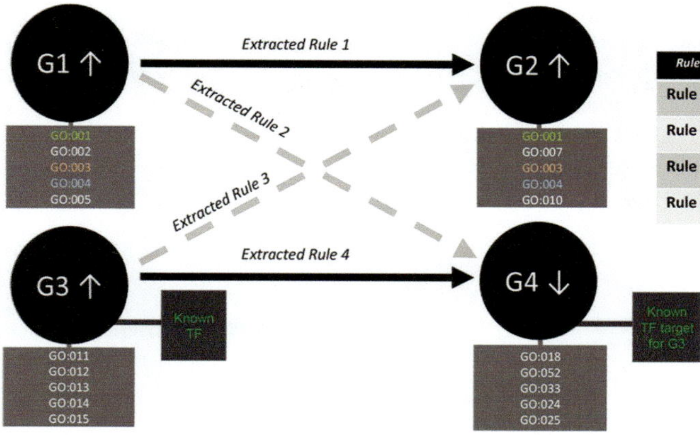


| Rule | Support | Confidence | BP | TF |
|---|---|---|---|---|
| Rule 1 | 0.9 | 0.85 | 1.001 | 0 |
| Rule 2 | 0.9 | 0.85 | 5 | 0 |
| Rule 3 | 0.9 | 0.85 | 5 | 0 |
| Rule 4 | 0.9 | 0.85 | 5 | 2 |

**Figure 5.7** Biological quality metrics' importance in determining each gene–gene connection's functional significance was revealed [29].

#### 5.2.2.4 Toxicology

Explainability is seen as the first principle to understand the effects of toxicology studies, mortality rate determination, and risk factors on mortality rates. Many ML model frameworks have been presented to explore and visualize the contribution of known risk factors to lung and bronchial cancer. In a study in which XAI was applied, five essential learners, namely generalized linear model (GLM), RF, gradient boosting machine (GBM), extreme gradient boosting machine (XGBoost), and deep neural network (DNN), were used to develop models. A permutation-based technique is used to interpret and visualize the output of the models. This critical technique showed that smoking and poverty had significant effects on these cancers. The impact of risk factors on mortality may vary spatially, but the contribution of each of the features is significant in toxicology studies. On the other hand, XAI can demonstrate these contributions [30].

#### 5.2.2.5 Pathology

The field of pathology, which usually deals with diagnosis and slide images, has begun to evolve into a new area called computational pathology with AI and ML. AI, which has an important place in increasing the accuracy and efficiency of pathologists, has some concerns about its trust due to its black-box feature. XAI methods are used to address these concerns. XAI aims to increase the reliability of AI by revealing the reasons behind the decisions. To understand the problems of a learned model based on data, causality should be asked Figure 5.8. In the case of a benign breast lesion, how does the spatial organization of the duct change from ordinary to atypia or from carcinoma in

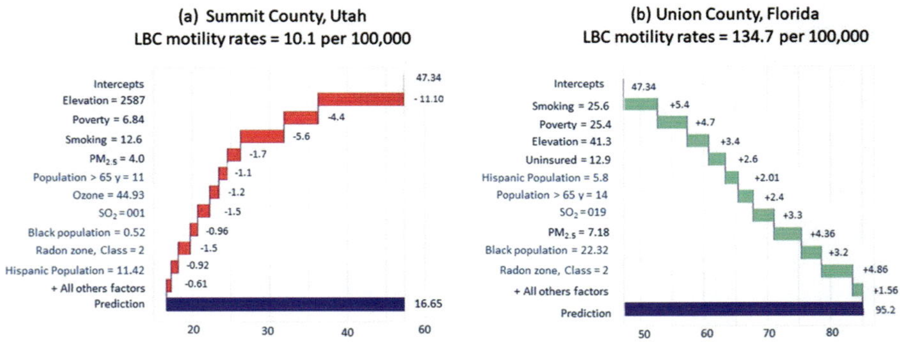


**Figure 5.8** The stack-ensemble model's breakdown plots for (a) Summit County, Utah, and (b) Union County, Florida [30].

situ to invasive cancer? Such questions are based on the principle of causality. Some data may not be visible and may be incorrect. Knowing these limits is related to the security policy. Can computational pathology systems and expert pathologists achieve the same accuracy by knowing biases to avoid unbalanced training datasets [31], or can more computational pathology achieve a better outcome? The principle of transparency should be adopted so that pathologists can clearly explain decisions that affect patients. All necessary information should be provided to make decisions based on XAI recommendations. The complexity of computational pathology applications and the interaction of pathologists are the main factors for patient safety, especially in pathology. This is not only about reducing bias with XAI or providing transparency but also about real-time monitoring of patient samples. To provide different and new perspectives on pathology, XAI can also enable pathologists to understand new disease mechanisms that will allow them to make meaningful therapeutic advances. These reasons are critical for the field of pathology [32].

#### 5.2.2.6 Drug discovery and protein–ligand scoring

Protein–ligand scoring is an essential computational method in a drug design process [33–38]. It is a sub-route to determine correct and incorrect binding modes by scoring according to drug design rules and determining the probability of the candidate molecule being active. The wealth of protein–ligand affinity data is generated by cutting systems based on machine learning. Convolutional neural networks (CNNs) are used to recognize strong interactions because the CNN method has been quite successful in similar image recognition problems [39, 40]. Unlike force field and scoring functions, which are designed to represent known physical interactions such as hydrogen bonding or steric interactions, both model structures and parameters can

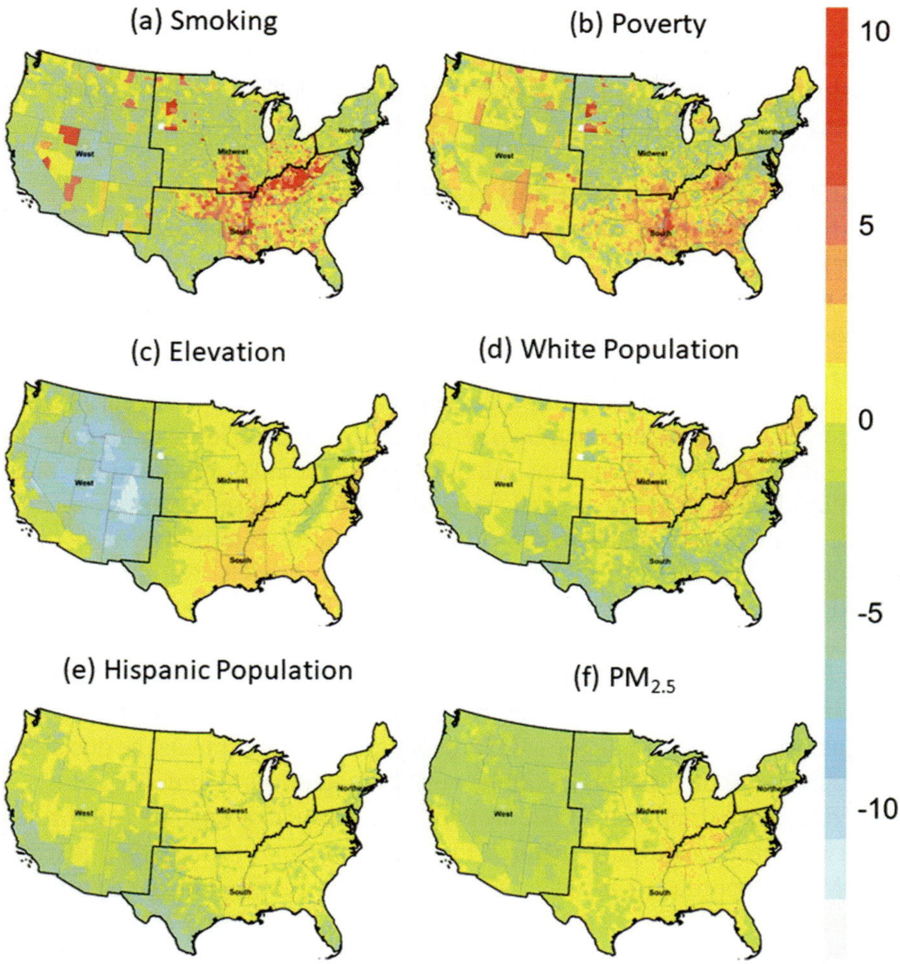


**Figure 5.9** The impact of (a) smoking, (b) poverty, (c) elevation, (d) white population, (e) Hispanic population, and (f) PM2.5 on the prediction of LBC mortality rates vary by location. Stack-ensemble models' "break-down plots" were used to calculate the contribution of risk factors in each county [30].

be derived from data in ML methods. This increase in model expression also increases model interpretability. During the interpretation of CNN models and development of score function, training and test sets need to be managed, and optimal parameters must be determined. Black-box treatment of models is not sufficient for such decisions. Therefore, additional visualizations and interpretable insights are required. In a study that complies with these definitions, convolution filters are visualized to gain insights into the first learned features Figure 5.9. Various methods are introduced and compared to give an atom-based approach to specific network decisions [41]. In this way, more accurate affinity results and explainable interpretations are provided by computationally intervening in the complex and long path of the drug discovery process.

#### 5.2.2.7 Model prediction and classification

This section presents examples from real-world research that uses at least one interpretability approach mentioned in the previous section to demonstrate their use in different areas of biomedical services and future opportunities in model prediction. Studies in the biomedical field have been used for more than 20 years. Linear regression and naive Bayesian models are used in many areas such as urology, toxicology, endocrinology, neurology, and cardiology. In addition, these models can be interpreted at a limited level in non-homogeneous or non-linear situations. Model-specific methods that focus on interpretation based on KNN or decision trees have been used for performance in the prediction of many health-related conditions. Interpretability, which is model-independent and local, can interpret DL models. An XAI method, SHAP, was used to analyze the predictions for the prevention of intraoperative hypoxemia. This increased the hypoxemia expectation of anesthetists by 15% [42]. Some methods used to achieve interpretability simply cannot be classified. Therefore, an approach focusing on subspaces has been proposed by Lakkaraju et al. [43]. In the MUSE technique, which explains the decisions taken from the three-level neural network in diagnosing depression, clusters are created to explain the model decisions. This is also a separate set of rules for a subspace containing features that the healthcare professional selects. The MUSE approach can select actionable features and generate optimized practices. Classibility is an essential factor in interpretability approaches. In making a model-independent interpretation, classification is made, and the subspace area is narrowed with the end-user's input.

A classic approach to global interpretability does not consider that datasets have more exciting features than others, as the patient and healthcare professional can influence their value by making some interventions. Therefore, MUSE can be classified as a global model-free interpretability approach. Still, it also demonstrates the characteristics of courses focused on personalized interpretation by narrowing the subdomain of search to end-user input [44].

Creating explicable models on medical data leads to rapid progress in the biomedical field. Model-independent annotations were used in a study in which tumor tissue detection was performed. Two open evolutionary neural networks on Patch Camelyon Benchmark were analyzed. Three segmentation

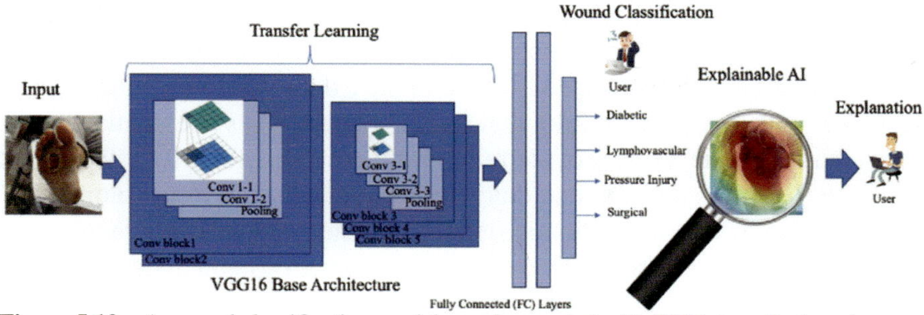


**Figure 5.10** A wound classification model may be created with DNN, transfer learning, and an explainable AI tool [46].

algorithms have been proposed to increase pixel quality. In accurate positive estimates, CNN estimates have been found to follow at least some aspects of expert knowledge [45].

Using XAI, a classification study used a hybrid approach using chronic wound transfer learning and fully connected layers. As shown in Figure 5.10, the benefits of this hybrid approach to clinicians can be seen, and AI has been shown to assist in interpreting and understanding decision-making processes. This work provided new insights into predictions, providing a new perspective on wound classifications. This hybrid model proposed for classifying wound types in the health and biomedical field has an essential role in describing and classifying chronic wounds. With more data collected, such studies will perform better. It is thought that such studies will give an idea about the use of XAI potentials in healthcare and will benefit researchers and clinical workers [46].

## 5.3 Limitations and Future Direction

With the emerging biomedical data science, AI techniques are used in many of the appropriate strategies to access and discover information, reveal the behavior of confidential data, and make new decisions with new insights. As mentioned in the beginning of the chapter, different AI techniques have been proposed and developed in biomedical fields such as drug discovery, medical records, early disease, wound diagnosis, and health analytics. AI has not only made progress in the field of biomedicine but has also dealt with and produced big data. The black-box feature of AI has been a big problem in all areas. Various approaches have also been proposed for this problem. The explainability of AI enables the system to bring better results and be well interpretable. It is helpful in showing users which way will be better. Having problems with reliability and transparency, AI was supported by XAI studies. While analysis and interpretation of bioimages can be complex with the deep learning model, accuracy, speed, and complex dataset can be more understandable with XAI. The development of XAI approaches is essential so that users and researchers can provide reliable explanations for why it works. At the same time, it is difficult and dangerous to believe data in the biomedical and health field. To overcome this situation, higher standards are required.

However, getting biomedical data to XAI can be difficult. Non-linear data and biases are critical perspectives. While computer vision, image analysis, statistics are used, cutting-edge AI approaches for biomedical data are advancing slowly. Therefore, datasets should be customized or modified for better performance and interpretations. It may not be easy and short, but there is no doubt about its necessity. Due to the complexity and problems of high-dimensional omic data, low-performance models emerge. Therefore, the development of AI approaches is necessary. The biases that cause the minimal interpretation of AI methods create the learning bias problem. This may indicate that the AI results are entirely wrong [47]. Incorrect parameter settings, unstable data, and complex issues cause learning bias. Technically, it can be caused by artifacts in AI models and uncontrollable results. XAI should be built to ensure that AI methods can give better results and have no security issues. The security problem in AI is, in some cases, more important than explainability. For example, reliability should be at the forefront rather than explained [48]. Rule-based learning and visualization assessments have made great strides in improving AI explainability in recent times [49]. XAI can increase the security and efficiency of AI, but the important thing here is that the AI methods must be well made [2]. Explainability will also mature when AI learning efficiency is accurate enough, and security issues are clarified and resolved. In this way, the age of AI will evolve, and new perspectives will emerge.

## 5.4 Conclusion

This book chapter demonstrates the need for clarity in biomedical studies and interpretability in decision-making. AI-specific terms and interpretations may not be apparent to biomedical professionals. The use of cross-disciplines, the knowledge of the medical environment and medical professionals, and the use of AI will increase explainability and interpretation. Explanation and understanding of individual fields alone may not be possible. The development of XAI in the biomedical field may result in the synergistic operation of these two fields. The term SVM or SHAP is unfamiliar to the medical professional, while a cancer diagnosis is remote to the computer science professional. However, both have the task of ensuring that the other specialist understands them and transfers them to the patient.

## References

[1] T. Miller, "Explanation in artificial intelligence: Insights from the social sciences," *Artificial intelligence,* vol. 267, pp. 1–38, 2019.

[2] J. Lötsch, D. Kringel, and A. Ultsch, "Explainable Artificial Intelligence (XAI) in Biomedicine: Making AI Decisions Trustworthy for Physicians and Patients," *BioMedInformatics,* vol. 2, no. 1, pp. 1–17, 2022. [Online]. Available: https://www.mdpi.com/2673-7426/2/1/1.

[3] A. Holzinger, "Explainable AI and Multi-Modal Causability in Medicine," *i-com,* vol. 19, no. 3, pp. 171–179, 2020, doi: doi:10.1515/icom-2020-0024.

[4] S. Bach, A. Binder, K.-R. Müller, and W. Samek, "Controlling explanatory heatmap resolution and semantics via decomposition depth," in *2016 IEEE International Conference on Image Processing (ICIP),* 2016: IEEE, pp. 2271–2275.

[5] G. Montavon, "Gradient-based vs. propagation-based explanations: An axiomatic comparison," in *Explainable AI: Interpreting, Explaining and Visualizing Deep Learning*: Springer, 2019, pp. 253–265.

[6] S. Thiebes, S. Lins, and A. Sunyaev, "Trustworthy artificial intelligence," *Electronic Markets,* vol. 31, no. 2, pp. 447–464, 2021.

[7] J. Lötsch and S. Malkusch, "Interpretation of cluster structures in pain-related phenotype data using explainable artificial intelligence (XAI)," *European Journal of Pain,* vol. 25, no. 2, pp. 442–465, 2021.

[8] A. B. Arrieta *et al.*, "Explainable Artificial Intelligence (XAI): Concepts, taxonomies, opportunities and challenges toward responsible AI," *Information fusion,* vol. 58, pp. 82–115, 2020.

[9] J. Lötsch, R. Sipilä, V. Dimova, and E. Kalso, "Machine-learned selection of psychological questionnaire items relevant to the development of persistent pain after breast cancer surgery," *British Journal of Anaesthesia,* vol. 121, no. 5, pp. 1123–1132, 2018.

[10] Q. V. Liao, D. Gruen, and S. Miller, "Questioning the AI: informing design practices for explainable AI user experiences," in *Proceedings of the 2020 CHI Conference on Human Factors in Computing Systems,* 2020, pp. 1–15.

[11] E. Loh, "Medicine and the rise of the robots: a qualitative review of recent advances of artificial intelligence in health," *BMJ leader,* pp. leader-2018-000071, 2018.

[12] X.-Y. Zhou, Y. Guo, M. Shen, and G.-Z. Yang, "Application of artificial intelligence in surgery," *Frontiers of medicine,* vol. 14, no. 4, pp. 417–430, 2020.

[13] R. Kavya, J. Christopher, S. Panda, and Y. B. Lazarus, "Machine Learning and XAI approaches for Allergy Diagnosis," *Biomedical Signal Processing and Control,* vol. 69, p. 102681, 2021.

[14] N. Amoroso *et al.*, "A roadmap towards breast cancer therapies supported by explainable artificial intelligence," *Applied Sciences,* vol. 11, no. 11, p. 4881, 2021.

[15] C. Dindorf *et al.*, "Classification and automated interpretation of spinal posture data using a pathology-independent classifier and explainable artificial intelligence (Xai)," *Sensors,* vol. 21, no. 18, p. 6323, 2021.

[16] S. El-Sappagh, J. M. Alonso, S. Islam, A. M. Sultan, and K. S. Kwak, "A multilayer multimodal detection and prediction model based on explainable artificial intelligence for Alzheimer's disease," *Scientific reports,* vol. 11, no. 1, pp. 1–26, 2021.

[17] J. Peng *et al.*, "An explainable artificial intelligence framework for the deterioration risk prediction of hepatitis patients," *Journal of Medical Systems,* vol. 45, no. 5, pp. 1–9, 2021.

[18] S. Sarp, M. Kuzlu, E. Wilson, U. Cali, and O. Guler, "The enlightening role of explainable artificial intelligence in chronic wound classification," *Electronics,* vol. 10, no. 12, p. 1406, 2021.

[19] H. Wu, W. Chen, S. Xu, and B. Xu, "Counterfactual Supporting Facts Extraction for Explainable Medical Record Based Diagnosis with Graph Network," in *Proceedings of the 2021 Conference of the North American Chapter of the Association for Computational Linguistics: Human Language Technologies*, 2021, pp. 1942–1955.

[20] Y. Zhang, Y. Weng, and J. Lund, "Applications of Explainable Artificial Intelligence in Diagnosis and Surgery," *Diagnostics,* vol. 12, no. 2, p. 237, 2022. [Online]. Available: https://www.mdpi.com/2075-4418/12/2/237.

[21] T. K. Yoo *et al.*, "Explainable machine learning approach as a tool to understand factors used to select the refractive surgery technique on the expert level," *Translational vision science & technology,* vol. 9, no. 2, pp. 8–8, 2020.

[22] N. Mirchi, V. Bissonnette, R. Yilmaz, N. Ledwos, A. Winkler-Schwartz, and R. F. Del Maestro, "The Virtual Operative Assistant: An explainable artificial intelligence tool for simulation-based training in surgery and medicine," *PloS one,* vol. 15, no. 2, p. e0229596, 2020.

[23] H. Ismail Fawaz, G. Forestier, J. Weber, L. Idoumghar, and P.-A. Muller, "Accurate and interpretable evaluation of surgical skills from kinematic

data using fully convolutional neural networks," *International journal of computer assisted radiology and surgery,* vol. 14, no. 9, pp. 1611–1617, 2019.

[24] B. Van der Velden, H. Kuijf, K. Gilhuijs, and M. Viergever, *Explainable artificial intelligence (XAI) in deep learning-based medical image analysis*. 2021.

[25] J. Sun, S. Lapuschkin, W. Samek, and A. Binder, "Explain and improve: LRP-inference fine-tuning for image captioning models," *Information Fusion,* vol. 77, pp. 233–246, 2022/01/01/ 2022, doi: https://doi.org/10.1016/j.inffus.2021.07.008.

[26] E. Tjoa and C. Guan, "A Survey on Explainable Artificial Intelligence (XAI): Toward Medical XAI," *IEEE Transactions on Neural Networks and Learning Systems,* vol. 32, no. 11, pp. 4793–4813, 2021, doi: 10.1109/TNNLS.2020.3027314.

[27] B. Kim, M. Wattenberg, J. Gilmer, C. Cai, J. Wexler, and F. Viegas, "Interpretability beyond feature attribution: Quantitative testing with concept activation vectors (tcav)," in *International conference on machine learning*, 2018: PMLR, pp. 2668–2677.

[28] M. Raghu, J. Gilmer, J. Yosinski, and J. Sohl-Dickstein, "Svcca: Singular vector canonical correlation analysis for deep learning dynamics and interpretability," *Advances in neural information processing systems,* vol. 30, 2017.

[29] A. Anguita-Ruiz, A. Segura-Delgado, R. Alcalá, C. M. Aguilera, and J. Alcalá-Fdez, "eXplainable Artificial Intelligence (XAI) for the identification of biologically relevant gene expression patterns in longitudinal human studies, insights from obesity research," *PLOS Computational Biology,* vol. 16, no. 4, p. e1007792, 2020, doi: 10.1371/journal.pcbi.1007792.

[30] Z. U. Ahmed, K. Sun, M. Shelly, and L. Mu, "Explainable artificial intelligence (XAI) for exploring spatial variability of lung and bronchus cancer (LBC) mortality rates in the contiguous USA," *Scientific Reports,* vol. 11, no. 1, p. 24090, 2021/12/16 2021, doi: 10.1038/s41598-021-03198-8.

[31] W. Samek, T. Wiegand, and K.-R. Müller, "Explainable Artificial Intelligence: Understanding, Visualizing and Interpreting Deep Learning Models," *ArXiv,* vol. abs/1708.08296, 2017.

[32] A. B. Tosun, F. Pullara, M. J. Becich, D. L. Taylor, J. L. Fine, and S. C. Chennubhotla, "Explainable AI (xAI) for Anatomic Pathology," *Advances in Anatomic Pathology,* vol. 27, no. 4, pp. 241–250, 2020, doi: 10.1097/pap.0000000000000264.

[33] G. L. Warren *et al.*, "A critical assessment of docking programs and scoring functions," *Journal of medicinal chemistry,* vol. 49, no. 20, pp. 5912–5931, 2006.

[34] D. B. Kitchen, H. Decornez, J. R. Furr, and J. Bajorath, "Docking and scoring in virtual screening for drug discovery: methods and applications," *Nature reviews Drug discovery,* vol. 3, no. 11, pp. 935–949, 2004.

[35] R. Wang, Y. Lu, and S. Wang, "Comparative Evaluation of 11 Scoring Functions for Molecular Docking," *Journal of Medicinal Chemistry,* vol. 46, no. 12, pp. 2287-2303, 2003/06/01 2003, doi: 10.1021/jm0203783.

[36] T. Cheng, X. Li, Y. Li, Z. Liu, and R. Wang, "Comparative assessment of scoring functions on a diverse test set," *Journal of chemical information and modeling,* vol. 49, no. 4, pp. 1079–1093, 2009.

[37] T. Cheng, Q. Li, Z. Zhou, Y. Wang, and S. H. Bryant, "Structure-based virtual screening for drug discovery: a problem-centric review," (in eng), *AAPS J,* vol. 14, no. 1, pp. 133–141, 2012, doi: 10.1208/s12248-012-9322-0.

[38] R. D. Smith *et al.*, "CSAR benchmark exercise of 2010: combined evaluation across all submitted scoring functions," *Journal of chemical information and modeling,* vol. 51, no. 9, pp. 2115–2131, 2011.

[39] C. Szegedy, V. Vanhoucke, S. Ioffe, J. Shlens, and Z. Wojna, "Proceedings of the IEEE conference on computer vision and pattern recognition," 2015.

[40] A. Krizhevsky *et al.*, "Advances in neural information processing systems," 2012.

[41] J. Hochuli, A. Helbling, T. Skaist, M. Ragoza, and D. R. Koes, "Visualizing convolutional neural network protein-ligand scoring," (in eng), *J Mol Graph Model,* vol. 84, pp. 96–108, 2018, doi: 10.1016/j.jmgm.2018.06.005.

[42] S. M. Lundberg *et al.*, "Explainable machine-learning predictions for the prevention of hypoxaemia during surgery," *Nature biomedical engineering,* vol. 2, no. 10, pp. 749–760, 2018.

[43] H. Lakkaraju, E. Kamar, R. Caruana, and J. Leskovec, "Faithful and customizable explanations of black box models," in *Proceedings of the 2019 AAAI/ACM Conference on AI, Ethics, and Society*, 2019, pp. 131–138.

[44] G. Stiglic, P. Kocbek, N. Fijacko, M. Zitnik, K. Verbert, and L. Cilar, "Interpretability of machine learning-based prediction models in healthcare," *WIREs Data Mining and Knowledge Discovery,* vol. 10, no. 5, p. e1379, 2020, doi: https://doi.org/10.1002/widm.1379.

[45] I. Palatnik de Sousa, M. Maria Bernardes Rebuzzi Vellasco, and E. Costa da Silva, "Local Interpretable Model-Agnostic Explanations for Classification

of Lymph Node Metastases," *Sensors,* vol. 19, no. 13, p. 2969, 2019. [Online]. Available: https://www.mdpi.com/1424-8220/19/13/2969.

[46] S. Sarp, M. Kuzlu, E. Wilson, U. Cali, and Ö. Güler, *A Highly Transparent and Explainable Artificial Intelligence Tool for Chronic Wound Classification: XAI-CWC*. 2021.

[47] J. Lötsch and A. Ultsch, "Machine learning in pain research," *Pain,* vol. 159, no. 4, p. 623, 2018.

[48] K. P. Murphy, *Machine learning: a probabilistic perspective*. MIT press, 2012.

[49] V. Dhar, "Data science and prediction," *Communications of the ACM,* vol. 56, no. 12, pp. 64–73, 2013.

# 6

# What Makes Survival of Heart Failure Patients? Prediction by the Iterative Learning Approach and Detailed Factor Analysis with the SHAP Algorithm

**A. Çifci[1], M. İlkuçar[2], and İ. Kırbaş[3]**

[1]Department of Electrical-Electronics Engineering, Faculty of Engineering and Architecture, Burdur Mehmet Akif Ersoy University, Turkey
[2]Department of Management Information Systems, Faculty of Management, Muğla Sıtkı Koçman University, Turkey
[3]Department of Computer Engineering, Faculty of Engineering and Architecture, Burdur Mehmet Akif Ersoy University, Turkey
Email: acifci@mehmetakif.edu.tr; muhammerilkucar@mu.edu.tr; ismailkirbas@mehmetakif.edu.tr

## Abstract

Cardiovascular disease is the leading cause of global death and disability. There are many types of cardiovascular diseases. The diagnosis of heart failure, one of the cardiovascular disease types, is a challenging task and plays a significant role in guiding the treatment of patients. However, machine learning approaches can be helpful for assisting medical institutions and practitioners in predicting heart failure in the early phase. This study is the first application that analyzes the dataset containing clinical records of 299 patients with heart failure using a feedforward backpropagation neural network (NN). The aim of this study is to predict the survival of heart failure patients based on the clinical data and to identify the strongest factors influencing heart failure disease development. We adopted the Shapley additive explanations (SHAP) values, which have been used to interpret model findings. From the study, it is observed that the best and highest accuracy of 91.11% is obtained compared to previous studies and it is found that feedforward backpropagation

NN performed better than the previous approaches. Also, this study revealed that time, ejection fraction (EF), serum creatinine, creatinine phosphokinase (CPK), and age are the strongest risk factors for mortality among patients suffering from heart failure.

## 6.1 Introduction

Cardiovascular diseases are the main cause of death globally [1, 2]. According to the World Health Organization (WHO), cardiovascular diseases are liable for the deaths of nearly 18 million people globally per year; in other words, 31% of annual global deaths. Heart attack and stroke, on the other hand, constitute approximately 85% of death causes due to these cardiovascular diseases. It is estimated that deaths due to cardiovascular diseases will increase by approximately 30% in 2030 [3].

The heart, arteries, and veins are all known as the cardiovascular system (also called the circulatory system). The cardiovascular system is essential for life and health. To supply oxygen to the body, it carries blood from the heart to the lungs and from there to all the other parts of the body. The body cannot perform the necessary important tasks in people with cardiovascular disease. Cardiovascular disease is a common term for a range of diseases, including high blood pressure (hypertension), atherosclerosis (hardening of the arteries), coronary heart disease, and stroke [4]. Cardiovascular disease may be associated with a person's heart failing to pump blood effectively, valves not functioning the way they should, or narrowing or hardening of the arteries. Cardiovascular disease is examined under four main headings: coronary heart disease, also known as coronary artery disease manifested as congestive heart failure, heart attack, and angina; cerebrovascular disease associated with stroke and transient ischemic attack; peripheral artery disease (also called peripheral arterial disease) affecting the arteries that supply the arms and legs; aortic atherosclerosis and chest or abdominal aortic aneurysm. Coronary heart disease, which refers to blockage or progressive narrowing of the vessels that feed the heart, has a separate significance since it accounts for one-third of all cardiovascular diseases [5].

The heart is the key organ that pumps blood throughout the body, supplying oxygen and nourishment to the vital tissues and organs. In the presence of heart failure due to various reasons, the heart cannot pump the amount of blood the body needs. As a result, fluid accumulation occurs in different parts of the body, especially in the lungs. Heart failure, which can develop acutely, can also be seen chronically. Heart failure, which indicates that the heart is not contracting with enough strength or is not filled with enough blood, often develops as a result of diseases such as cardiovascular diseases, heart attack, myocarditis (inflammation of the heart muscle), high blood pressure, and diabetes [6–8].

There is an increasing interest in using machine learning algorithms in the medical field, especially in heart failure research [9, 10]. The most common research areas using machine learning approaches in heart failure are diagnosis, classification, estimation of treatment compliance, and estimation of hospital admission or re-hospitalization of patients [11]. The bispectrum-related features to analyze heart rate variability signals of congestive heart failure are studied where recognition accuracy is achieved as 98.79% with support vector machine (SVM) classifier and genetic algorithm (GA) [12]. In [13], Austin et al. applied bootstrap aggregation (bagging), boosting, random forests, and SVMs to classify heart failure subtypes. They found that the use of tree-based methods will have better results than the regression models. Guidi et al. [14] made a comparison between machine learning approaches of NN, SVM, fuzzy genetic system, classification and regression tree (CART), and random forest for the analysis of heart failure patients. They concluded that the CART method was more appropriate. See also [15], where the authors compared the effectiveness of boosting, random forests, and logistic regression to predict readmissions caused by heart failure. An automated ECG signals identification approach is proposed where decision tree (DT) and *k*-nearest neighbor (*k*-NN) classifiers were performed for automatic differentiation of congestive heart failure and normal ECG signals with an identification accuracy of 99.86 [16]. A comparative study for heart failure disease prediction using machine learning methods such as DT, naïve Bayes, random forest, SVM, and logistic regression was presented by Alotaibi in [17]. He applied 10-fold cross-validation process during the learning of the model and showed that the DT algorithm achieved the highest success rate of 93.19%. A recent study on congestive heart failure detection was presented by Porumb et al. [18], where they used convolutional NNs on ECG signals. They achieved 100% congestive heart failure detection accuracy.

The remainder of this study is structured as follows. Section 6.2 provides an overview of related research. Section 6.3 describes the dataset and explains artificial neural networks (ANNs) in general. The results are given and discussed in Section 6.4. Conclusion and future work are presented in the Section 6.5.

## 6.2 Related Works Using Heart Failure Dataset

This section reviews research using the heart failure clinical records dataset for heart failure patients' survival prediction and the strongest feature identification.

In this study, we analyze a dataset containing clinical records of patients with heart failure, published by Ahmad et al. [19]. They used Kaplan Meier plot and Cox regression to predict mortality and identify the essential factors of heart failure patients. They found that age, renal dysfunction, EF, high blood pressure, and anemia were the essential factors contributing to an increased risk of death among heart failure patients. Zahid et al. [20] investigated the same dataset to identify the informative risk factors for both genders and to create gender-based survival prediction models. They found a significant difference in the survival prediction models for female and male patients having heart failure. Chicco and Jurman [21] showed that only serum creatinine and EF were good enough to predict heart failure patients' survival from clinical records, and also using these two features alone could lead to more accurate predictions than using all other original dataset features. In [22], Le et al. utilized multilayer perceptron (MLP) NN for predicting heart failure and achieved 88% accuracy. Moreno-Sanchez [23] explored the same dataset and developed a heart failure survival prediction model. The author employed different ensemble tree machine learning techniques and compared their performance. With 83% accuracy, extreme gradient boosting (XGBoost) performed the best. Moreover, the features that most influence the results of the model were found to be serum creatinine, anemia, EF, and time. The authors in [24] sought to identify key features and machine learning algorithms that could improve the accuracy of predicting heart failure. To this end, the authors trained five machine learning classifiers, namely SVM, logistic regression, DT, naïve Bayes, and *k*-NN. The results showed that the best-performing model achieved an accuracy of 80% in terms of heart failure prediction, and they found serum creatinine and EF to be critical risk factors for mortality in heart failure patients. In one very recent study on the same dataset, Giridhar et al. [25] ignored the unnecessary and lesser correlated features in the dataset. They used a random forest model trained on the main dominant seven features which were EF, time, serum sodium, serum creatinine, age, CPK, and platelets. According to the results, the model performed effectively, with an accuracy level of 90% and the model results highlighted time as the most important feature for heart failure survival.

In this study, we used a dataset, containing heart failure clinical records collected by Ahmad et al. [19]. Compared with the existing studies, the main contributions of this study include the following:

- We developed a predictive model for assessing the survival of heart failure patients using iterative training approach over a feedforward backpropagation NN.

- We used SHAP to identify the strongest key features that have an impact on the development of heart failure disease.
- We applied SHAP to explain how each feature influences heart failure disease and thus makes them more acceptable for physicians.
- Feedforward backpropagation NN achieved the highest accuracy of 91.11% among all previous models, which is encouraging.

## 6.3 Materials and Methods

### 6.3.1 Heart failure dataset

The current study is based on the heart failure clinical records dataset, available at the University California Irvine (UCI) Machine Learning Repository [21]. The clinical records dataset of 299 patients (194 men and 105 women) was obtained from two main hospitals of Faisalabad, Pakistan between April and December 2015. All the patients had left ventricular systolic dysfunction in classes III or IV of the New York Heart Association (NYHA) classification scheme [26]. All 299 patients were of age 40 or older. The follow-up time was between 4 and 285 days with a mean of 130 days.

The dataset includes the following potential risk factors: platelets, serum creatinine, age, anemia, CPK, diabetes, EF, high blood pressure, serum sodium, sex, and smoking. Anemia in patients was evaluated according to their hematocrit level. Patients with a hematocrit of less than 36% were considered as anemic. The detailed information about each feature in the dataset is presented in Table 6.1.

Data types and sizes are different from each other. It has been pre-processed to organize data such as missing, corrupt, empty, and endpoints. Standardization has been applied to pull the data into a certain range. The proposed framework is depicted in Figure 6.1.

The correlation information of the features with each other is given in Table 6.2. According to the table, the highest positive correlation between heart failure and death comes from serum creatinine with 0.294 and age with 0.254.

### 6.3.2 Overview of artificial neural networks

ANNs are a special type of machine learning algorithms based on the working principle of biological neurons of the human brain [27, 28]. The first ANNs were introduced by McCulloch and Pitts in 1943 [29]. However, until 1974, when Werbos developed the backpropagation learning algorithm method, it

**Table 6.1** Description of each feature [21].

| Feature | Explanation | Measurement | Range |
|---|---|---|---|
| Age | Age of the patient | Years | [40, ..., 95] |
| Anemia | Decrease of red blood cells or hemoglobin | Boolean | 0, 1 |
| CPK | Level of the CPK enzyme in the blood | mcg/L* | [23, ..., 7861] |
| Diabetes | If the patient has diabetes | Boolean | 0, 1 |
| EF | Percentage of blood leaving the heart at each contraction | Percentage | [14, ..., 80] |
| High blood pressure | If a patient has hypertension | Boolean | 0, 1 |
| Platelets | Platelets in the blood | kiloplatelets/mL | [25.01, ..., 850.00] |
| Serum creatinine | Level of creatinine in the blood | mg/dL* | [0.50, ..., 9.40] |
| Serum sodium | Level of sodium in the blood | mEq/L* | [114, ..., 148] |
| Sex | Woman or man | Binary | 0, 1 |
| Smoking | If the patient smokes | Boolean | 0, 1 |
| Time | Follow-up period | Days | [4, ..., 285] |
| (Target) Death event | If the patient died during the follow-up period | Boolean | 0, 1 |

*mcg/L: micrograms per liter, mg/dL: milligrams per deciliter, mEq/L: milliequivalents per liter.

was not so popular [30]. The backpropagation learning algorithm method had a big effect upon increasing the success of ANNs and became ground for being the most popular machine learning algorithm today. Nowadays, ANN is being used to solve many different problems such as clustering, classification, prediction, time series, etc. As shown in Figure 6.2, ANN is basically a network structure that consists of interconnected nodes and weights. This structure has three layers: an input layer, where data input is provided, hidden layer, and output layer, where the results are transferred to the external environment.

Input has one layer and the number of nodes is equal to the number of attributes of the dataset. The hidden layer can be one or more. The number of nodes in each hidden layer can be different. There is no rule related to how many hidden layers and this layer's nodes have to be. According to characteristic features of the problem, the number of the hidden layers and the number of these layers' nodes can be different. The performance of the network can be increased by trying a different number of hidden layers and different number of these layers' nodes. The output consists of one layer. The output layer must have qualifications that allow us to see properly that the

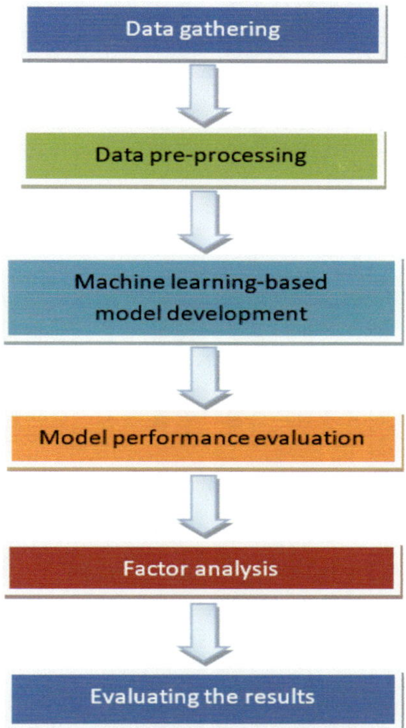


**Figure 6.1** Block diagram of our framework.

result will be obtained by a number of the output layer's nodes. For example, if the output data is positive/negative, it is sufficient for the output layer to be a single node.

ANN learning is the process of optimizing weight values to minimize output error. This learning process involves forward computations and back-propagation of the error from the output to the weights. It is a feedforward process that uses the dataset and weights to adjust the weight values in a way that reduces the amount of error.

Figure 6.3 shows the structure of a node. To generate an output, a node in an ANN takes inputs x, multiplies each input by a weight w, adds a bias term, and then applies a transfer function f(x). To operate the system in a certain threshold value, it has to be given +1 (called bias value) to all nodes. A node output could be the input of the next node/nodes. In order for these output nodes to not repress other input nodes, the output must be taken to a set interval by passing through a transfer function ($f(x)$). There are different transfer functions used for this in literature.

**Table 6.2** Correlation matrix for features.

| | Age | Anemia | CPK | Diabetes | EF | High blood pressure | Platelets | Serum creatinine | Serum sodium | Sex | Smoking | Time | Death event |
|---|---|---|---|---|---|---|---|---|---|---|---|---|---|
| Age | 1.0 | 0.088 | −0.082 | −0.101 | 0.06 | 0.093 | −0.052 | 0.159 | −0.046 | 0.065 | 0.019 | −0.224 | 0.254 |
| Anemia | 0.088 | 1.0 | −0.191 | −0.013 | 0.032 | 0.038 | −0.044 | 0.052 | 0.042 | −0.095 | −0.107 | −0.141 | 0.066 |
| CPK | −0.082 | −0.191 | 1.0 | −0.01 | −0.044 | −0.071 | 0.024 | −0.016 | 0.06 | 0.08 | 0.002 | −0.009 | 0.063 |
| Diabetes | −0.101 | −0.013 | −0.01 | 1.0 | −0.005 | −0.013 | 0.092 | −0.047 | −0.09 | −0.158 | −0.147 | 0.034 | −0.002 |
| EF | 0.06 | 0.032 | −0.044 | −0.005 | 1.0 | 0.024 | 0.072 | −0.011 | 0.176 | −0.148 | −0.067 | 0.042 | −0.269 |
| High blood pressure | 0.093 | 0.038 | −0.071 | −0.013 | 0.024 | 1.0 | 0.05 | −0.005 | 0.037 | −0.105 | −0.056 | −0.196 | 0.079 |
| Platelets | −0.052 | −0.044 | 0.024 | 0.092 | 0.072 | 0.05 | 1.0 | −0.041 | 0.062 | −0.125 | 0.028 | 0.011 | −0.049 |
| Serum creatinine | 0.159 | 0.052 | −0.016 | −0.047 | −0.011 | −0.005 | −0.041 | 1.0 | −0.189 | 0.007 | −0.027 | −0.149 | 0.294 |
| Serum sodium | −0.046 | 0.042 | 0.06 | −0.09 | 0.176 | 0.037 | 0.062 | −0.189 | 1.0 | −0.028 | 0.005 | 0.088 | −0.195 |
| Sex | 0.065 | −0.095 | 0.08 | −0.158 | −0.148 | −0.105 | −0.125 | 0.007 | −0.028 | 1.0 | 0.446 | −0.016 | −0.004 |
| Smoking | 0.019 | −0.107 | 0.002 | −0.147 | −0.067 | −0.056 | 0.028 | −0.027 | 0.005 | 0.446 | 1.0 | −0.023 | −0.013 |
| Time | −0.224 | −0.141 | −0.009 | 0.034 | 0.042 | −0.196 | 0.011 | −0.149 | 0.088 | −0.016 | −0.023 | 1.0 | −0.527 |
| Death event | 0.254 | 0.066 | 0.063 | −0.002 | −0.269 | 0.079 | −0.049 | 0.294 | −0.195 | −0.004 | −0.013 | −0.527 | 1.0 |

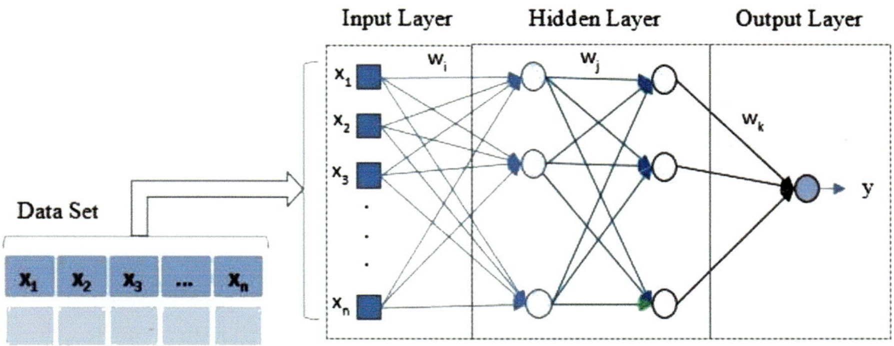


**Figure 6.2** ANN structure.

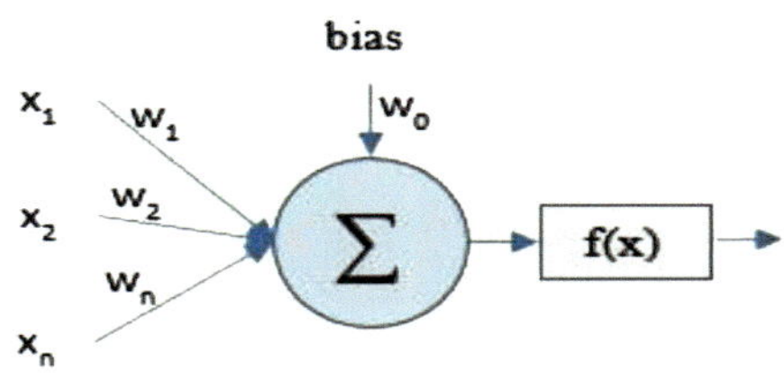


**Figure 6.3** A node structure.

In Figures 6.4(a), 6.4(b), and 6.4(c), some transfer functions that are frequently used in the literature are given. The transfer function to be selected, according to the characteristic features of the problem, can affect the system performance. In the study, the rectified linear unit (ReLU) transfer function was used in all layers. In this function, if the result on one node is equal and greater than zero ($f(x) \geq 0$), the output value is $f(x)$; otherwise (smaller than zero, $f(x) < 0$), it is 0. This means that if the value is negative, it cannot be transferred to the next nodes.

Training the network is the process of determining the weight values that minimize the amount of output error. For this, the difference between incoming data from network output and expected data gives the number of errors. This difference is reflected in the backward weights and the learning of the network is realized. There are too many functions used for loss function in the literature. The mean squared error (MSE) loss function was considered in this study. The MSE loss function is defined by the following equation:

$$\text{MSE} = \frac{1}{n}\sum (z_i - y_i)^2, \tag{6.1}$$

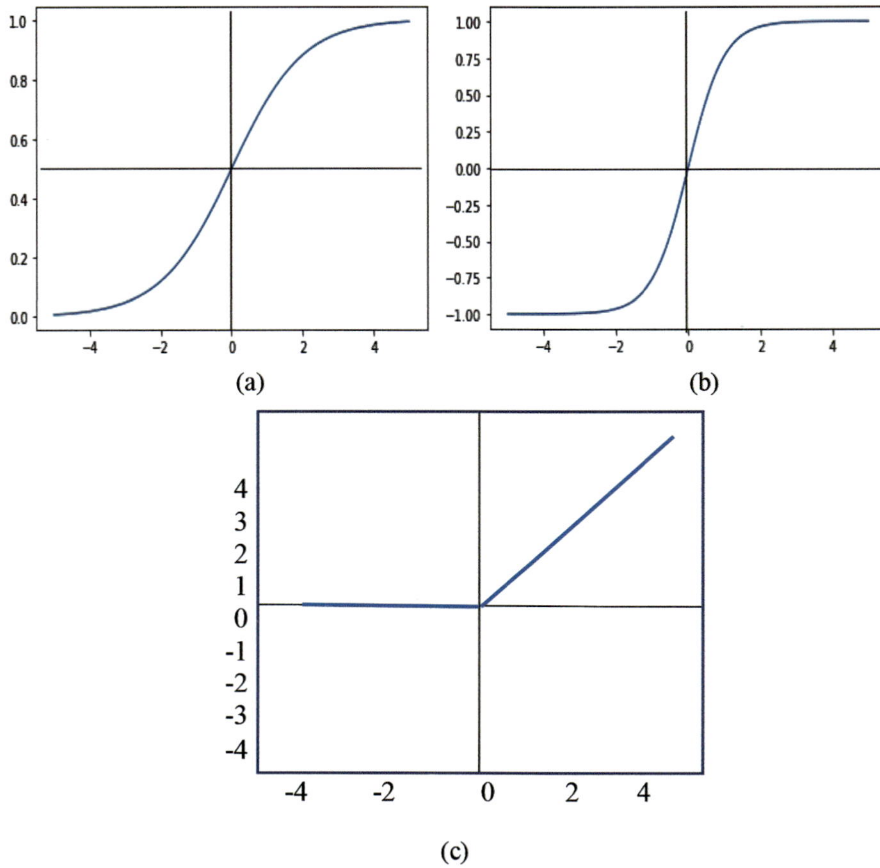


**Figure 6.4** Transfer functions. (a) Sigmoid. (b) Hyperbolic tangent. (c) ReLu.

where $n$, $y_i$, and $z_i$ state the number of samples, the output value obtained from the network, and the expected output value, respectively.

## 6.4 Results

Machine learning using a feedforward backpropagation ANN was performed in data of 299 heart failure patients with different features (age, anemia, CPK, etc.) obtained from the UCI Machine Learning Repository. Figure 6.5 summarizes the modeling development process. 70% of the data was used for the training set (the validation set was taken from the training data itself for 10%) and the remaining 30% was reserved for the test set.

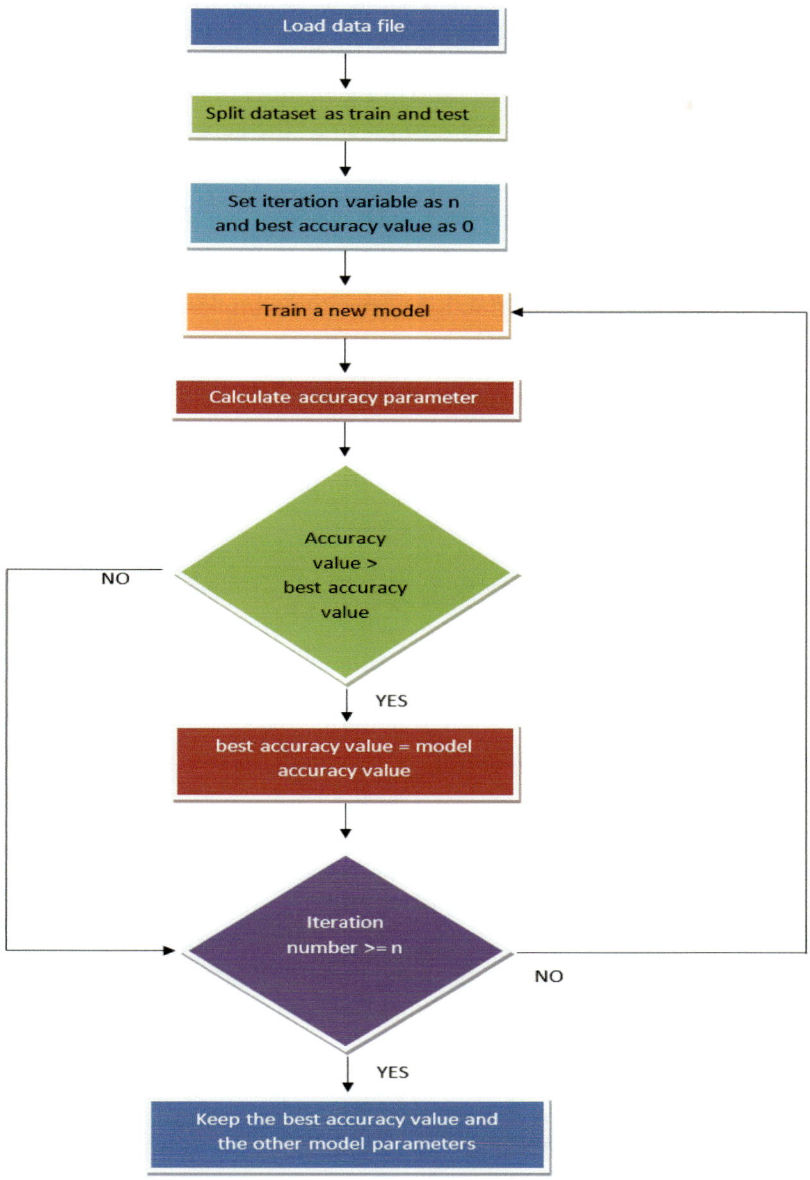


**Figure 6.5** Flowchart of the modeling development process.

The metrics and formulas listed below were used to measure the prediction and classification performance of the model.

**Accuracy:** Accuracy value is the ratio of the number of correct predictions to the total number of samples. It is also given as the success of the algorithm in most applications.

$$\text{Accuracy} = \frac{\text{TP} + \text{TN}}{\text{TP} + \text{TN} + \text{FP} + \text{FN}}. \tag{6.2}$$

**Sensitivity:** Sensitivity is the fraction of positive samples correctly predicted by the classifier.

$$\text{Sensitivity} = \frac{\text{TP}}{\text{TP} + \text{FN}}. \tag{6.3}$$

**Specificity:** It is the fraction of negative samples correctly predicted by the classifier.

$$\text{Specificity} = \frac{\text{TN}}{\text{TN} + \text{FP}}. \tag{6.4}$$

**Precision:** It is the fraction of records that actually turn out to be positive among the predicted positive class.

$$\text{Precision} = \frac{\text{TP}}{\text{TP} + \text{FP}}. \tag{6.5}$$

In the above equations, TP, FP, TN, and FN represent the true positive, false positive, true negative, and false negative, respectively.

ANN consists of a 12-node input layer, an output layer, and a hidden layer, as illustrated in Figure 6.2. Different network topologies were created with hidden layer node numbers between 1 and 20, and network testing training was performed in this way and the best network structure was tried to be determined according to the test accuracy rates. Test accuracy rates are shown in Table 6.3.

According to Table 6.3, the best performing network model is ANN with a hidden layer with 11 nodes giving 91% accuracy. While the number of hidden layer nodes was 1, the test accuracy rate was as high as 0.88. However, the coordination between validation and training graphic, as depicted in Figure 6.6, deteriorated after 30–40 iterations. This indicates that the network has a tendency to memorize. A memorized network is undesirable as it does not have the ability to generalize for different data.

The ANN optimization algorithm used in this study is stochastic gradient descent (SGD). The following network hyperparameters are used: transfer

**Table 6.3** Test accuracy rates for hidden layer nodes.

| Hidden layer nodes | 1 | 2 | 3 | 4 | 5 | 6 | 7 | 8 | 9 | 10 | **11** | 12 | 13 | 14 | 15 | 16 | 17 | 18 | 19 | 20 |
|---|---|---|---|---|---|---|---|---|---|---|---|---|---|---|---|---|---|---|---|---|
| Test accuracy | 0.88 | 0.75 | 0.75 | 0.87 | 0.83 | 0.87 | 0.88 | 0.87 | 0.84 | 0.85 | **0.91** | 0.86 | 0.88 | 0.86 | 0.87 | 0.88 | 0.87 | 0.86 | 0.87 | 0.90 |

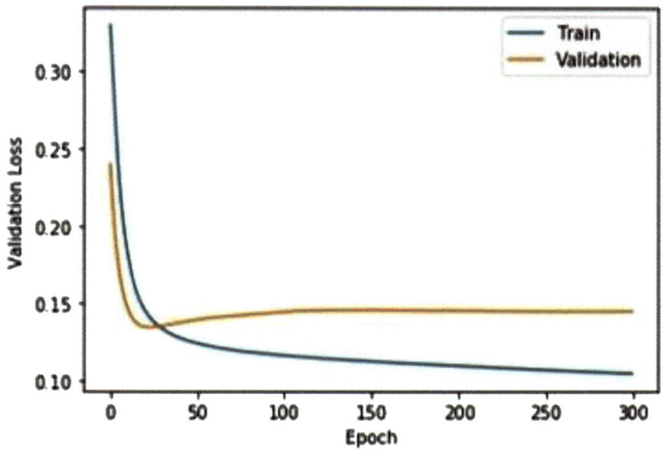


**Figure 6.6** Validation and training graph for network structure with hidden layer node number 1.

function of hidden and output layers is ReLU, the value of the learning rate is 0.001, momentum is 0.2, decay is 1e-4, batch size is 10, and the number of epochs is 300. Accordingly, the training accuracy rate is 0.87, and the value of training error is 0.1. The test accuracy rate and the value of test error are obtained as 0.91 and 0.08, respectively. The graphs of accuracy, loss, and validation of the training process are given in Figures 6.7(a), 6.7(b), and 6.7(c).

The confusion matrix is given in Table 6.4 for the best performing network model (12-11-1).

SHAP is an acronym for SHapley Additive exPlanations and is one of the most recent approaches to interpret the predictions of any machine learning model. This algorithm was first proposed by Lundberg and Lee [31] in 2017 and is known as an effective approach to reverse-engineer the output of any predictive algorithm.

SHAP values indicate the impact of each feature to the final prediction and can efficiently explain models' predictions. SHAP values calculate the change in the expected model prediction by associating it for each input factor when conditioning on the output feature of the model. Figure 6.8(a) depicts the risk factors evaluated by the average absolute SHAP value. Features with

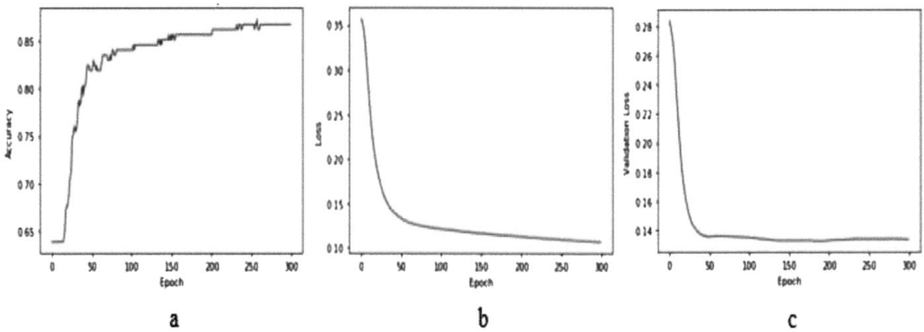


**Figure 6.7** ANN training performance graphics. (a) Accuracy. (b) Loss function. (c) Validation.

**Table 6.4** Test confusion matrix.

| | **Predicted positive** | **Predicted negative** |
|---|---|---|
| Actual positive | 62 | 6 |
| Actual negative | 2 | 20 |

large absolute SHAP values are important. Figure 6.8(b) displays the most important features in the ANN model. The vertical axis ($y$-axis) indicates the feature name, in the order of importance from top to bottom. On the horizontal axis ($x$-axis) is the SHAP value. The red dots represent high-risk values, whereas the blue dots represent low-risk values.

Since identifying the most influential features is the main goal of this study, we will focus on the top five features (in descending order of influence according to the mean SHAP values). As shown in Figure 6.8(a), the top five features are time, EF, serum creatinine, CPK, and age. Time is the most influential feature, contributing on average ±0.24 to heart failure survival. By contrast, the least informative feature, smoking, contributes only ±0.01. However, Figure 6.8(a) provides no additional information as to whether a feature is positively or negatively related to heart failure. Figure 6.8(b) can be used to understand this directional relationship. As shown in Figure 6.8(b), lower values of time and EF have positive SHAP values (the dots extending toward the right are increasingly blue) and higher values of time and EF have negative SHAP values (the dots extending toward the left are increasingly red). This indicates a negative correlation of time and EF with heart failure risk. The reverse is seen for serum creatinine, CPK, and age – older age, elevated serum creatinine, and CPK lead to higher heart failure risk. The results obtained from Figure 6.8 are consistent with the results from the existing literature [32–36].

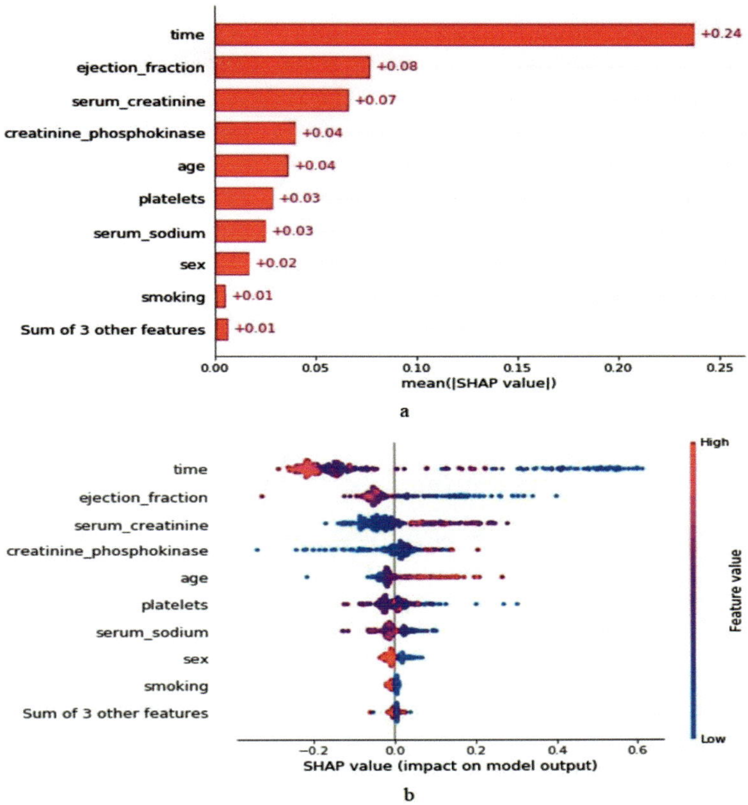


**Figure 6.8** Feature importance based on SHAP values. (a) Mean absolute SHAP values. (b) SHAP summary plot for ANN model trained on the heart failure dataset.

Figure 6.9 shows the SHAP waterfall plot for the heart failure survival prediction made by the ANN model. The color of each arrow represents the impact of the feature on model output. The red color refers to the positive impact of the feature, while the blue color represents the negative impact of the feature. In other words, the positive impact of the feature pushes the prediction higher from the base value, while the negative impact pushes the prediction lower. The base value ($E[f(X)]$) of the model indicated below the $x$-axis is 1.321. The final prediction value (the base value + sum of all the SHAP values) is $f(x) = 2.104$. Time, EF, serum creatinine, age, and CPK have the highest overall impact on the heart failure dataset. The features time, EF, and serum creatinine push the predictions 0.42, 0.18, and 0.1 higher, respectively. The features platelets and sex have negative effects of 0.03 and 0.02, respectively.

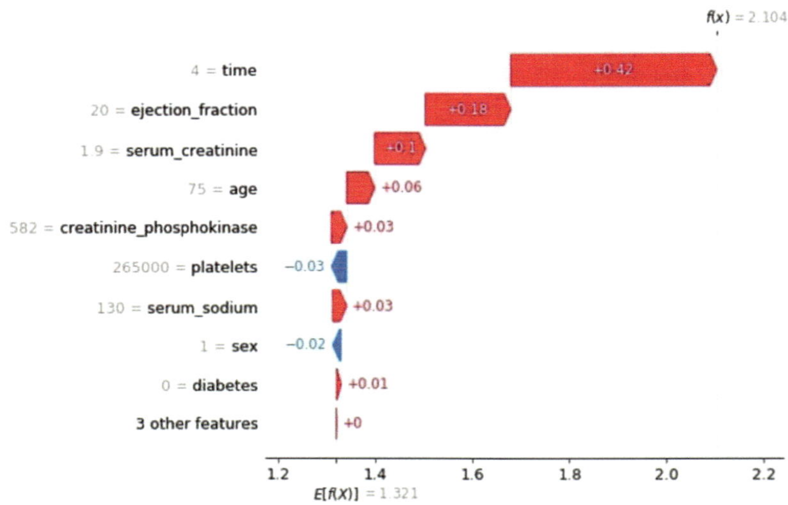


**Figure 6.9** SHAP waterfall plot for ANN model trained on the heart failure dataset.

The comparison of results with other previous studies over the heart failure database is given in Table 6.5. The results presented in Table 6.5 indicate that the feedforward backpropagation NN produced a remarkable performance as compared to the other methods, yielding an accuracy of 91.11%. With our study, a maximum sensitivity of 96.88% with a specificity of 76.92% was achieved.

Chicco and Jurman [21] classified the data using 10 different ML models – random forests, DT, XGBoost, linear regression, one rule, ANN, naïve Bayes, two SVMs, and *k*-NN. The best results were obtained using random forests with an accuracy of 74% and a sensitivity of only 49.1%. Le et al. [22] used an MLP NN with an accuracy of 88.23%. Moreno-Sanchez [23] employed ensemble machine learning trees (DT, XGBoost, random forest, adaptive boosting, gradient boosting, and extra trees). The model performance with XGBoost was the best, with an accuracy of 83% over the other ensemble trees. Hasan et al. [24] performed *k*-NN, logistic regression, SVM, DT, and naïve Bayes. The highest accuracy of 80% was achieved with the DT classifier. Giridhar et al. [25] trained random forest to predict the chances of heart failure in a patient and random forest obtained the best performance with an accuracy of 90%. Based on these results, our study outperformed those in the literature.

**Table 6.5** Comparison of results on the heart failure dataset.

| Author(s) (Year) | Methods | Accuracy (%) | Sensitivity (%) | Specificity (%) | Precision (%) |
|---|---|---|---|---|---|
| Chicco and Jurman (2020) [21] | Random forests | 74 | 49.1 | 86.4 | 65.7 |
| Le et al. (2020) [22] | MLP NN | 88.23 | 87.75 | Not mentioned | 90.38 |
| Moreno-Sanchez (2020) [23] | XGBoost | 83 | 83 | 92 | 83 |
| Hasan et al. (2021) [24] | DT | 80 | 51.72 | 93.44 | Not mentioned |
| Giridhar et al. (2021) [25] | Random forest | 90 | 90.2 | Not mentioned | 90.5 |
| Our study | Feedforward backpropagation NN | 91.11 | 96.88 | 76.92 | 91.18 |

## 6.5 Conclusion

In this study, machine learning by using feedforward backpropagation NN was performed on the clinical records dataset that belongs to heart failure of 299 patients. In the study, with the help of the software, different ANN topologies were tested automatically and the best performance network structure was tried to be obtained. Out of the different ANN models developed, a feedforward ANN model trained with the backpropagation algorithm having a network topology of 12-11-1 showed an accuracy of 91.11%. In comparison with the previous studies, this study achieved the highest accuracy of predicting heart failure patients' survival. Furthermore, the results from our study show which parameters can be considered as the best predictors of an accurate model predicting the survival of heart failure patients based on the clinical data. Accordingly, time, EF, serum creatinine, CPK, and age are the five most important features for survival prediction. The findings of this study demonstrated that the SHAP-identified important features were consistent with the recent related studies. The main limitations of the study are the size of the dataset and the age of patients. The dataset has a limited number of patient's clinical records, and only patients aged 40 and over were considered. Future works can be focused on improving the accuracy of the study with modified features.

## References


[1] H. Ritchie, M. Roser, Causes of Death. Published Online at OurWorldInData.org. 2018. https://ourworldindata.org/causes-of-death, (accessed 10 December 2021).

[2] H. Chen, C. Tan, Z. Lin, T. Wu, Y. Diao, 'A feasibility study of diagnosing cardiovascular diseases based on blood/urine element analysis and consensus models', Comput. Biol. Med. 43 (7) (2013) 865–869. https://doi.org/10.1016/j.compbiomed.2013.03.012.

[3] World Health Organization (WHO), Key facts about cardiovascular diseases (CVDs), Available at: https://www.who.int/news-room/fact-sheets/detail/cardiovascular-diseases-(cvds). (accessed 10 December 2021).

[4] T. Vivekanandan, S.J. Narayanan, 'A hybrid risk assessment model for cardiovascular disease using cox regression analysis and a 2-means clustering algorithm', Comput. Biol. Med. 113 (2019) 1–10. https://doi.org/10.1016/j.compbiomed.2019.103400.

[5] E.O. Lopez, B.D. Ballard, A. Jan, Cardiovascular Disease. In: StatPearls [Internet]. Treasure Island (FL): StatPearls Publishing; 2021. https://www.ncbi.nlm.nih.gov/books/NBK535419/, (accessed 12 January 2022).

[6] E. Tanai, S. Frantz, 'Pathophysiology of Heart Failure'. Comprehensive Physiology. 6(1) (2015) 187–214. https://doi.org/10.1002/cphy.c140055.

[7] C.D. Kemp, J.V. Conte, 'The pathophysiology of heart failure', Cardiovascular Pathology, 21(5) 2012, 365–371. https://doi.org/10.1016/j.carpath.2011.11.007.

[8] J. Špinar, 'Hypertension and ischemic heart disease'. Cor et Vasa, 54(6) (2012) e433–e438. https://doi.org/10.1016/j.crvasa.2012.11.002.

[9] E.E. Tripoliti, T.G. Papadopoulos, G.S. Karanasiou, K.K. Naka, D.I. Fotiadis, 'Heart failure: Diagnosis, severity estimation and prediction of adverse events through machine learning techniques'. Comput. Struct. Biotechnol. J. 15 (2017) 26–47. https://doi.org/10.1016/j.csbj.2016.11.001.

[10] S.E. Awan, F. Sohel, F.M. Sanfilippo, M. Bennamoun, G. Dwivedi, 'Machine learning in heart failure: Ready for prime time', Current Opinion in Cardiology 33 (2018) 190–195. https://doi.org/10.1097/HCO.0000000000000491.

[11] G. Lorenzoni, S.S. Sabato, C. Lanera, D. Bottigliengo, C. Minto, H. Ocagli, P. De Paolis, D. Gregori, S. Iliceto, F. Pisanò, 'Comparison of machine learning techniques for prediction of hospitalization in heart failure patients', J Clin Med. 8(9) (2019) 1–13. https://doi.org/10.3390/jcm8091298.

[12] S.N. Yu, M.Y. Lee, 'Bispectral analysis and genetic algorithm for congestive heart failure recognition based on heart rate variability', Comput. Biol. Med. 42 (2012) 816–825. https://doi.org/10.1016/j.compbiomed.2012.06.005.

[13] P.C. Austin, J.V. Tu, J.E. Ho, D. Levy, D.S. Lee, 'Using methods from the data-mining and machine-learning literature for disease classification and prediction: A case study examining classification of heart failure subtypes', J. Clin. Epidemiol. 2013, 66, 398–407. https://doi.org/10.1016/j.jclinepi.2012.11.008.

[14] G. Guidi, M.C. Pettenati, P. Melillo, E. Iadanza, 'A machine learning system to improve heart failure patients assistance', IEEE Journal of Biomedical and Health Informatics, 18(6) (2014) 1750–1756. https://doi.org/10.1109/JBHI.2014.2337752.

[15] B.J. Mortazavi, N.S. Downing, E.M. Bucholz, K. Dharmarajan, A. Manhapra, S.X. Li, S.N. Negahban, H.M. Krumholz, 'Analysis of machine learning techniques for heart failure readmissions', Circ Cardiovasc Qual Outcomes 9 (2016) 629–640. https://doi.org/10.1161/CIRCOUTCOMES.116.003039.

[16] V.K. Sudarshan, U. Acharya, S.L. Oh, M. Adam, J.H. Tan, C.K. Chua, K.P. Chua, R.S. Tan, 'Automated diagnosis of congestive heart failure using dual tree complex wavelet transform and statistical features extracted from 2s of ECG signals', Computers in Biology and Medicine, 83 (2017), 48–58. https://doi.org/10.1016/j.compbiomed.2017.01.019.

[17] F.S. Alotaibi, 'Implementation of machine learning model to predict heart failure disease', International Journal of Advanced Computer Science and Applications, 10 (6) (2019) 261–268. https://doi.org/10.14569/IJACSA.2019.0100637.

[18] M. Porumb, E. Iadanza, S. Massaro, L. Pecchia, 'A convolutional neural network approach to detect congestive heart failure', Biomedical Signal Processing and Control, 55 (2020) 1–9. https://doi.org/10.1016/j.bspc.2019.101597.

[19] T. Ahmad, A. Munir, S.H. Bhatti, M. Aftab, M.A. Raza, 'Survival analysis of heart failure patients: a case study', PLoS ONE. 12(7) (2017) 1–8. https://doi.org/10.1371/journal.pone.0181001.

[20] F.M. Zahid, S. Ramzan, S. Faisal, I. Hussain, 'Gender based survival prediction models for heart failure patients: a case study in Pakistan', PLoS ONE. 14(2) (2019) 1–10. https://doi.org/10.1371/journal.pone.0210602.

[21] D. Chicco, G. Jurman, 'Machine learning can predict survival of patients with heart failure from serum creatinine and ejection fraction alone', BMC Med Inform Decis Mak 20(16) (2020) 1–16. https://doi.org/10.1186/s12911-020-1023-5.

[22] M.T. Le, M.T. Vo, L. Mai, S.V. Dao, 'Predicting heart failure using deep neural network', 2020 International Conference on Advanced Technologies for Communications (ATC), IEEE (2020), Nha Trang, Vietnam, 8-10 Oct. 2020, pp. 221–225. https://doi.org/10.1109/ATC50776.2020.9255445.
[23] P.A. Moreno-Sanchez, 'Development of an explainable prediction model of heart failure survival by using ensemble trees', 2020 IEEE International Conference on Big Data (Big Data), IEEE (2020), Atlanta, GA, USA, 10–13 Dec. 2020, pp. 4902–4910. https://doi.org/10.1109/BigData50022.2020.9378460.
[24] M.A.M. Hasan, J. Shin, U. Das, A. Yakin Srizon, 'Identifying prognostic features for predicting heart failure by using machine learning algorithm', 11th International Conference on Biomedical Engineering and Technology, Tokyo, Japan, 17–20 March 2021, pp. 40–46. https://doi.org/10.1145/3460238.3460245
[25] U.S. Giridhar, Y. Gotad, H. Dungrani, A. Deshpande, D. Ambawade, 'Machine learning techniques for heart failure prediction: an exclusively feature selective approach', IEEE International Conference on Communication information and Computing Technology (ICCICT), Mumbai, India, 25–27 June 2021, pp. 1–5. https://doi.org/10.1109/ICCICT50803.2021.9510091
[26] The Criteria Committee of the New York Heart Association. Nomenclature and criteria for diagnosis of diseases of the heart and great vessels. 9th ed. Boston, Mass: Little, Brown & Co; 1994, 253–256.
[27] J. Zou, Y. Han, S.S. So, Overview of Artificial Neural Networks. In: Livingstone D.J. (Eds.) Artificial Neural Networks. Methods in Molecular Biology™, 458, 2008 14–22. Humana Press. https://doi.org/10.1007/978-1-60327-101-1_2.
[28] Z.R. Yang, Z. Yang, Artificial Neural Networks. Comprehensive Biomedical Physics, Elsevier. Editor(s): Anders Brahme, 2014, pp. 1–17, https://doi.org/10.1016/B978-0-444-53632-7.01101-1.
[29] W.S. McCulloch, W. Pitts, 'A logical calculus of the ideas immanent in nervous activity', The Bulletin of Mathematical Biophysics, 5(4) (1943) 115–133. https://doi.org/10.1007/BF02478259.
[30] P. Werbos, Beyond regression: New tools for prediction and analysis in the behavioral sciences, Ph.D. dissertation, Committee on Applied Mathematics, Harvard Univ., Cambridge, MA, Nov. 1974.
[31] S.M. Lundberg, S.-I. Lee, 'A unified approach to interpreting model predictions', 31st Conference on Neural Information Processing Systems (NIPS 2017), Long Beach, CA, USA.

[32] S.G. Wannamethee, A.G. Shaper, I.J. Perry, 'Serum creatinine concentration and risk of cardiovascular disease: a possible marker for increased risk of stroke', Stroke 1997; 28 (3): 557–563. doi: 10.1161/01.str.28.3.557

[33] P.C. Austin, J.V. Tu, J.E. Ho, D. Levy, D.S. Lee, 'Using methods from the data-mining and machine-learning literature for disease classification and prediction: a case study examining classification of heart failure subtypes', Journal of Clinical Epidemiology 2013, 66 (4): 398–407. doi: 10.1016/j.jclinepi.2012.11.008

[34] S. Angraal, B.J. Mortazavi, A. Gupta, R. Khera, T. Ahmad, N.R. Desai, D.L. Jacoby, F.A. Masoudi, J.A. Spertus, H. M. Krumholz, 'Machine learning prediction of mortality and hospitalization in heart failure with preserved ejection fraction', JACC Heart Fail 2020, 8 (1): 12–21. doi: 10.1016/j.jchf.2019.06.013

[35] R.S. Aujla, R. Patel, Creatine Phosphokinase. In: StatPearls [Internet]. Treasure Island (FL): StatPearls Publishing, available at https://www.ncbi.nlm.nih.gov/books/NBK546624/, 2021.

[36] S. Hajouli, D. Ludhwani, Heart Failure and Ejection Fraction. In: StatPearls [Internet]. Treasure Island (FL): StatPearls Publishing, available at https://www.ncbi.nlm.nih.gov/books/NBK553115/, 2021.

# 7

# Class Activation Mapping and Deep Learning for Explainable Biomedical Applications

**Prasath Alias Surendhar S.[1], R. Manikandan[2], and Ambeshwar Kumar[3]**

[1]Department of Biomedical Engineering, Aarupadai Veedu Institute of Technology (AVIT), India
[2]School of Computing, SASTRA Deemed University, India
[3]Dayananda Sagar University, India
Email: prasath179@hotmail.com; srmanimt75@gmail.com; ambeshwar.kumar@gmail.com

## Abstract

For a number of medical diagnostic tasks, deep learning (DL) methods have proven to be quite successful, sometimes even outperforming human experts. The algorithms' black-box nature has, however, limited their therapeutic application. Recent studies on explainability seek to identify the factors most responsible for a model's choice. In the biomedical domain, deep neural networks (DNNs) now represent most successful machine learning (ML) technologies. The various topics of interest in this field include BBMI (study of interface between the brain as well as body's mechanical systems), bioimaging (the study of biological cells and tissues), medical imaging (study of human organs through the creation of visual representations), and public and medical health management (PmHM). This study provides an overview of explainable artificial intelligence (XAI) applied in class activation mapping-based DL medical picture analysis. For the purpose of categorizing DL-based medical image analysis (MIA) techniques, a framework of XAI criteria is presented. The papers are then surveyed and categorized in accordance with framework as well as based on anatomical location for use in MIA.

## 7.1 Introduction

A possible technique to improve the effectiveness and accessibility of the diagnosis process is through computer-aided diagnostics (CAD), which uses AI. The most effective AI technique for a variety of challenges, including those involving medical imaging, is DL. It is utilized for medical imaging jobs like categorization of Alzheimer's, the detection of lung cancer, the detection of retinal diseases, etc. [1]. It is state-of-the-art for many computer vision applications. Although AI-based technologies have shown impressive outcomes in the medical field, they have not been widely used in clinics. This is caused by the DL algorithms' inherent black-box character, as well as other factors including high computing costs. It results from the inability to clearly represent knowledge for a particular task carried out by a DNN, despite existence of the underlying statistical principles. Decision boundary utilized for classification may be shown in a few dimensions utilizing method specifications, making simpler AI techniques like linear regression as well as decision trees self-explanatory [2]. These, however, are not complex enough to do jobs like classifying most 2D and 3D medical images. The adoption of DL in numerous fields, including finance and autonomous driving, where explainability as well as reliability are crucial components for end-user trust, is hampered by absence of tools to examine the behavior of black-box methods. DL is now a potent method for resolving image classification issues and is frequently applied to the study of medical images. CNNs have potential to automatically classify various cancerous lesions, including breast, skin, and lung cancer. But CNNs are harder to understand because they are not interpretable or explicable. More rigorous neural network models and training techniques must be created in order to give analysis that is both visually comprehensible and explicable in order to advance CNN-based medical diagnostic techniques [3].

In fact, the most effective ML techniques in a number of fields, including image analysis and defect diagnostics, are artificial neural networks (ANNs) and DL. All medical levels are covered by the DL applications in the biomedical sectors, starting with genomic applications like gene expression and ending with public medical health management like forecasting demography data or infectious disease epidemics. We can observe that during the past three years, a number of research publications has enhanced exponentially. Majority of these papers are in two primary sub-fields of medical/bioimaging and genomics [4].

A significant area of research in computer vision is semantic image segmentation, which involves giving a semantic class label to every pixel of an image. Weakly supervised training approaches were proposed to lessen the annotation effort because gathering completely annotated training data poses a significant bottleneck for improving segmentation models. CAM is a visualization approach that draws attention to discriminative picture regions that are pertinent to a specific class and where a model uses these image regions to identify the specified class [5]. A layer known as global average pooling (GAP) must be present after the last convolutional layer of a specific method in order to produce a class activation map. A GAP layer of this type generates a single number by adding up all of the values in a feature map. Usage of a global max pooling (GMP) layer, for example, only considers activation of a certain image region. Weights applied explicitly show how significant every image region is in identifying the class of interest. The location of the most informative picture areas is identified by overlaying generated heatmap on the input image in question after heatmap has been up-sampled to fit the size of input image in question [6].

**Taxonomy of explainability approaches:**
In literature, a number of taxonomies are developed to categorize various explainability methodologies [7]. Generally speaking, classification approaches are not absolute; they can differ greatly depending on features of techniques and are divided into multiple overlapping or distinct classes at once. Here, many taxonomies and categorization techniques are briefly addressed. A more thorough analysis of taxonomies may be found in [8].

**Model specific vs. model agnostic:**
These techniques are built around unique method specifications. A unique form of model-specific interpretability called the graph neural network (GNN) explainer (GNNExplainer) [9] is required due to the complexity of data representation. It is not restricted to a particular method architecture and is typically applicable in *post-hoc* analysis. The structural parameters or internal model weights cannot be accessed directly by these methods.

**Global methods vs. local methods:**
A single model result is applicable to local interpretable techniques. This can be accomplished by developing techniques that can provide an explanation for the basis of a specific forecast or result. For instance, it is intrigued by particular features and their traits. Global approaches, on the other hand, focus on internal workings of a method by taking advantage of the general understanding of model, training, and related data. It aims to provide a general explanation for the model's behavior. This strategy, which seeks to identify features that are generally accountable for methods that improved

performance among all other features, is shown well by the concept of feature importance.

**Pre-model vs. in-model vs. post-model:**
These techniques are autonomous and applied to any model architecture. Examples of these techniques that are often used include principal component analysis (PCA) and t-distributed stochastic neighbor embedding (t-SNE). In this technique PCA is embedding technique which can be improved into autonomous model. Some techniques are used after creating a model; hence, they are referred to as post-model techniques. These techniques have the ability to produce insightful conclusions regarding the precise lessons that a model acquired during training.

**Surrogate methods vs. visualization methods:**
Surrogate methodologies use an ensemble of many models to examine other black-box models. By comparing the judgments made by black-box design and surrogate model, it is possible to interpret decisions made by the black-box design more clearly. An illustration of a surrogate approach is the decision tree [10]. Although the visualization techniques do not create a new model, they do make some aspects of the models easier to understand visually, such as activation maps. It should be emphasized that these classification techniques do not overlap much because they are based on various logical intuitions. For instance, since most *post-hoc* models, such as attributions, are not reliant on a model's structure, they can also be viewed as model agnostic. However, several of the attribution approaches do have criteria with regard to the restrictions on model layers or the activation functions.

According to Stiglic et al. [11], explainability is the capacity to communicate how an AI decision has been reached to a wider range of end-users in a language that humans can comprehend. The various end-users concentrate on the various explainability vantage points. The model's or algorithm's explicability is of more significance to data scientists or professionals in AI. Clinical inference and prediction are, however, of more relevance to medical professionals or doctors. Interpretability is a related concept to explainability. The ability to explain an abstract concept's meaning is referred to as interpretability [12]. Explainability refers to how predictions are interpreted in the presence of novel cases, whereas interpretability refers to how a method is interpreted after being trained on data [13]. Additionally, there are two categories of XAI methods: *post-hoc* and intrinsic [14]. A decision-making method or underlying principles of a method can be understood without the need for additional information using an intrinsic method. Linear regression

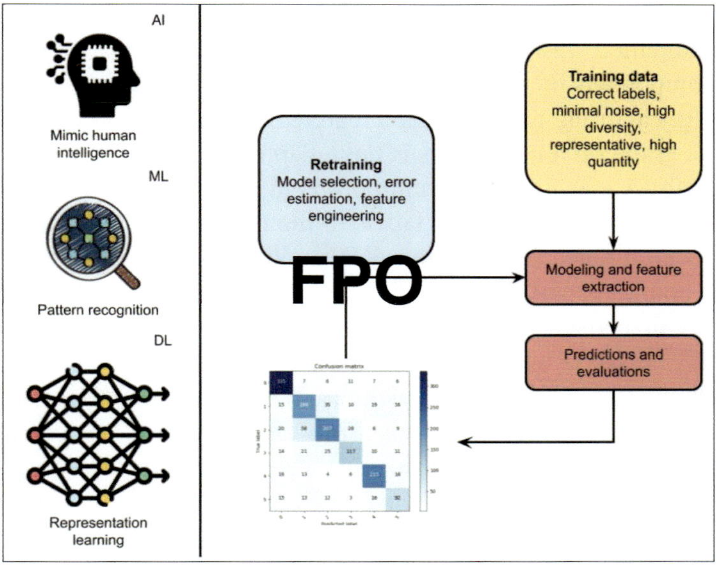


**Figure 7.1** Relationship between explainable Machine learning and Deep Learning.

(LR), logistic regression, *k*-nearest neighbor, rule-based learners, GAM, Bayesian methods, and decision trees are examples of common intrinsic approaches. AI is a subset of ML, which is a subset of DL. Additionally, we think that XAI is a subset of AI and that its fundamental technique is ML. As a result, Figure 7.1 depicts connection between explainable AI, DL, and ML. By employing this technique, we may determine what portion of the input data contributes to the categorization choice made by any classifier. Principal component analysis (PCA), Shapley additive explanations (SHAP), class activation mapping (CAM), and gradient-weighted class activation mapping (Grad-CAM) are other *post-hoc* techniques [15]. Dimension reduction, attention mechanisms, constrained NN method, text explanation, local explanation, explanation by example, explanation by simplification, and feature relevance are some categories for *post-hoc* explainability methodologies, according to Kavya et al. [16].

## 7.2 Background Study

Previous studies [17] on weakly supervised learning demonstrate that a classification network's output can estimate object positions in addition to label predictions. In [18], a new loss function is put forth that enhances a segmentation system by using location, classes, and border priors. A spectral clustering method was utilized in the work [19] to divide coarsely segmented picture components into communities. Then, a network driven by communities is built, capturing the spatial and feature associations between communities, and a graph driven by labels is built, capturing the correlations between image labels. A convex optimization problem is then developed to represent the mapping of the image-level labels to the relevant communities. In [20], class activation maps (CAMs) for CNNs with GAP are described. With no need for bounding box annotations, classification-trained CNNs may now learn to localize visual objects.

CheXNet, a 121-layered CNN created by Friedman [21], is used to detect pneumonia in chest X-ray pictures. When compared to the traditional techniques that seasoned radiologists rely on, CheXNet is more effective. CheXNet can, in fact, accurately identify pathology and calculate the likelihood of having pneumonia. The most likely area of pathology in a particular input image is also located using CAM as a qualitative assessment. Similar to this, Sarp et al. [22] suggested using MRNet, a DL method, to shorten the time it takes to analyze knee MRI data and eliminate diagnostic mistakes. In fact, automatic analyses using deep learning techniques, which learn features from input photos provided during training, can help with diagnosis as well as help to prioritize high-risk patients. Additionally, the work by [23] made use of CAM as a visualization tool, enabling researchers to see which elements of an input image have the most impact on the predictions made. ResNet-152, a DL method for early skin cancer screening that was developed by work [24], allows for the classification of 12 different skin-related disorders. By utilizing the gradient data flowing into final convolutional layer, Grad-CAM is utilized as a tool to better comprehend method predictions and to produce visual explanations. Chen et al. [25] created a segmentation method that combines ResNet as well as U-Net, two CNNs, for precise diagnosis, as well as treatment planning of eye cancers. The segmentation model that has been built is utilized to do quantitative analysis on eye tumor tissues, assisting medical professionals in creating effective treatment plans for patients. The location and segmentation of malicious tissue in input pictures is done using CAM. In particular, class activation maps created for CNNs designed to identify ocular cancers are improved, and segmentation models based on U-Net are trained using these maps. DL-based assistant was developed by Rucco et al. [26] to assist pathologists in classifying liver cancer, resulting in an easily usable diagnostic tool. A review of the impact of model efficacy on pathologists' diagnoses is also included in this paper. Additionally, CAM serves as an explanation tool for the forecasts that are produced.

The term "CAM" was initially used to describe CNNs with a global average pooling layer following last convolutional layer in [27]. In this instance, the weights of the top classification layer were designated as weights *k*. Later, a number of more complex methods for determining *k* were put forth. Grad-CAM is generic enough to work with any network architecture. Grad-sensitivity CAMs and conservation have recently been enhanced by the introduction of an axiom-based version [28]. In contrast, Grad-CAM++ [4] computes a real weighted average of gradients. To account for the significance of each activation map position, each weight of the average is obtained as a weighted average of partial derivatives along spatial axes. A smoothening mechanism has been added to the gradient computation, substantially extending the strategy in [29]. Finally, Score-CAM [33] does away with gradients in favor of computing the weights αk using a channel-wise increase in confidence. This enhance the network security based on the security of feeding network with input *x* multiplied by αk as well as that of a baseline input

Researchers have made contributions to the field of computerized tongue diagnosis throughout the last few decades, including the development of tongue examination systems and tongue analysis. A computerized approach for examining the tongue was developed by Wei et al. [34] with the goal of quantifying the tongue's characteristics for traditional Chinese medical diagnoses. The association between tongue appearances and diseases was discovered by Chang et al. [35] using Bayesian network classifiers based on quantitative data. Additionally, numerous publications have put forth methods for tongue segmentation, color analysis, and shape analysis [36].

The threshold of tongue concavity is a crucial criterion for categorizing the tooth-marked tongue in studies on the condition. Cho et al. [37] noted that tongue images frequently feature a tongue with visible teeth. The tongue is paler, thicker, and more delicate than the typical tongue. An approach to extract features of tooth-marked tongues was put forth in the work [38] and was based on particular thresholds. First, the author established a threshold for the change in curvature of the tongue edge in order to locate suspicious tooth-marked areas. Second, he used a diamond-shaped box to scan the tongue's edge. Finally, a feature to categorize the tongue with dental marks was defined using the *R*-value of the box, which indicates the color of the tongue picture. Krizhevsky et al. [39] computed the slope and the length of the tongue picture and applied this data as a threshold to distinguish tongues with dental marks. Rajpurkar et al. [40] outlined the characteristics of tongues, focusing on changes in brightness and curvature. By thresholding these feature values, they were able to categorize tongues with dental marks.

Recently, some studies have extracted tooth-marked features using CNN features. A technique for feature extraction using CNN and final classification using a multi-instance classifier was proposed in [41].

Many computer vision applications, including object detection as well as image classification, have seen a dramatic improvement in performance because of CNN. Recent studies investigating CNN visuals are numerous. Deconvolutional networks were utilized in the work [42] to display the patterns that activate each unit and to identify the performance contribution of various model layers. Nguyen et al. [43] improved the quality of "raw" gradients by applying guided backpropagation to the changes. A CNN learns object detectors while being trained to recognize scenes, according to Kiani et al. [44]. They demonstrated that the same network can carry out object categorization and object localization in a single forward pass. The features of several convolutional layers were reversed by Kim et al. [45], who also examined the visual coding of CNN. They demonstrated that some CNN layers, such as those with different degrees of geometric characteristics, maintain accurate information. Ronneberger et al. [46] proposed class activation mapping (CAM). By altering the image classification CNN architecture, this method highlighted the regions that are specifically discriminative for each class. Convolutional layers and global average pooling were utilized in place of fully connected layers and projected category score was mapped back to the first convolutional layer to create the CAM. These techniques are utilized for many different medical imaging tasks, including categorization of cancer and detection of pneumonia, in addition to standard datasets.

The studies' pertinent data were then extracted and evaluated after we included articles that satisfied the review's selection criteria. We also explain how XAI can be used in medical applications by using an experimental showcase on breast cancer diagnosis. The obstacles that the researchers have faced are outlined, along with the future research directions, and we conclude by summarizing the XAI techniques used in the medical XAI applications. According to the survey results, medical XAI is a promising area for research, and the purpose of this study is to provide guidance for medical professionals as well as AI researchers when developing medical XAI applications.

A multiclass XGBoost method to choose laser surgery choice at an expert level is described in [47]. The suggested method was tested on patients who underwent refractive surgery at B&VIIT Eye Center, and the accuracy rate on the external validation dataset was 78.9%, according to the authors. Additionally, it gives a clinical explanation of how the SHAP methodology is used in machine learning. A framework for surgical training with automated educational visual feedback was developed in [48]. The accuracy, specificity, and sensitivity of the SVM model that the authors trained and assessed on simulated medical and surgical data were 92%, 82%, and 100%, respectively. Additionally, they identified the teachable metrics that contribute to categorization, which gave a complete explanation of the suggested ML technique. Otsu [49] trained an FCN network to categorize surgical skill levels utilizing surgical kinematics, resulting in an accurate and understandable medical application for assessing surgical expertise.

The term "Omics" is frequently used in the literature to refer to this field of study, but other terms, such as "bioinformatics" or "biomedicine," have also been used. The aim of the Omics is to explore and comprehend biological processes at a molecular level in order to forecast and prevent diseases by including patients in the development of a more significant as well as tailored treatment. Data from genetics and (gen/transcript/epigen/prote/metabol/pharmacogen/multi) Omics are covered by the Omics [50]. In the realm of Omics, predictions of human drug targets as well as their interactions, as well as predictions of protein function, all play a crucial role. We suggest reading the work [51], which presented a thorough summary of genomics and significant difficulties in real-world ML tasks.

The examination of the cell (cytopathology) and the tissue comes next, following the DNA and protein levels (histopathology). Histopathology and cytopathology are frequently utilized in the diagnosis of inflammatory disorders, cancer, and several infectious diseases. Under a microscope, histological as well as cytopathological slides – typically produced by fine-needle aspiration biopsies – are analyzed [52]. The primary study area for DL in biomedical applications is bioimaging, as it is known in the literature. Medical imaging studies human organs by examining several types of imaging (medical, clinical, and health) [53]. Today, there are major medical high-resolution image acquisition methods available, including parallel MRI, multi-slice CT, digital PET, and 2D/3D X-ray. There is some dispute among translators because of the quantity of information contained in these medical photos [54]. The makers of medical imaging systems make an effort to offer applications, workstations, and solutions for picture archiving, viewing, and analysis. The accuracy of a disease's diagnosis and/or assessment in bio and medical imaging depends on both picture acquisition and image interpretation. The improvement of the technology in recent years has greatly enhanced image acquisition. Physicians interpret medical images most often; however, interpreters' abilities might vary greatly and become fatigued. In fact, computer-aided picture interpretation and analysis is a major focus of DL applications in bio as well as medical imaging [55]. In both bio and medical imaging, segmentation, localization, and classification of nuclei and mitosis, as well as lesions and anatomical objects, are the main topics of DL studies published in these fields.

GANs can create manipulated visuals, such as the numerous retinal images synthesized from Lundberg and Lee's [56] unseen tubular structured annotation that contains binary vascular morphology. In [57], adversarial examples in medical imaging are investigated and constructively used to test model performance on data that has been intentionally manipulated in addition to clean and noisy data. To increase robustness of progressive holistically nested network (P-HNN) method for diseased lung segmentation of CT scans, a conditional GAN is investigated in [58] to supplement artificially produced lung nodules. In [59], a novel GIN is proposed to extract features from real patients as well as create virtual patients using the features that are both esthetically and pathophysiologically plausible. The GIN is a combination of a CNN and GANs [60]. CNNs and a GAN are the cornerstones of the deep generative multi-task. A model that has been trained using one type of data can be applied to another using transfer learning. By basing the formation of a conditional generative adversarial network on a genuine picture sample, Eliza Yingzi [61] uses it to create realistic chest X-ray images with various illness features. By creating samples that are actually informative, this method offers the advantage of getting around the restrictions of tiny training datasets. Ramprasaath [62] developed a two-stage DL architecture for diagnosing Alzheimer's disease utilizing partial multi-modal imaging data to address the issue of missing data in multi-modal investigations. A 3D cycle consistent GAN method is employed in the first step to impute missing PET data utilizing associated MRI data. The second step uses a landmark-based multi-modal multi-instance NN for classifying brain diseases.

## 7.3 Discussion

Recent advancements in artificial intelligence have revolutionized several aspects of healthcare, including diagnosis and surgery. These methods have proven successful in these sectors. Some diagnosis tasks based on DL are even more accurate than those performed by human doctors. The black-box aspect of the DL model, however, restricts the models' ability to be explained and prevents their widespread application in medicine. Numerous researchers in interdisciplinary field of AI and medicine have understood that explainability of the AI model, not its accuracy, is the key to its deployment in the clinical setting. Before being accepted and included into the medical practice, medical AI applications should be explained. Therefore, there is a drive

| S. No. | Year | Aim | AI method | AI simulation parameters | XAI technique | XAI technique type | XAI evaluation |
|---|---|---|---|---|---|---|---|
| 1 | 2021 | Allergy diagnosis | KNN, SVM, C5.0, MLP, AdaBag, and RF | Accuracy: 86.39%<br>Sensitivity: 75% | IF–THEN rules | Rule based | No |
| 2 | 2021 | Breast cancer therapies | Cluster analysis | N/A | Adaptive dimension reduction | Dimension reduction | No |
| 3 | 2021 | Spine | One-class SVM and binary RF | *F*1: 80+12%<br>MCC: 57+23%<br>BSS: 33+28% | LIME | Explanation by simplification | No |
| 4 | 2021 | Alzheimer's disease | Two-layer method with RF | First layer accuracy: 93.95%;<br>*F*1_score: 93.94%<br>Second layer: 87.08%<br>*F*1_Score: 87.09% | SHAP and fuzzy | Feature relevance rule | No |
| 5 | 2021 | Hepatitis | LR, DT, KNN, SVM, and RF | Accuracy: 91.9% | SHAP, LIME, and partial dependence plots (PDP) | Feature relevance explanation by simplification | No |
| 6 | 2021 | Chronic wound | CNN-based method: pretrained VGG_16 | Precision: 95%<br>Recall: 94%<br>*F*1_Score: 94% | LIME | Explanation by simplification | No |
| 7 | 2021 | Fenestral otosclerosis | CNN-based method: proposed otosclerosis LNN method | AUC: 99.5%<br>Sensitivity: 96.4%<br>Specificity: 98.9% | Visualization of learned deep representations | Visual explanation | No |
| 8 | 2021 | Lymphedema | Counterfactual multi-granularity graph | Precision: 99.04%<br>Recall: 99.00%<br>*F*1_Score: 99.02% | GNN counterfactual reasoning | RNN architecture | No |

| S. No. | Year | Aim | AI method | AI simulation parameters | XAI technique | XAI technique type | XAI evaluation |
|---|---|---|---|---|---|---|---|
| 9 | 2020 | Clinical diagnosis | ECNNs | Top-3 Sensitivity: 88.8% | Bayesian network ensembles | Bayesian methods | Yes |
| 10 | 2020 | GBM diagnosis | VGG16 | Accuracy: 97% | LIME | Explanation by simplification | No |
| 11 | 2020 | Pulmonary nodule diagnostic | CNN | Accuracy: 82.15% | VINet, LRP, CAM, and VBP | Visual explanation | No |
| 12 | 2020 | Alzheimer's disease diagnosis | NB and grammatical evolution | ROC: 0.913<br>Accuracy: 81.5%<br>*F*1_Score: 85.9%<br>Brier: 0.178 | CFG | Rule-based | No |
| 13 | 2020 | Lung cancer diagnosis | NN and RF | N/A | LIME and natural language explanation | Explanation by simplification text explanation | No |
| 14 | 2020 | TBI identification | *k*-means, spectral clustering, and Gaussian mixture | N/A | Quality assessment of clustering features | Feature relevance | No |
| 15 | 2020 | COVID-19 chest X-ray diagnosis | CNN-based method: proposed COVID-Net | Accuracy: 93.3%<br>Sensitivity: 91.0% | GS Inquire | RNN architecture | No |
| 16 | 2020 | Colorectal cancer diagnosis | CNN | Accuracy: 91.08%<br>Precision: 91.44%<br>Recall:91.04%<br>*F*1_Score: 91.26% | X-CFCMC | Visual explanation | Yes |

| S. No. | Year | Aim | AI method | AI simulation parameters | XAI technique | XAI technique type | XAI evaluation |
|---|---|---|---|---|---|---|---|
| 17 | 2020 | Diagnosis of thyroid nodules | NN | Accuracy: 93.15%<br>Sensitivity: 92.29%<br>Specificity: 93.62% | CAM | Visual explanation | No |
| 18 | 2020 | Phenotyping psychiatric disorders diagnosis | DNN | White matter<br>Accuracy: 90.22%<br>Sensitivity: 89.21%<br>Specificity: 91.23% | EDNN | Visual explanation | No |
| 19 | 2020 | PD diagnosis | CNN | Accuracy: 95.2%<br>Sensitivity: 97.5%<br>Specificity: 90.9% | LIME | Explanation by simplification | No |
| 20 | 2019 | Post-stroke hospital discharge disposition | LR, RF, RF with adaboost, and MLP | Test accuracy: 71%<br>Precision: 64%<br>Recall: 26%<br>*F*1_Score: 59% | LR and LIME | Intrinsic, explanation by simplification | No |
| 21 | 2019 | Breast cancer diagnostic decision as well as therapeutic decisions | WKNN and RBIA | Accuracy: 80.3% | CBR method | Explanation by example | Yes |
| 22 | 2019 | Alzheimer's diagnosis | RF, SVM, and DT | Sensitivity: 84%<br>Specificity: 67%<br>AUC: 0.81% | An interpretable ML method: SHIMR | Rule-based | No |

to survey the medical XAI because the acceptance of medical AI applications demands explainable AI.

Even if the subject benefits from the advent of quantitative assessment methods, many of the suggested metrics fall short in terms of offering a suitable and inexpensive evaluation for explainability. Comparing various methodologies becomes difficult from a numerical perspective when there are multiple metrics used rather than a single score. Second, although average increase is too discrete to accurately assess gain in method confidence, average reduction by itself is easily capable of producing an inaccurate assessment. We have discussed a number of XAI techniques and how they might be applied to medical image analysis, but how can one determine whether a given XAI method offers a solid justification? Success criteria for explanation are more challenging to establish than performance metrics usually employed in medical image analysis, such as accuracy, Dice coefficient, or ROC analysis. Explainability, and especially the attribution techniques that may be used for a number of business use cases, are becoming more and more of a commercial interest. For the two different user groups, the explainability approaches have two distinct but overlapping purposes. By examining the model characteristics and comprehending how the model interacts with the data, DL practitioners can use them to develop better systems. In order to increase confidence as well as trust in method decision and to help uncover potentially dubious decisions, clinical end-users might be given explanations as justification for decision. A new study assessed how well data scientists understood explanations. Common difficulties including missing data as well as redundant features were added in this study, and the data scientists were given descriptions of trained methods to help them spot flaws. The study found that there was a lack of trust in methods since they tried to justify problems as important characteristics. Contrary to end consumers' lower levels of acceptance and trust who are suspicious of black-box nature. It is noteworthy that skilled data scientists were able to make use of them well to comprehend method as well as data challenges.

## 7.4 Conclusion

Significant progress has been made in explaining DL models' judgments, particularly those that are employed for medical diagnosis. In order to address dependability issues and help end-users build trust and make better decisions, it is helpful for model designers to understand the features that contribute to a given decision. The majority of these techniques focus on local explainability, or discussing the choices made for a single example. In cases when images have same spatial orientation, this is then extrapolated to a global level by averaging highlighted features. However, cutting-edge techniques like idea vectors offer a more comprehensive perspective on the choices made for every class in terms of domain concepts. In recent years, XAI techniques have advanced swiftly to fulfill the changing demands of AI researchers and end-users of their models. Although it is simple to fall into the trap of thinking that more contemporary methods are objectively superior to its more traditional counterparts, it is crucial to realize that every method was created to further our comprehension of various aspects of artificial intelligence solutions. For instance, KNN interpolation as well as other traditional methods are frequently employed in place of more sophisticated modern techniques in the process of data augmentation. This is partially due to the more traditional approach's longer history and well-known drawbacks. Because there aren't many examples of the current approach's triumphs and failures in the real world, it is possible that it will produce data bias, which may be challenging to understand. To more accurately design underlying data distribution of samples, the tendency for data augmentation is to enhance the number of parameters taken into account and the complexity of data transformations.

The biological explanation may be one of XAI's future directions in medical image analysis. Several researchers have used DL to predict biological processes from imaging characteristics. In these analyses, NN was trained using a biological target. However, conducting a similar study in the opposite direction, for instance, by performing a route analysis on imaging phenotypes, could offer an intriguing biological explanation. Aside from helping doctors with diagnosis, XAI may also be effective for extracting unknown data from medical photos. For instance, a study on diagnosis of tuberculosis on chest X-rays revealed that assessing chest X-rays with an XAI that provided a visual explanation was more accurate for 10 out of the 13 participating doctors (or 77%) than analyzing chest X-ray without an XAI.

## References

[1] Jo, T. Nho, K. Saykin, A.J,'Deep learning in Alzheimer's disease: Diagnostic classification and prognostic prediction using neuroimaging data', Front. Aging Neurosci., 11, 220, 2019.

[2] Hua, K.L. Hsu, C.H. Hidayati, S.C.Cheng, W.H. Chen, Y.J,'Computer-aided classification of lung nodules on computed tomography images via deep learning technique',OncoTargetsTher., 8, 2015–2022, 2015.

[3] Sengupta, S. Singh, A. Leopold, H.A. Gulati, T. Lakshminarayanan, V, 'Ophthalmic diagnosis using deep learning with fundus images–A critical review',Artif. Intell. Med., 102, 101758, 2020.

[4] Leopold, H. Singh, A. Sengupta, S. Zelek, J. Lakshminarayanan, V., 'Recent Advances in Deep Learning Applications for Retinal Diagnosis using OCT', In State of the Art in Neural Networks; El-Baz, A.S., Ed.; Elsevier: New York, NY, USA, 2020.

[5] Holzinger, A. Biemann, C. Pattichis, C.S. Kell, D.B,'What do we need to build explainable AI systems for the medical domain?', arXiv 2017, arXiv:1712.09923.

[6] Stano, M. Benesova, W. Martak, L.S,'Explainable 3D convolutional neural network using GMM encoding', In Proceedings of the Twelfth International Conference on Machine Vision, Amsterdam, The Netherlands, 11433, p. 114331U, 2019.

[7] Moccia, S. Wirkert, S.J. Kenngott, H. Vemuri, A.S. Apitz, M. Mayer, B. De Momi, E. Mattos, L.S. Maier-Hein, L,'Uncertainty-aware organ classification for surgical data science applications in laparoscopy', IEEE Trans. Biomed. Eng., 65, 2649–2659, 2018.

[8] Adler, T.J. Ardizzone, L.Vemuri, A. Ayala, L. Gröhl, J. Kirchner, T. Wirkert, S. Kruse, J. Rother, C. Köthe, U. 'Uncertainty-aware performance assessment of optical imaging modalities with invertible neural networks', Int. J. Comput. Assist. Radiol. Surg., 14, 997–1007, 2019.

[9] Meyes, R. de Puiseau, C.W. Posada-Moreno, A. Meisen, T,'Under the Hood of Neural Networks: Characterizing Learned Representations by Functional Neuron Populations and Network Ablations', arXiv 2020, arXiv:2004.01254.

[10] Arrieta, A.B. Díaz-Rodríguez, N. Del Ser, J. Bennetot, A. Tabik, S. Barbado, A. García, S. Gil-López, S. Molina, D. Benjamins, R. 'Explainable Artificial Intelligence (XAI): Concepts, taxonomies, opportunities and challenges toward responsible AI', Inf. Fusion, 58, 82–115, 2020.

[11] Stiglic, G. Kocbek, P. Fijacko, N. Zitnik, M. Verbert, K. Cilar, L,'Interpretability of machine learning based prediction models in healthcare', arXiv 2020, arXiv:2002.08596.

[12] Arya, V. Bellamy, R.K. Chen, P.Y. Dhurandhar, A. Hind, M. Hoffman, S.C. Houde, S. Liao, Q.V. Luss, R.; Mojsilovi´c, A,'One explanation does not fit all: A toolkit and taxonomy of ai explainability techniques', arXiv 2019, arXiv:1909.03012.

[13] Ying, Z. Bourgeois, D. You, J. Zitnik, M. Leskovec, J. Gnnexplainer, 'Generating explanations for graph neural networks', In Proceedings of

the Advances in Neural Information Processing Systems 32, Vancouver, BC, Canada, 32, 9240–9251, 2019.

[14] Yang, G. Ye, Q. Xia, J,'Unbox the black-box for the medical explainable AI via multi-modal and multi-centre data fusion: A mini-review, two showcases and beyond', Inf. Fusion, 77, 29–52, 2022.

[15] Tjoa, E.; Guan, C. 'A Survey on Explainable Artificial Intelligence (XAI): Toward Medical XAI. IEEE Trans', Neural Netw. Learn. Syst., 14, 1–21, 2020.

[16] Kavya, R. Christopher, J. Panda, S. Lazarus, Y.B, 'Machine Learning and XAI approaches for Allergy Diagnosis', Biomed. Signal Process. Control, 69, 102681, 2021.

[17] Amoroso, N. Pomarico, D. Fanizzi, A. Didonna, V. Giotta, F. La Forgia, D. Latorre, A. Monaco, A. Pantaleo, E. Petruzzellis, N, 'A roadmap towards breast cancer therapies supported by explainable artificial intelligence', Appl. Sci, 11, 4881, 2021.

[18] Dindorf, C. Konradi, J. Wolf, C. Taetz, B. Bleser, G. Huthwelker, J. Werthmann, F. Bartaguiz, E. Kniepert, J. Drees, P, 'Classification and automated interpretation of spinal posture data using a pathology-independent classifier and explainable artificial intelligence (Xai)', Sensors, 21, 6323, 2021.

[19] El-Sappagh, S. Alonso, J.M. Islam, S.M.R. Sultan, A.M. Kwak, K.S, 'A multilayer multimodal detection and prediction model based on explainable artificial intelligence for Alzheimer's disease', Sci. Rep., 11, 1–26, 2021

[20] Peng, J. Zou, K. Zhou, M. Teng, Y. Zhu, X. Zhang, F. Xu, J, 'An Explainable Artificial Intelligence Framework for the Deterioration Risk Prediction of Hepatitis Patients', J. Med. Syst., 45, 1–9, 2021.

[21] Friedman, J.H. 'Greedy function approximation: A gradient boosting machine', Ann. Stat., 29, 1–10, 2001.

[22] Sarp, S. Kuzlu, M. Wilson, E. Cali, U. Guler, O, 'The enlightening role of explainable artificial intelligence in chronic wound classification. Electronics, 10, 1406, 2021.

[23] Tan, W. Guan, P. Wu, L. Chen, H. Li, J. Ling, Y. Fan, T. Wang, Y. Li, J. Yan, B, 'The use of explainable artificial intelligence to explore types of fenestral otosclerosis misdiagnosed when using temporal bone high-resolution computed tomography', Ann. Transl. Med., 9, 969, 2021.

[24] Wu, H. Chen, W. Xu, S. Xu, B, 'Counterfactual Supporting Facts Extraction for Explainable Medical Record Based Diagnosis with Graph Network', In Proceedings of the 2021 Conference of the North American Chapter of the Association for Computational Linguistics: Human

Language Technologies, Online, 6–11 June 2021; Association for Computational Linguistics: Stroudsburg, PA, USA, 1942–1955, 2021.
[25] Chen, J. Dai, X. Yuan, Q. Lu, C. Huang, H, 'Towards Interpretable Clinical Diagnosis with Bayesian Network Ensembles Stacked on Entity-Aware CNNs', In Proceedings of the 58th Annual Meeting of the Association for Computational Linguistics; Association for Computational Linguistics: Stroudsburg, PA, USA, 3143–3153, 2020.
[26] Rucco, M. Viticchi, G. Falsetti, L, 'Towards personalized diagnosis of glioblastoma in fluid-attenuated inversion recovery (FLAIR) by topological interpretable machine learning', Mathematics, 8, 770, 2020.
[27] Gu, D. Li, Y. Jiang, F. Wen, Z.Liu, S. Shi, W. Lu, G. Zhou, C, 'VINet: A Visually Interpretable Image Diagnosis Network. IEEE Trans. Multimed', 22, 1720–1729, 2020.
[28] Kroll, J.P. Eickhoff, S.B. Hoffstaedter, F. Patil, K.R, 'Evolving complex yet interpretable representations: Application to Alzheimer's diagnosis and prognosis', In Proceedings of the 2020 IEEE Congress on Evolutionary Computation (CEC), Glasgow, UK, 19–24 July 2020.
[29] Meldo, A. Utkin, L. Kovalev, M. Kasimov, E, 'The natural language explanation algorithms for the lung cancer computer-aided diagnosis system',Artif. Intell. Med., 108, 101952, 2020.
[30] Yeboah, D. Steinmeister, L. Hier, D.B. Hadi, B. Wunsch, D.C. Olbricht, G.R. Obafemi-Ajayi, T, 'An Explainable and Statistically Validated Ensemble Clustering Model Applied to the Identification of Traumatic Brain Injury Subgroups', IEEE Access, 8, 180690–180705, 2020.
[31] Wang, L. Lin, Z.Q. Wong, A, 'COVID-Net: A tailored deep convolutional neural network design for detection of COVID-19 cases from chest X-ray images', Sci. Rep., 10, 19549, 2020.
[32] Wong, A. Shafiee, M.J. Chwyl, B. Li, F, 'FermiNets: Learning generative machines to generate efficient neural networks via generative synthesis', arXiv 2018, arXiv:1809.05989.
[33] Sabol, P. Siňcák, P. Hartono, P. Kŏcan, P. Benetinová, Z. Blichárová, A. Verbóová, L'. Štammová, E. Sabolová-Fabianová, A. Jašková, A, 'Explainable classifier for improving the accountability in decision-making for colorectal cancer diagnosis from histopathological images', J. Biomed. Inform., 109, 103523, 2020.
[34] Wei, X. Zhu, J. Zhang, H. Gao, H. Yu, R. Liu, Z. Zheng, X. Gao, M. Zhang, S, 'Visual Interpretability in Computer-Assisted Diagnosis of Thyroid Nodules Using Ultrasound Images', Med. Sci. Monit., 26, e927007, 2020.

[35] Chang, Y.-W. Tsai, S.-J. Wu, Y.-F. Yang, A.C, 'Development of an Al-Based Web Diagnostic System for Phenotyping Psychiatric Disorders', Front. Psychiatry, 11, 1–10, 2020.

[36] Magesh, P.R. Myloth, R.D.Tom, R.J, 'An Explainable Machine Learning Model for Early Detection of Parkinson's Disease using LIME on DaTSCAN Imagery', Comput. Biol. Med., 126, 104041, 2020.

[37] Cho, J. Alharin, A. Hu, Z. Fell, N. Sartipi, M, 'Predicting Post-stroke Hospital Discharge Disposition Using Interpretable Machine Learning Approaches', In Proceedings of the 2019 IEEE International Conference on Big Data (Big Data), Los Angeles, CA, USA, 9–12 December 2019; IEEE: New York, NY, USA, 4817–4822, 2019.

[38] Lamy, J.B. Sekar, B. Guezennec, G. Bouaud, J. Séroussi, B, 'Explainable artificial intelligence for breast cancer: A visual case-based reasoning approach', Artif. Intell. Med., 94, 42–53, 2019.

[39] Krizhevsky, A, Sutskever, I, and Hinton, G. E., 'ImageNet Classification with Deep Convolutional Neural Networks,' in [Advances in Neural Information Processing Systems 25], Pereira, F., Burges, C. J. C., Bottou, L., and Weinberger, K. Q., eds., Curran Associates, Inc. (2012).

[40] Rajpurkar, P, Irvin, J, Zhu, K, Yang, B, Mehta, H, Duan, T, Ding, D, Bagul, A., Langlotz, C., Shpanskaya, K., 'CheXNet: Radiologist-Level Pneumonia Detection on Chest X-Rays with Deep Learning', arXiv preprint arXiv:1711.05225, 2017.

[41] Bien, N., Rajpurkar, P., Ball, R. L., Irvin, J., Park, A., Jones, E., Bereket, M., Patel, B. N., Yeom, K. W., Shpanskaya, K., et al., 'Deep-learning-assisted diagnosis for knee magnetic resonance imaging: Development and retrospective validation of MRNet', PLoS Medicine 15(11), e1002699, 2018.

[42] Han, S., Kim, M., Lim, W., Park, G., Park, I., and Chang, S., 'Classification of the Clinical Images for Benign and Malignant Cutaneous Tumors Using a Deep Learning Algorithm,' Journal of Investigative Dermatology 138(7), 1529–1538, 2018.

[43] Nguyen, H.-G., Pica, A., Hrbacek, J., Weber, D. C., La Rosa, F., Schalenbourg, A., Sznitman, R., and Cuadra, M. B., 'A novel segmentation framework for uveal melanoma in magnetic resonance imaging based on class activation maps', in [International Conference on Medical Imaging with Deep Learning ], 370–379, 2019

[44] Kiani, A., Uyumazturk, B., Rajpurkar, P., Wang, A., Gao, R., Jones, E., Yu, Y., Langlotz, C. P., Ball, R. L., Montine, T. J., et al., 'Impact of a deep learning assistant on the histopathologic classification of liver cancer', npj - Digital Medicine 3(1), 1–8 2020.

[45] Kim, M., Han, J., Hyun, S., Janssens, O., Van Hoecke, S., Kee, C., and De Neve, W., 'Medinoid: ComputerAided Diagnosis and Localization of Glaucoma Using Deep Learning', Applied Sciences 9(15), 3064, 2019.

[46] Ronneberger, O., Fischer, P., and Brox, T., 'U-Net: Convolutional Networks for Biomedical Image Segmentation', in [Medical Image Computing and Computer-Assisted Intervention – MICCAI 2015], 234–241, Springer International Publishing, 2015.

[47] Zhang, Y., Weng, Y., & Lund, J. (2022). Applications of Explainable Artificial Intelligence in Diagnosis and Surgery. *Diagnostics*, 12(2), 237

[48] Milletari, F., Navab, N., and Ahmadi, S.-A., 'V-Net: Fully Convolutional Neural Networks for Volumetric Medical Image Segmentation', in [2016 Fourth International Conference on 3D Vision (3DV], 565–571, 2016.

[49] Otsu, N., 'A Threshold Selection Method from Gray-Level Histograms', IEEE Transactions on Systems, Man, and Cybernetics 9(1), 62–66, 1979.

[50] Johnson, J. M. and Khoshgoftaar, T. M., 'Survey on deep learning with class imbalance', Journal of Big Data 6, 27, 2019.

[51] He, K., Zhang, X., Ren, S., and Sun, J., 'Deep Residual Learning for Image Recognition', in Proceedings of IEEE International Conference on Computer Vision, 770–778, 2016.

[52] Huang, G., Liu, Z., Van Der Maaten, L., and Weinberger, K. Q., 'Densely Connected Convolutional Networks', in Proceedings of IEEE International Conference on Computer Vision, 4700–4708, 2017.

[53] Chattopadhay, A., Sarkar, A., Howlader, P., and Balasubramanian, V. N., 'Grad-CAM++: Generalized Gradient-Based Visual Explanations for Deep Convolutional Networks', in [2018 IEEE Winter Conference on Applications of Computer Vision (WACV) ], 839–847, 2018.

[54] Li, K., Wu, Z., Peng, K.-C., Ernst, J., and Fu, Y., 'Tell Me Where to Look: Guided Attention Inference Network', in Proceedings of the IEEE Conference on Computer Vision and Pattern Recognition, 9215–9223, 2018.

[55] Ribeiro, M. T., Singh, S., and Guestrin, C., 'Why Should I Trust You?": Explaining the Predictions of Any Classifier', in Proceedings of the 22nd ACM SIGKDD International Conference on Knowledge Discovery and Data Mining, KDD '16, 1135–1144, Association for Computing Machinery, New York, NY, USA, 2016.

[56] Lundberg, S. M. and Lee, S.-I., 'A Unified Approach to Interpreting Model Predictions', in [Advances in Neural Information Processing Systems, Guyon, I., Luxburg, U. V., Bengio, S., Wallach, H., Fergus, R.,

Vishwanathan, S., and Garnett, R., eds., 30, 4765–4774, Curran Associates, Inc., 2017.

[57] Smadi, O., Hawkins, N., Hans, Z., Bektaş, B., Knickerbocker, S., Nlenanya, I., & Hallmark, S., 'Naturalistic driving study: development of the Roadway Information Database', 2015.

[58] Ghasemzadeh, Ali, 'Complementary methodologies to identify weather conditions in naturalistic driving study trips: Lessons learned from the SHRP2 naturalistic driving study & roadway information database'," Safety Science 119, 21-28, 2019.

[59] Pantangi, SarvaniSonduru, 'Do high visibility crosswalks improve pedestrian safety? A correlated grouped random parameters approach using naturalistic driving study data', Analytic methods in accident research 30,100155, 2021

[60] Sheykhfard, Abbas, 'Analysis of the occurrence and severity of vehicle-pedestrian conflicts in marked and unmarked crosswalks through naturalistic driving study', Transportation research part F: traffic psychology and behaviour 76, 178-192, 2021.

[61] Du, Eliza Yingzi, 'Pedestrian behavior analysis using 110-car naturalistic driving data in USA', 23rd International Technical Conference on the Enhanced Safety of Vehicles (ESV), 2013.

[62] Selvaraju, Ramprasaath R, 'Grad-cam: Visual explanations from deep networks via gradient-based localization', Proceedings of the IEEE international conference on computer vision, 2017.

[63] Ramaswamy, Harish Guruprasad,'Ablation-cam: Visual explanations for deep convolutional network via gradient-free localization', Proceedings of the IEEE/CVF Winter Conference on Applications of Computer Vision, 2020.

# 8

# Pragmatic Study of IoT in Healthcare Security with an Explainable AI Perspective

**Adrija Mitra, Yash Anand, and Sushruta Mishra**

Kalinga Institute of Industrial Technology, Deemed to be University, India
Email: adrijamitra01@gmail.com; yashanand1605@gmail.com; sushruta.mishrafcs@kiit.ac.in

## Abstract

The Internet of Things (IoT) is the concept of connecting any device to the Web and other connected gadgets. IoT resembles a ubiquitous network, with the exception that any electrical equipment connected to it has internet connectivity. IoT in the health industry is a great example of this pervasive computing. With the rise of explainable AI, security in IoT using predictive methods is an important concern that needs to be taken care of. If IoT in healthcare is to be successful, serious security issues must be resolved. Medical professionals and society handling IoT devices must ensure that the data collected by IoT devices is appropriately protected and it can be achieved through proper interpretation of results through explainable AI approaches. The main objective of this work is to draw a comparative analysis of two IoT security healthcare strategies in the context of explainable AI aspect. To achieve these objectives, we have discussed two distinct models in this study. The first model takes into account security in intelligent healthcare leveraging block-chain and explainable intelligence. The second model offers a healthcare security method based on easily interpretable deep learning. Also included is a table that compares the two models.

## 8.1 Introduction

A network of linked devices that send and receive data via the internet is known as the Internet of Things (IoT). The IoT is now widely employed to

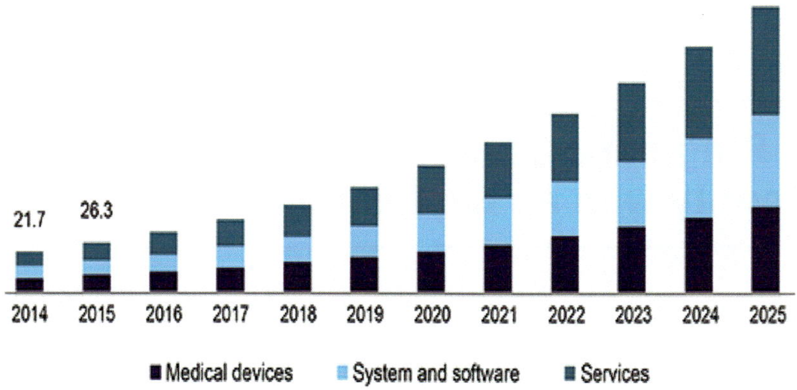


**Figure 8.1** IoT in healthcare market size, by component, 2014–2025 (USD Billion) (data missing).

reduce human stress. The IoT has evolved into an industry-agnostic lexicon to explain how technology is presently being implanted in numerous areas, including healthcare, and changing the way businesses are performed [1] as shown in Figure 8.1. The Internet of Things has changed the way stakeholders interact with front-line healthcare workers and will proceed in this manner going forward. By redefining the relationship between technology and human touch in the delivery of healthcare solutions, the IoT is certainly transforming the healthcare industry. IoT applications in healthcare are advantageous for patients, families, doctors, hospitals, and insurance providers [2].

The Internet of Medical Things (IoMT) is revolutionizing healthcare, but security is the biggest obstacle to adoption. The security of the data generated by IoT devices must be properly safeguarded, according to healthcare professionals, IoT device managers, and developers [3]. The majority of the information gathered by medical devices is considered protected health data under HIPAA and other laws. Therefore, if they are not appropriately protected, IoT devices might be used as entry points for stealing important data. According to 82% of healthcare organizations, hackers have hacked their IoT hardware. The creation of secure Internet of Things (IoT) hardware and software is one step toward overcoming this challenge. Equally crucial is ensuring that IoT devices used in healthcare are appropriately controlled to prevent data from unsupervised devices from getting into the wrong hands. For instance, if patient monitoring equipment is not securely decommissioned once it is no longer needed or utilizes obsolete software or firmware, hackers may gain access to the network or be able to steal confidential health information.

## 8.2 Objective

As we all know, the IoT is enabling the integration of the physical world with the internet with many specialized devices and technologies. Examples of some tools used in the healthcare domain are medical data transferring tools, air quality sensors, devices for capturing the vitals of the patient and remote care biometric scanners, and a great number of other devices, which has made healthcare a lot more convenient for the doctors as well as the patients. The facilities that are provided by these devices are well taken care of and if any issue arises in the functionality of the devices, we immediately go through the problem. But what we least focus on is the security concerns of the devices in use. Many IoT devices are vulnerable to security due to a number of reasons listed below:

- The computational capacities of the devices are inadequate.
- Having an inefficient built-in security system.
- The access controls of the devices are very poor.
- The testing of the devices is not done properly because the security issues are not considered to be as important as wasting their budget on it.

If the IoT does not prefer security measures, then they can be easily hacked, and once the hackers have control over the devices, they can easily steal and misuse the users' data to threaten them and may also use the people's data to manipulate them.

## 8.3 Motivation

Given the current scenario and whatever happened around the globe related to COVID-19, we realized how IoT enabled healthcare. It provided customized attention to the people when there were less number of healthcare workers and the number of patients was increasing rapidly [4]. COVID-19 created havoc in the society as it was a transmissible disease and people were scared of going near COVID patients. In the scenario, the technologies used in IoT did the blood pressure check, the pulse rate check, the oximeter check, exercise check, disease condition check, etc. The major impact of IoT in the healthcare industry is the cost reduction. It enables patients to check their vitals in real time and it significantly reduces unnecessary visits to the doctors. It also enables the doctors to make decisions based on evidence, thus bringing absolute transparency. But there is a saying that all pros come with a set of their own cons. While it is benefiting the doctors to use the real-time vitals remotely, which is reducing the transportation cost and speeding up the treatment with constant communication, it also reduces the use of hospital resources. But we must ensure that the IoT devices that are being used or those that are to be purchased are secure and the device security has been adequately configured. These are additional concerns that arise when the devices are connected to the patients i.e., the doctors and the hospitals might have access to the confidential data of the patient and this data can be misused later. The authentication and identification of the devices used are the major security concerns in IoT. The security check in the IoT of healthcare has been given the least importance, which has many future repercussions. Thus, we chose this topic to bring attention toward the security issues in IoT of healthcare.

## 8.4 Standards for Cybersecurity

The stated standards are necessary to make cybersecurity precautions apparent. The generic sets of guidelines for the best use of certain measures are referred to as cybersecurity standards [5]. The standards may include procedures, rules, frameworks for comparison, etc. It makes security more effective, makes integration and interoperability easier, allows for meaningful comparisons between different security methods, lessens complexity, and provides the framework for new improvements.

| Cybersecurity requirements | | |
|---|---|---|
| | **Features** | **Description** |
| CIA | Confidentiality | The IoT system's confidentiality assures that no unauthorized users or devices are allowed to access medical information [6]. |
| | Integrity | Integrity describes the correctness and completeness of data over a system's full lifespan. Integrity makes sure that patients' medical information is not changed, deleted, or distorted by an enemy, preventing an incorrect diagnosis or prescription [7]. |
| | Availability | Availability makes sure that authorized users may access medical information and equipment when they need to [8]. It refers to maintaining the continuity of security services and avoiding device malfunctions and operational outages [9]. In particular, during the course of therapy, physicians should have access to patient data. |

| Cybersecurity requirements | | |
|---|---|---|
| | **Features** | **Description** |
| Non-CIA | Identification and authentication | Before allowing any entities (patients, physicians, devices, etc.) to interact with the resources of the IoT system, identification ensures their identities [10]. Verifying a person's or device's identity before use is called authentication of a system's resources [11]. Applications and device authentication can demonstrate that the interacting systems are not enemies, and networked data sharing is allowed. |
| | Authorization (access control) | After confirming the user's identification, access privileges or rights should be established for resources so that different users may only access those that are necessary for their duties [12]. For instance, a physician should have greater access to patient information than other medical professionals [13]. |
| | Privacy | Privacy means that patient secrets and personal information should not be shared without permission. IoT systems should adhere to privacy regulations that let users manage their personal data [14]. |
| | Accountability | Accountability should guarantee that the business or person is required to respond to or bear responsibility for their actions in the event of theft or an abnormal occurrence in a health IoT system. |
| | Non-repudiation | Someone cannot retract an action that has already been taken because of non-repudiation [15]. In fact, it gives consumers the ability to demonstrate whether an event occurred or not. |
| | Auditing | A system's capacity to continually track and monitor actions is known as auditing. All user behaviors in an IoT-based healthcare system, such as system login time and data modification, should be logged in sequential sequence. |
| | Data freshness | Data freshness refers to the need that data be current to prevent the repetition of out-of-date messages. For instance, a doctor has to be aware of his present patient's electrocardiography (ECG) information. |

## 8.5 Comparison of Existing Relevant Models

The number of connected devices is growing, which raises worries about cybersecurity. Every industry is using the technology, which improves connection and makes our life simpler. There are drawbacks to this, too, and as hackers look to take advantage of ever-increasing connection, the issue is becoming worse. Perhaps, the medical sector, where client data protection is of the highest concern, is where this is most readily apparent. Patient data security breaches are common, despite the fact that healthcare providers place a high focus on it. To avoid harmful vulnerabilities and implement numerous security-related processes, it is crucial to protect IoT medical equipment. Let us examine the specifications for protecting IoT medical devices in more detail.

### 8.5.1 Secure explainable intelligent model for smart healthcare under block-chain framework

Block-chain technology has been existing since 1991. Block-chain was initially only used for financial transactions, but in 2014, researchers looked at the most recent developments and potential applications in other financial and inter-organizational transaction domains. And during the past several years, the use of block-chain has multiplied across all sectors for a wide range of use cases and implementations. Block-chain is made up of cloud service providers (CSPs), edge service providers (ESPs), and Internet of Things (IoT) devices with limited computing, storage, and power. Lightweight clients (LCs) are used to describe IoT devices in this study. In general, the cloud server generates and sends to the edge server a trusted code for each service. The service is requested and received by the lightweight client from the closest edge server [16]. Block-chain methodology is established in order to ensure that the service and its provider are not phony and that there is trustworthiness. The arbitration node and lightweight node are the authors' two primary elements in their block-chain network.

Let us look at a medical sector security architecture that uses block-based information between systems to protect sensitive data on cloud servers. The notion of block-chain (BC) technologies was established in the healthcare systems since any data available on the Internet is susceptible to several assaults and patient health records include sensitive data that must not be exposed to any unauthorized or unauthentic person. Several healthcare models based in British Columbia have been proposed in the system in recent years [17]. These models are decentralized, which is a feature of block-chain technology, but as the number of chains increases, this attribute has led to an issue known as illness duplication in several applications, notably in healthcare. This study employs a BC-based architecture to address the problem, which might result in the creation of a new block if the patient's condition, allergies, new symptoms, prescriptions, etc., change. A distributed network

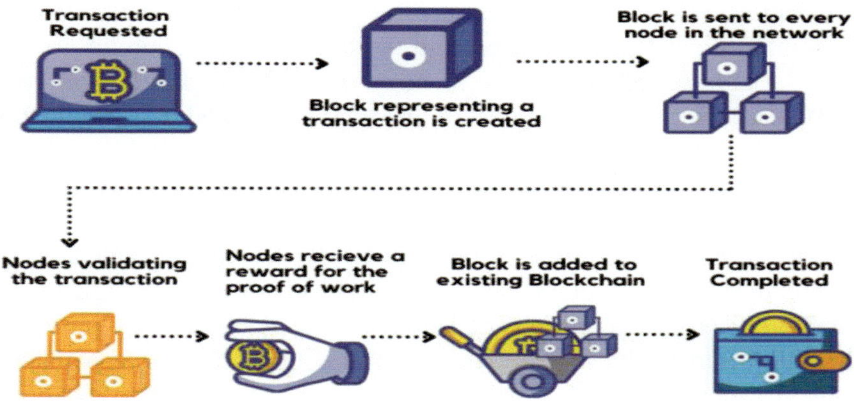


**Figure 8.2** Working of block-chain.

called a "block-chain" enables information to be decentralized, boosting security system and making manipulation more difficult. To keep and process data, companies can join this decentralized public ledger system via nodes. The originating entity that wishes to store or manage the data may access the data in blocks through verification, verification, and consensus.

As in Figure 8.2, anytime a user requests a transaction using a block-chain-based application, a block is produced in the block-chain network to store the transaction's contents. The transaction is then validated by sending that block to each node in the distributed peer-to-peer network. After the validation, the network's nodes are rewarded for the proof of work (also known as distributed consensus). The user then receives a successful transaction when the block is added to the current block-chain. Additionally, block-chain enables data analysis with little to no human involvement, which lowers the chance of human mistake [18]. Compared to preceding block-chain models, the block-chain model is more secure. This feature results in a problem known as sickness overlapping when the number of chains is increased. Because it provides an additional layer of data protection, which increases patient confidence, the framework is effective and successful. Combining wearable smart technologies with block-chain technology is another way to use it in healthcare. Considering how many individuals are using wearable technology, giving healthcare providers a safe mechanism to communicate this data would enable them to treat and monitor their patients more effectively. Even though their patients are at a higher risk for health issues, doctors may be able to let them live normal lives by remotely monitoring their data. By providing patients and experts with a new means to monitor their development, this technology may also aid clinical studies.

Patients are hesitant to disclose their personal information because of the hazards of hacker/attackers and the Internet's susceptibility to these threats. The term "block-chain technology" refers to the decentralized digital database that is used to protect online transactions and data lists that are continually growing. It is made up of interconnected, immutable key referencing information pieces. By keeping patient data in encrypted data, the security architecture described in this study will boost security by protecting sensitive medical data transported over networks. By utilizing an encryption algorithm and a public block-chain, the block-chain-based IoT framework's primary objective is to establish a safe and dependable security procedure. The project's main objective is to develop an IoT block-chain system that will increase patient data's safety and scalability because data security is one of the biggest issues with IoT health systems that cannot be ignored [19].

As a consequence, patients will feel more at ease disclosing their private medical information to doctors and informational facilities, improving the dependability and credibility of the entire process. This study intends to propose a framework for managing the health system and ensuring the security of sensitive information for IoT cloud-based database servers in order to achieve these goals. Data are often sent from the real world to the remote server through three stages in any IoT-based block-chain system. Sensors or actuators are utilized to collect data at the base layer. These data are transported straight to the second division and separated into a number of blocks, where it is then received by the cloud server in the third layer. Since patient dataset shows sensitive data that should only be accessed or shared by the patient, securing this data inside the IoT architecture is crucial. In this study, modifications are made to the IoT system's second layer to protect this information against unauthorized and unverified access. The dependability and trust among patients and resource centers are improved by incorporating an additional data security feature in the second layer. To gather data, the framework works with patients, physicians, and even hospitals [20]. Kaggle.com's real-time data collecting was utilized to assuage concerns over complexity and dimensionality. Private patient information collected as part of this data collection includes details like age, sex, chest discomfort, heart rate, S.C., H.R.A., P.E., thal, and more.

In order to support SHA-256 hashing technique, the suggested solution generates a 128-bit AES key. To protect data from illegal access, each user's data are encrypted and divided into chunks. To show the recommended model's practical use in healthcare, an interface-based system is being created. The effectiveness of the recommended approach is then verified in the MATLAB program in terms of MAE, RMSE, MSE, encryption time, and

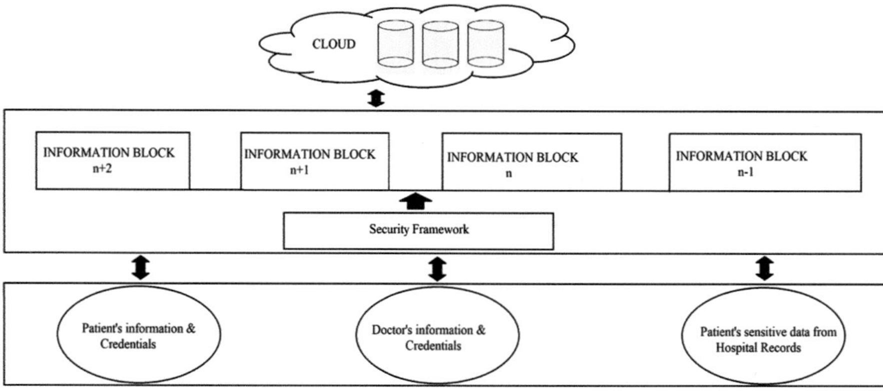


**Figure 8.3** Framework for IoT block-chain system.

decryption time. The most used encryption algorithms are RSA and DSA. Patients are reluctant to provide their personal information online due to the Internet's susceptibility to various hacker/attacker dangers. Block-chain technology refers to the distributed digital database that is used to secure constantly expanding data lists and online transactions. It is composed of linked chunks of non-modifiable key referencing information. The security architecture presented in this study will protect sensitive medical data transmitted across networks and will increase security by storing patient data in encrypted form. The experimental findings reveal that the suggested framework has the shortest encryption and decryption times, indicating that its performance is more effective and reliable [21]. It is also more efficient and durable. Block-chain technology depends on a wide range of contemporary encryption methods, including RSA, AES, triple DES, two-fish, and others, propelling block-chain cryptography to the fore. For block-chain to become more appealing, safety of consumer and transactional data must be provided.

By entering their credentials in an application-oriented way, users may register themselves. Figure 8.4 shows the recommended IoT–block-chain approach for healthcare systems.

The recommended block-chain-based IoT healthcare system is divided into four sections: registration, login, authentication form, and data center. In this section, we will go through each component in detail, step by step.

To utilize the system, the user must first register. This user may be a doctor or patient. During this procedure, crucial information is captured and kept, such as the user's name, phone number, user ID, password, user type, and picture. Depending on the user type, you can tell if someone enrolling is a patients or a doctor. The image is further stored in a database so that it may

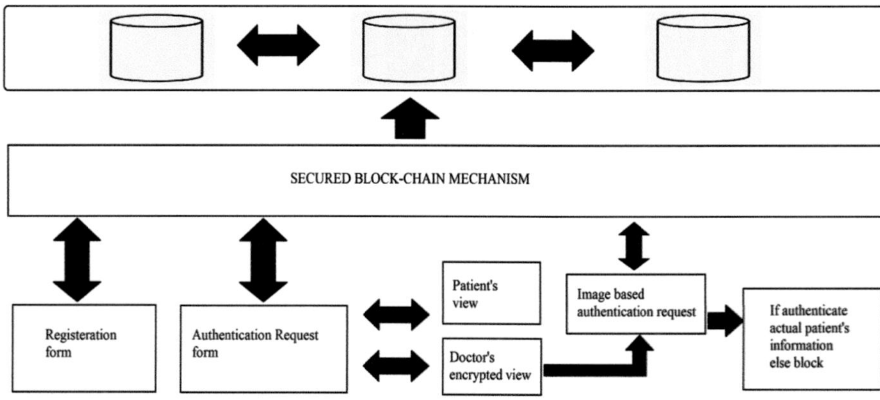


**Figure 8.4** Interface of the block-chain-based IoT healthcare system.

later be used for verification. The user uploads and stores all required data on the cloud.

- Users can connect to the system by entering their login information after registering. The user must first provide their user name, password, and user type before clicking the login button to gain access to the proposed IoT system. When a user clicks the login button, the login module immediately sends a request to the cloud storage, where the credentials are checked against those already saved there. The login module receives a response, enabling the user to access the system if the entered credentials match any of the registered users. It rejects the access request and only grants access to authorized and authentic users if the credentials do not match anybody in the cloud. As previously stated, the user can be a doctor or a patient. Different information may be seen and entered by both parties.
- The name, phone number, age, and sex of the user must be provided or observed when the user is a patient. Their medical information is also presented, including BP, SC, HRA, PENMV, and the patient's appointed doctor.
- After logging in and entering his credentials, a screen allowing the doctor to view and assess the patient's health by selecting his name appears. The doctor will not have simple access to the patient data, though, as the information previously obtained was encrypted.
- Image-based authentication: The doctor must submit decoding credentials, which include a photo, in order to study the patient's private

information. The system verifies the decoding credentials and tries to authenticate the request with the cloud storage; if they match, the patient's medical information is decoded and made available to the designated doctor; if not, access to the data is prohibited, adding another degree of protection.

Block-chain technology in healthcare has the drawback that in some applications, notably healthcare, this feature has led to an issue known as sickness overlapping as the number of chains expands. Patients worry that unauthorized and fraudulent persons may have access to their private and sensitive medical data, which may then be used against them. The problem with these technologies was that each hospital or healthcare facility needed to customize them, which took a lot of time. The earlier medical information is not accessible when a patient transfers to another hospital for treatment of any sickness due to the different BCs, and new knowledge on the patient's allergies, symptoms, and medicines cannot be entered to the records. This results in illnesses that overlap, which results in discrepancies that stymie therapy.

The effectiveness of healthcare IoT systems may be improved and protected with the use of block-chain technology [22]. A multi-layer IoT healthcare system built on block-chain is suggested in this article. The AES key generation function for encryption and the SHA256 for chain construction are both used to preserve and protect the patient data. The proposed framework is effective and valuable because it offers an additional degree of data protection that increases patient confidence. The MATLAB program is used to evaluate the performance of the suggested framework using a number of encryption measurements, such mean absolute error (MAE), root mean square error (RMSE), mean squared error (MSE), and encryption and decryption durations.

### 8.5.2 Secure IoT healthcare with access control based on explainable deep learning

Recent years have seen a rapid advancement in artificial intelligence technology, and deep learning is now widely used in many different industries. The performance of deep learning in photo recognition is quite amazing. This study offers a method for deep neural network based efficient photo identification with less data, which might be applied to home access control systems. Among the recognized objects are animals and human faces. The embedded device may get inference models based on data from incredibly effective training servers. The testing results demonstrate that picture identification is quite accurate. Consumer goods and sophisticated home access control systems may both employ artificial intelligence.

The storing and processing of enormous volumes of medical data is required by the present health service, which is centered on conventional administration. The Internet of Things (IoT) has evolved into Internet-of-Things healthcare with amazing data processing powers and enormous data storage as a result of its inclusion and continual development. The resultant system intends to construct an artificial healthcare system that can continuously monitor a patient's medical state via a wearable device, thanks to advancements in the industrial Internet of Things (IIoT). The cloud server where the wearable IoT module keeps the data it has collected is vulnerable to assaults and data leak from unauthorized individuals and outsiders [23]. This paper presents an IoT-based, deep-learning-based, data analytics approach to address this security issue. Data about the user are captured, and private information is separated and isolated. Health-related data are analyzed in the cloud using a convolutional neural network (CNN), which do not include any personal data about the consumers. As a consequence, a user-based secure access system that creates again for IoT healthcare system is introduced. A connection between system adoption and attributes is found using the recommended study. The proposed CNN classifier has a 95% $F1$ score, 95% recall, and 95% precision. As the size of the training set is expanded, performance improves. With data augmentation, the system operates more effectively than it would have without it. Additionally, accuracy of approximately 98% may be attained with additional users. The recommended system's effectiveness and durability in terms of minimum privacy violations and high integrity of data are demonstrated through experimental inquiry.

In recent years, processing of data, portability, scalability, accessibility, and applications for wireless sensor networks have all increased significantly. Combining this technological advancement with advancements in mobile networks, wireless communications, and radio frequency identification (RFID), the Internet of Things now has a solid foundation (IoT). One of the technologies utilized to do this research and offer a workable solution to the current issue is machine learning. According to the findings, using techniques for machine learning has enhanced the country economically as a whole.

The healthcare sector has seen a number of issues with storage and processing of data as a result of the recent corona-virus. This consensus states that the Internet of Things (IoT) is indeed the ideal approach for addressing the growth of smart healthcare. With the aid of artificial intelligence, data networks, and sensor technology, it is feasible to comprehend data processing, security systems, and intelligent identification for the administration for healthcare and link and exchange information. This agreement opens the door for a real-time, secure, and dependable healthcare system. The main problems in the IoT healthcare industry, however, have been recognized as data manipulation and leaking [24].

This demonstrates the significance of safe access control while working with medical data. By utilizing more seasoned centralized computing systems like access-control lists and job access control, these security vulnerabilities may be substantially mitigated. The edge entry control plane, which is mainly composed of access control computers and confidence generation servers and is used to handle data user access using machine learning techniques, supports a number of Internet-of-Things healthcare applications. As a consequence, the idea includes a secure access control mechanism (SACM) for IoT healthcare that is federated and attribute-based on deep learning. The system architecture is thoroughly covered in this section. In order to guarantee data integrity and secure consumer privacy in IoT-based health systems, the user, trust generation servers, and access control web server are the three organizations that are essential to trust-based access control. In order to convey just non-speech body noises and information while blocking ambient noise and speech-related noises, the user constructs a privacy-isolating zone. The confidentiality zone identifies the stride signal as well as other health information at the user end depending on the acceleration stream. The security modules and data extraction using a non-privacy component are implemented at the cloud end. In IoT-based healthcare systems, unauthorized employees frequently change medical data, resulting in data leaks and privacy violations. When dealing with sensitive medical data, securing safe network access at all levels is crucial. Information about the level of trustworthiness of a group of users is sent from the trust generating servers to the access control firewall, which authorizes access. In order to establish trust and manage access, server-based data is viewed as semi-trusted, while new users are recognized as being unreliable. Figure 8.5 depicts the advised system design.

At the source, a privacy-isolation zone is constructed to receive non-speech body sound and data. This ensures that data transport and cloud-based storage are both secure. At the cloud end, a security module with servers for access control and trust creation is employed to extract the data using a customized deep CNN approach. This ensures the confidentiality of medical information throughout. The system is assessed under scenarios of data tampering and privacy leaks in order to predict performance. The wearable device frequently integrates the user's identification and any linked information about their gait with touch, mobility, and other wellness data acquired at the patient's end.

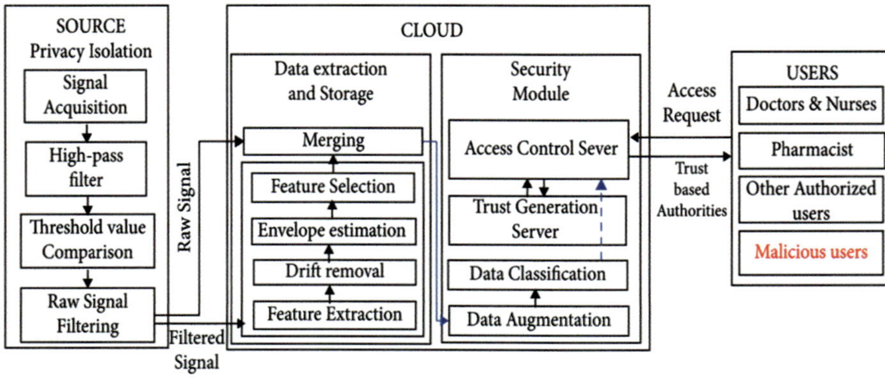


**Figure 8.5** Framework of access control system based on deep learning.

The signal can be retrieved inside the border depending on an upper limit. In the data that are gathered, there is also gravity information provided alongside the gait information. The fixed downward force gravity value is 9.8 m/s$^2$. It is difficult to identify a fixed threshold with the user's movements since the gravity projection will change on each axis. The gait signals interact with the data obtained, resulting in a low signal-to-noise ratio (SNR) that makes it challenging to distinguish between the data. Additionally, the data are aliased based on the time domain. As a result, utilizing a window function to separate the aliased signals is not an option. From the various behavior data, distinct frequency features are detected. For data separation, the Fourier transform is employed to analyze signals in the frequency domain. In the frequency domain, gravity is seen as a DC component. The gait changes in a relatively high range of 1.4–2.1 Hz as compared to gravity. A low-pass filter is used to filter the gait data, while a high-pass filter is used to filter the gravity data. Building low-pass and high-pass filtering functions can make use of wavelet, elliptic, Chebyshev, and Butterworth filters. The wavelet filter cannot be used on a user terminal with limited resources because of the time-consuming wavelet-based procedure. The Butterworth filter has more persistent amplitude–frequency characteristics than the elliptic and Chebyshev filters. Additionally, it boasts the most flat stopband attenuation and the flattest band-pass frequency response curve. Average SNR values for elliptic, Chebyshev, and Butterworth filters are 11.9, 11.5, and 12, respectively. A greater SNR value improves the retrieval signal's accuracy. As a result, the Butterworth filter is the optimum option for implementation.

The cloud is used for data extraction and archiving. Drift reduction, envelope estimation, and feature selection are used to process the filtered signal and extract features. It is then transferred to the security module after being mixed with the raw signal. After the security module has completed data categorization and augmentation, the trust generating server and access control server determine whether to provide access to the user based on the users requesting access to the data. Cost and time restrictions place limitations on the collecting of all sample data. As a result, extra training samples are created via data augmentation to improve the module's generalization. The time warping procedure is used to change the signal's time-domain location and gather data at different rates. Additionally, data collecting at different pressures is subjected to amplitude distortion, which results in a random change in the amplitude of the data. The signal breadth, time location, variable wearing angles of the data collecting device, and noise environments are depicted using time scaling, permutation, rotation processing, and random noise addition.

In the case of outliers and intrinsic sensor noise, the signal variance increases. As a result, signal drift occurs. With the amplification of variation, the drift becomes more intense. When the signal is projected, PCA yields the greatest variance in the orthogonal direction. Each component's drift is removed using the linear regression fitting approach. The squared sum of errors between both the actual and fitting components is computed for each component, and the actual and fitting components are estimated for each component. After that, the component is removed from the trend term update. As a result, the study's main emphasis is on information fluctuation in general.

The trust-generating server is creating a social network. Users' social similarity is determined by their social participation. The link probability at the associated edge for the formation of the user's social graph is determined based on users' social similarity. Deep restoration learning (DRL) technology enables social data- and trust-based access control. Social data are used in the susceptible infected recovered (SIR) and graph convolutional network (GCN) algorithms to evaluate trust. The influence of each user node is calculated in traditional models using the GCN. The eigenvector, closeness, adjacency, and degrees centrality indicating the properties of each node are examined using InfGCN, an effect identification model.

The training data, rate of infection, and buffering capacity must all be continually adjusted to the user access threshold in order to ensure maximum integrity of data and a low number of privacy violations. The twin delayed deep deterministic (TD3) policy gradient approach is used by existing local access control models to learn the construction threshold. The universal access management paradigm uses the TD3 algorithms and federated training architecture to allow user privacy preservation. In the unique machine learning method known as federated learning, each member needs a trained model. This does away with the requirement for a private dataset to protect the privacy of the participants by acting as a user access server and aiding in the development of a universal model.

Whenever you want to have a deep knowledge about anything, it will require an enormous amount of dataset and the collection of the data is going to be a tedious and very time consuming process and will also be extremely expensive to store, monitor, and study the humongous amount of data. As the data size is increased, the model used to run this great amount of data will also become more complex that is again something that nobody is willing to do. There are no standard parameters set to select the trend or area of focus from where we can extract the data. This deep learning is a very resource demanding technology that is going to require very powerful GPUs and graphics with high performing processing units.

This paper suggests a data processing and privacy preservation approach that makes use of deep learning in order to isolate and evaluate unstructured health data for IoT-based health systems, as well as to prevent access from being granted to risky users. Information that is important to privacy is separated from non-sensitive information through filters. Several numbers of scenarios are used to test the system's resiliency and effectiveness, and its performance is examined. This concept can be used to assist future smart healthcare systems. This system design may be developed to include a wide range of wearable IoT healthcare devices. To distinguish between authorized and malevolent users, the access control model uses social graphs. In the IoT healthcare setting, these graphs, in conjunction with CNN, aid in granting authorization to certain users. In order to more accurately generalize the system's performance, the next scope of work entails overcoming the work's financial and time constraints. User identity protection methods may be made even more stringent with the installation of a block-chain-based security module. The system's performance may be guaranteed to increase over time by enabling real-time sample collecting and system upgrades.

## 8.6 Comparative Analysis of the Models

The first step in developing a safe environment against cyber risks and assaults is building a secure IoT device. To prevent unmonitored devices from ending up in the wrong hands, it is equally crucial to ensure that IoT devices are monitored properly. It may be easier to steal protected information if a healthcare institution employs unprotected medical equipment with out-of-date operating systems.

| Model name | Aim of the work | Methods used | Benefits | Future scope |
|---|---|---|---|---|
| Secure model for IoT healthcare system under encrypted block-chain framework | In IoT-based healthcare systems, preserving data integrity and protecting user privacy with encrypted block-chain | Encrypted block-chain | IoT enables data flow from Internet-connected devices to private block-chain networks, which provide tamper-resistant records of shared transactions | The AES key generation capability is utilized for encryption, and SHA256 is used for chain formation to preserve and safeguard patient data. The added layer of data protection makes the suggested architecture more effective and efficient and increases patient trust |
| Secure IoT healthcare architecture with deep learning-based access control system | Deep-learning-based access control system for IoT-based healthcare systems: ensuring data integrity and protecting user privacy | Access control system based on deep learning | Security isolation Cloud security model | Filters distinguish between data that are sensitive to privacy and data that are not. The system's resiliency and efficacy are put to the test, and its performance is scrutinized. This idea might be used to future smart healthcare systems |

## 8.7 Using explainable AI in IoT security

It is exceedingly difficult to make up for the negative effects of healthcare decision-making since they directly affect individuals. As a result, AI models utilized in this industry should not only be effective but also trustworthy, open, understandable, and interpretable. This requirement should be given top consideration, particularly in IoT applications that offer monitoring, diagnosis, and health recommendations. For this, several investigations have been conducted. To allow content-based image processing techniques for use in surgical education, Chittajallu et al. suggested the XAI-CBIR human-assisted explainable AI system. By removing the semantic descriptors from the image in the query video, the CNN-based DL model in XAI-CBIR lists comparable images. It refines itself by iterative training using pertinent user feedback. By generating a visual saliency map, the proposed system assesses the explainability of images that are comparable to the image in the query. In order to tackle COVID-19-like pandemics, Hossain et al. [68] developed a tri (stakeholder layer, edge layer, and cloud layer) smart healthcare system. The framework is able to identify COVID-19 utilizing chest X-ray or CT scan pictures, as well as traits including social withdrawal, masks, and temperature regulation of the body. In the edge layer, the authors employed Inception v3, Deep Tree, and ResNet50 models. Utilizing local insights model agnostic (LIMA) on the datasets generated based on the learning variables of these DL models provides interactive explainability. In order to guarantee the dependability of AI systems deployed in the healthcare domain, Dave et al. concentrated in on the usefulness of feature- and example-based XAI algorithms on the cardiovascular disease dataset. The authors demonstrated how feature-based XAI techniques SHAP and LIME, as well as exemplar technique Anchors, Counterfactuals, Integrated gradients, CEM, and KernelSHAP, may be used to explain the behaviors of black box models. A unique Adaptive Weighted High-importance Path Particles (Ada-WHIPS) model was developed by Hatwell et al. to improve the AdaBoost model, which is used in computer-assisted diagnosis in the healthcare industry. Ada-WHISP explains the categorization of AdaBoost models using a novel formulation and straightforward classification methods. A risk assessment method was created by Pnevmatikakis et al. for experts in the health insurance industry. A digital coaching system that predicts people's lives and generates appropriate lifestyle advice is also part of the planned system. In this system, lifestyle predictions are made using the random forest and DNN algorithms. For the predictability of the outcome, SHAP was applied. A CNN-based hierarchy occlusion (HihO) model was presented by Monroe et al. [69] to significantly improve the comprehensibility of statistical data in medical imaging processes in Internet of Things (IoT) healthcare applications. On the Parkinson's progression markers initiative (PPMI) dataset, the authors compared the created approach to GRAD-CAM and the (Parkinson progression markers initiative) RISE methodologies. It has been demonstrated that the suggested model renders 20 and 200 times more quickly than the GRAD-CAM and RISE models, respectively. The explainability of IA models used to categorize hand motions based on EMG data was the main topic of Gozzi et al.'s study [73]. The authors especially looked at how XAI models may improve the quality of life for amputees who use myo-controlled prosthetics. In order to classify hand movements, the authors employed the SVM, LDA, XRT, CNN, and GRAD-CAM algorithms. GRAD-CAM and SHAP were used in the XAI process.

This section looks at the requirements and advantages of employing XAI techniques in the IoT-based healthcare industry:

- XAI techniques give additional information regarding the reasoning of machine learning outcomes in medical use cases where not only the output but also its factors are important.
- It investigates and controls the behavior of machine learning techniques used in individualized patient care. For instance, the medical data gathered from IoT wearable devices frequently contain missing or incorrect data and may result in erroneous choices. A seamless decision-making process is ensured by the use of XAI, which aids in identifying and fixing any unanticipated flaws or shortcomings.
- Due to its probabilistic interpretability feature, it is able to make local judgments on how it achieves the treatment outcome of patient illness using predictive methods. For instance, in a health service, in addition to the justification gathered from all patients, an explanation is also given concerning a specific patient.
- It facilitates the finding of obscure facts and data, particularly with the dangers of contracting diseases, as well as fresh viewpoints on ML issues. If we can understand the method, we could find significant new data and previously unnoticed patterns.
- Unexpected deviations might happen in the ML algorithm's training set. For instance, it may result in bias problems in a sickness prediction software, such as outright rejecting the outcome indicated by a certain sensory module. A method for identifying these inefficiencies in the model is provided by XAI.

## 8.8 Conclusion

Explainable AI is an emerging domain where the interpretation of results of predictive models can be analyzed. Recently, the healthcare sector has seen the development of a variety of advanced methodologies. Because they deal with private and sensitive information, including personal health information, attackers may target these devices. Understanding the features and guiding principles of security requirements in the IoT for healthcare is essential. In this study, academic works are reviewed that discussed the security requirements for IoT-based healthcare in explainable AI perspective. Researchers, information technology engineers, health practitioners, and policymakers concerned with IoT and healthcare technologies are likely to benefit from the findings of this study. This result provides impetus for additional research and the development of a robust IoT-based healthcare system.

As an example, despite the fact that healthcare providers and businesses have a plethora of rules in place for anything related to wearable devices, they must continue to improve them. There is a pressing need to reconsider their privacy rights, age restrictions, encryption methods, cloud services, and a variety of other issues. To establish a safe and comprehensive strategy, they would need to adapt and adjust their practices, as well as be able to network with the correct vendors. These Internet-connected IoT gadgets, especially wearable devices, have shown to be beneficial to everyone in terms of convenience, health, and networking, and there is now a large research effort to standardize data gathering and sharing by these devices.

## References

[1] Z.Xu, W. Liu, J. Huang, C. Yang, J. Lu, and H. Tan, "Artificial intelligence for securing IoT services in edge computing: a survey," Security and Communication Networks, vol. 2020, 13 pages, 2020.

[2] E. Mohamed, "The relationship between artificial intelligence and internet of things: a quick review," Journal of Cybersecurity and Information Management, vol. 1, no. 1, pp. 30–34, 2020

[3] Dutta, A., Misra, C., Barik, R. K., & Mishra, S. (2021). Enhancing mist assisted cloud computing toward secure and scalable architecture for smart healthcare. In Advances in Communication and Computational Technology (pp. 1515–1526). Springer, Singapore.

[4] Rath, M., & Mishra, S. (2020). Security approaches in machine learning for satellite communication. In Machine learning and data mining in aerospace technology (pp. 189–204). Springer, Cham.

[5] M. Masoud, Y. Jaradat, A. Manasrah, and I. Jannoud, "Sensors of smart devices in the internet of everything (IoE) era: big opportunities and massive doubts," Journal of Sensors, vol. 2019, 26 pages, 2019.

[6] Mekki N, Hamdi M, Aguili T, Kim TH. Scenario-based vulnerability analysis in IoT-based patient monitoring system. Proceeding of the 14th International Joint Conference on e-Business and Telecommunications. 2017 July 24–26; Madrid, Spain. 2017: 554–559.

[7] Jaigirdar FT, Rudolph C, Bain C, Acm. Can I Trust the Data I See? A Physician's Concern on Medical Data in IoT Health Architectures. Proceeding of Proceedings of the Australasian Computer Science Week Multiconference. 2019 Jan 29–31; Sydney, NSW, Australia. New York: Association for Computing Machinery (ACM); 2019: 1–10.

[8] Koutli M, Theologou N, Tryferidis A, Tzovaras D, Kagkini A, Zandes D, et al. Secure IoT e-Health Applications using VICINITY Framework and GDPR Guidelines. Proceeding of 15th International Conference on Distributed Computing in Sensor Systems (DCOSS). 2019 May 29–31; Santorini Island, Greece. IEEE; 2019: 263–270.

[9] Assiri A, Almagwashi H. IoT Security and Privacy Issues. Proceeding of 1st International Conference on Computer Applications and Information Security (ICCAIS). 2018 Aug 23; Riyadh, Saudi Arabia. IEEE; 2018: 1–5.

[10] Jaiswal S, Gupta D. Security Requirements for Internet of Things (IoT). Proceedings; Singapore. Springer Singapore; 2017: 419–427.

[11] Lin J, Yu W, Zhang N, Yang XY, Zhang HL, Zhao W. A Survey on Internet of Things: Architecture, Enabling Technologies, Security and Privacy, and Applications. IEEE Internet Things J. 2017; 4(5): 1125–1142.

[12] Sangpetch O, Sangpetch A. Security context framework for distributed healthcare IoT platform. Proceeding of Third International Conference on Internet of Things Technologies for HealthCare. 2016 Oct 18–19; Västerås, Sweden. Springer Verlag; 2016: 71–76.

[13] Alkeem EA, Yeun CY, Zemerly MJ. Security and privacy framework for ubiquitous healthcare IoT devices. Proceeding of 10th International Conference for Internet Technology and Secured Transactions (ICITST). 2015 Dec 14–16; London, UK. IEEE; 2015: 70–75.

[14] Mosenia A, Jha NK. A Comprehensive Study of Security of Internet-of-Things. IEEE Trans Emerg Top Comput. 2017; 5(4): 586–602.

[15] Islam SMR, Kwak D, Kabir MH, Hossain M, Kwak KS. The Internet of Things for Health Care: A Comprehensive Survey. IEEE Access. 2015; 3: 678–708.

[16] K. Saleem, I. S. Bajwa, N. Sarwar, W. Anwar, and A. Ashraf, "IoT healthcare: design of smart and cost-effective sleep quality monitoring system," Journal of Sensors, vol. 2020, 17 pages, 2020.

[17] Sahoo, S., Mishra, S., Mishra, B. K. K., & Mishra, M. (2018). Analysis and implementation of artificial bee colony optimization in constrained optimization problems. In Handbook of research on modeling, analysis, and application of nature-inspired metaheuristic algorithms (pp. 413–432). IGI Global.

[18] Mishra, S., Mahanty, C., Dash, S., & Mishra, B. K. (2019). Implementation of BFS-NB hybrid model in intrusion detection system. In Recent developments in machine learning and data analytics (pp. 167–175). Springer, Singapore.

[19] S.Shakya, "An efficient security framework for data migration in a cloud computing environment," Journal of Artificial Intelligence, vol. 1, no. 1, pp. 45–53, 2019.

[20] Sahoo, S., Das, M., Mishra, S., & Suman, S. (2021). A hybrid DTNB model for heart disorders prediction. In Advances in electronics, communication and computing (pp. 155–163). Springer, Singapore.

[21] Jena, L., Kamila, N. K., & Mishra, S. (2014). Privacy preserving distributed data mining with evolutionary computing. In Proceedings of the International Conference on Frontiers of Intelligent Computing: Theory and Applications (FICTA) 2013 (pp. 259–267). Springer, Cham.

[22] Jena, L., Mishra, S., Nayak, S., Ranjan, P., & Mishra, M. K. (2021). Variable optimization in cervical cancer data using particle swarm optimization. In Advances in electronics, communication and computing (pp. 147–153). Springer, Singapore.

[23] Mishra, S., Mallick, P. K., Tripathy, H. K., Jena, L., & Chae, G. S. (2021). Stacked KNN with hard voting predictive approach to assist hiring process in IT organizations. The International Journal of Electrical Engineering & Education, 0020720921989015.

[24] Mishra, S., Dash, A., & Mishra, B. K. (2020). An insight of Internet of Things applications in pharmaceutical domain. In Emergence of pharmaceutical industry growth with industrial IoT approach (pp. 245–273). Academic Press.

# 9

# Chest Disease Identification from X-rays using Deep Learning

**M. Hacibeyoglu and M.S. Terzi**

Department of Computer Engineering, Necmettin Erbakan University, Turkey
Email: hacibeyoglu@erbakan.edu.tr; msterzi@gmail.com

## Abstract

In the medical field, early diagnosis means the definition of the disease in the period when the clinical signs of the disease do not appear or there are symptoms that do not cause pain and distress to the person. Delayed diagnosis causes aggravation of the disease and even the disappearance of the possibility of treatment. The field of medical diagnostics contains a multitude of challenges that are very similar to classical machine learning problems. Particularly in the field of radiology, there are multi-label classification problems where medical images are interpreted to indicate multiple existing or suspected pathologies. Chest X-ray is preferred in the diagnosis of chest diseases because it is inexpensive, widely available, and uses low-dose radiation. However, in many countries, the insufficient number of radiologists and difficulties in making a diagnosis reduce the success rate. This shows the need for an artificial intelligence system that can diagnose from chest X-rays. In this study, a deep learning model has been developed that can diagnose from chest X-rays. Training and testing of the developed convolutional neural network model was carried out with the ChestX-ray14 dataset consisting of 112,120 chest X-rays taken from 30,805 different patients. As a result of the experimental studies, the developed deep learning model was compared with the literature and it was seen that it achieved successful results.

## 9.1 Introduction

Chest disease is a deadly illness caused by a virus or bacterium to which you have been exposed to in the environment [1]. Chest diseases are an infection of the lung; the lungs fill with liquid, which makes breathing difficult. It mainly affects the youth, the elderly, and immunocompromised people [2]. Chest disease is a very common disease all over the world because the infection can be transmitted among people with direct contact.

The number of visits to emergency services with thoracic disease as the primary diagnosis is more than 1.5 million each year in the United States alone [3]. According to the World Health Organization (WHO), chest disease kills approximately 1.4 million children worldwide every year, making it the leading cause of death among children [4]. Chest disease is a high-risk disease, particularly in developing countries where millions of people live in poverty and do not have access to medical facilities. Furthermore, in low- and middle-income countries, it remains the primary cause of infant mortality and the most common reason for hospitalization of adults [5].

Since its invention at the end of the 19th century, X-rays have been the primary modality in the investigation of chest infection [6]. Still, applying chest X-rays to diagnose pneumonia is the best available method [7]. The WHO recommends X-rays for all patients diagnosed clinically with severe chest disease [8]. In addition, many studies have pointed out the essential role of chest X-ray in clinical decision-making in pulmonary diseases [6, 9]. Even in developed countries, chest X-rays are commonly used for diagnosis. For example, there were 43.5 million imaging tests reported in England from March 2018 to March 2019 and 22.7 million of these tests were X-rays and more than half of it were chest X-rays [10].

The main reasons for applying chest X-rays in the diagnosis of chest disease are as follows: it is relatively inexpensive, widely available, less time-consuming, and has a low dose of radiation exposure [11]. However, it is true that there is a scarcity of radiologists in developing and developed countries. It is also known that with timely and accurate diagnosis and management, the mortality due to lung diseases can be reduced [12]. But especially in developing countries, the shortage of experienced radiologists is linked to alarming mortality rates in children with lung disease because of delayed diagnosis and treatment [13]. Around the world, in low-population residential areas, most health centers do not have access to radiologists for X-ray interpretation.

Chest X-ray has great potential to determine a wide range of possible chest diseases, but reading chest X-rays are an important, difficult, and challenging task. First of all, the resolution of chest X-rays is lower than those of magnetic resonance imaging and computerized tomography; therefore, even experienced radiologists cannot easily interpret them [14]. Second, X-ray images are often vague and diagnoses can overlap with each other [15]. Finally, the interpretation of chest X-rays is directly influenced by the radiologist's experiment and misinterpretation of chest X-rays could result in serious outcomes [16, 17]. For instance, a study in France, including 81 radiology residents from six university hospitals, found that there was a success rate of 47.4% for abnormal chest X-rays and of 79.6% for normal chest X-rays; the study concludes that radiology residents lack severe theoretical background in chest X-ray reading [18]. Another study in Ethiopia showed that radiologists found radiologic evidence in only 51.6% of children who were clinically diagnosed with WHO-defined severe chest disease. The results of the study indicate that improvements are required in the interpretation of chest X-rays [12].

Obviously detecting chest disease in X-rays is a challenging task for radiologists. In this respect, a high accuracy diagnosis of thoracic disease strongly requires automated detection of disease from chest X-rays. Automated disease detection using artificial intelligence (AI) technology promises great success in healthcare over the past decade [19–22]. Similarly, in chest disease detection, AI would reduce detection errors compared to human expertise, provide tremendous benefit in clinical settings, and it would be invaluable for healthcare delivery to populations with inadequate access to diagnostic imaging specialists [23, 24]. In addition, many studies on chest X-rays have been used in deep learning algorithms in recent years. Using the convolutional neural network (CNN) algorithm, nodules were detected in the lung from X-ray images in the dataset of the Japanese Society of Radiology Technologies [25]. Wang et al. [7] conducted studies with the ChestX-ray14 dataset, and chest diseases were detected using the ResNet-50 deep learning algorithm. Yao et al. [26] carried out tests with the OpenI dataset, and 71% of success was achieved in thoracic diseases with the recurrent neural network model. Rajpurkar et al. [27] developed a model called CheXNet using a dense convolutional network and achieved a 76% success rate on the ChestX-ray14 dataset.

In this study, we developed a CNN model for automated detection of chest disease from X-rays using deep learning techniques. The aim of this study was to rapidly detect chest disease from X-rays, exceed the average radiologist performance, and automate and simplify the pneumonia detection process.

## 9.2 Deep Learning

AI, which is currently one of the developing technologies, can be defined as an artificial operating system that exhibits behaviors such as perception, learning, thinking, problem solving, communication, and decision making. In other words, AI is the system that allows complex operations carried out by humans in daily life to be carried out by computers at higher speeds.

Machine learning (ML), which is a sub-theory of AI, is a science that addresses the processes of designing and developing algorithms that aim to make computers learn like a living organism. The focus of ML research is on giving computers the ability to detect complex trends and make rational decisions based on available data. The performance of ML approaches is directly proportional to the quality of the training set, the success of the data pre-processing techniques, and the determination of the correct parameters.

Deep learning, which is a subset of ML, is a neural network algorithm consisting of many layers that can be trained with a training dataset and predict unprecedented examples. Deep learning has a structure that lets you learn by converting big data into smaller data.

There are two important factors that enable the concept of deep learning to be born and used frequently today. The first of these is the reduction of the training time and costs of deep learning algorithms, thanks to the developing graphics processing units, and the other is the easy acquisition of the necessary arguments for the training of big data. The most important factor in the high performance of deep learning algorithms is that the deep network can be trained with a large number of data.

Deep learning architectures consist of different layers with different levels of abstraction for feature extraction, data transformation, classification, and regression operations. Each subsequent layer uses the output of the preceding layer as input for its own layer [28]. These inputs are transformed into new representations of the data with nonlinear transformation functions. A hierarchical network is created by gradually reducing the layers. This network is designed in a way similar to the functioning of the human brain. It creates a deep understanding by passing each new data it receives through different levels of hierarchical abstraction. In this way, the superior properties of the data are learned by increasing the abstraction at each layer [29]. The most important advantage of deep learning, which is a system based on learning from data representation, is that it uses efficient algorithms for hierarchical feature extraction instead of manually extracted features [30].

The deep learning architectures developed with the increase in the number and diversity of layers of neural networks, the acceleration of computers, and the use of graphics processing units (GPU) in the field of ML are shown below:

- Convolutional neural networks (CNN)
- Recurrent neural networks (RNN)
- Long short-term memory (LSTM)
- Limited Boltzmann machines (RBM)
- Deep belief networks (DBN)
- Deep auto-encoders (DAE)

In this study, the CNN architecture, which is the basis of the developed model, will be mentioned.

### 9.2.1 Convolutional neural networks

In recent years, there have been remarkable developments in CNN models in research and applications in the medical field. The most important factor that provides this is that CNN models can work with a huge amount of data produced today, which has become easier to access. As a result of the development and use of CNN models, classification and prediction processes can be performed with high accuracy by using pictures, videos, and similar data obtained from patients. Patient diagnosis methods developed with large amounts of data, high-performance GPUs, and new generation CNN models have opened a whole new page in the field of medicine.

CNN architecture, a product of multilayer perceptron, is inspired by the visual center of animals. It mimics the brain's way of processing visual information. The cells in the visual center are divided into sub-regions to cover the entire image. Simple cells concentrate on the edges, and complex cells concentrate on the entire image [31].

The most important benefit of CNN architecture is that it requires less training and has fewer parameters than fully connected networks. Traditional CNN architecture has five main layers: input, convolution, pooling, fully connected, and output layers. From these layers, many different CNN architectures can be created with the changes made in the number of convolutional layer, pooling layer, and fully connected layer [32]. A CNN architecture composed of input, one convolutional layer, one pooling layer, and one fully connected layer and output is shown in Figure 9.1.

As the name suggests, the first layer of the CNN architecture is the input layer. The raw data are given as input values to the deep learning network

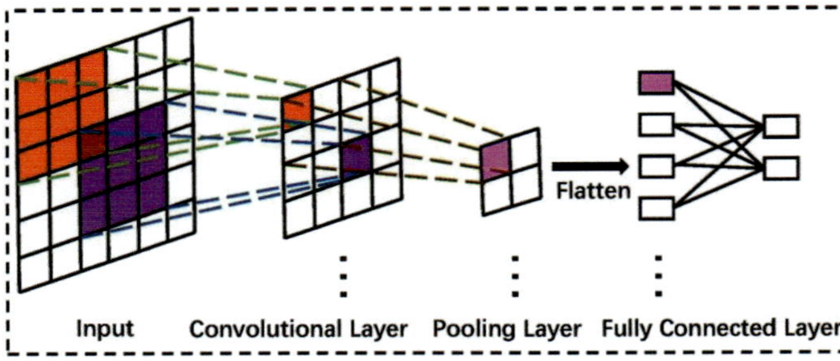


**Figure 9.1** A CNN architecture composed of input, one convolutional layer, one pooling layer, and one fully connected layer and output [33].

in this layer. The size of the data in the input layer becomes important for the CNN model to be created. Choosing a high input image size increases the memory requirement, training time, and testing time. In addition, it can increase the success of the model. Choosing a low input image size reduces memory requirements and training and testing times. In addition, since the depth of the created model decreases, its performance may decrease. In medical image processing studies, an optimum value for the input image size should be determined for the network depth and success, as well as the hardware computation cost.

| | | |
|---|---|---|
| 2 | 0 | 2 |
| 2 | 2 | 1 |
| 2 | 0 | 1 |

**Figure 9.2** A sample kernel of size 3 × 3.

The convolution layer, which is the most basic of CNN, can also be called the transform layer. The convolution operation is based on the process of circulating a certain filter over the entire image and is a specialized linear operation that can process input data of different sizes. Input data are usually a two-dimensional array. Kernel or filter is a two-dimensional array with learnable parameters that operate on the input matrix in the convolutional layer. Kernels can be of different sizes such as 3 × 3, 7 × 7, or 9 × 9. A sample kernel of size 3 × 3 is is shown in Figure 9.2.

The filters create the output data by applying the convolution operation to the images from the previous layer. The convolution operation is mathematically,

$$s[i,j] = (IxK)[i,j] = \textstyle\sum_m (\sum_n I[m,n]K[i-m,j-n]), \tag{9.1}$$

where $I$ is the input value for $m \times n$ size image, $K$ is the kernel, and $s$ is the resulting value with $i$ and $j$ coordinates.

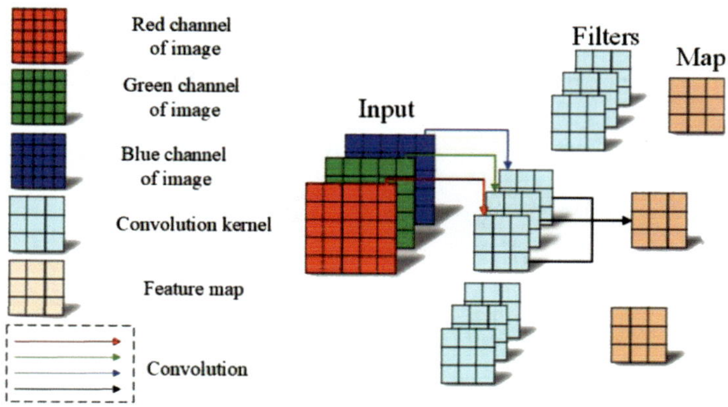


**Figure 9.3** Convolution process and feature maps [34].

The size of these kernels has a high impact on learning because the kernel size determines how large the data will affect each other. Convolution process is done by moving a certain step to the right or left on the input image with a kernel. During this movement, when the boundary of the input matrix is reached, it is continued by sliding down one step. This traversal is done over the entire image matrix. The filters are mathematically processed according to eqn (9.1) with the values in each color channel. A feature map is created by summing the results of the convolution operation on each color channel. An example of convolution process and feature mapsis shown in Figure 9.3. As a result of this convolution process, a feature map is formed where the features specific to each filter are discovered.

The activation function is performed as the last component of the convolutional layer in order to increase the nonlinearity in the output. The activation function analyzes the net information coming to the artificial nerve cell and calculates the output information. The activation function enables the CNN model to learn complex real-world data. A CNN without an activation function has difficulty in learning and detecting complex structures in the data and often falls short. For this reason, we need to use an appropriate activation function for a strong CNN. Although there are activation functions that are known to be more useful for certain problems, which activation function to use may vary according to CNN models. The important point to be considered when choosing the activation function is that the derivative of the selected function can be easily calculated because this will provide an advantage in terms of computational cost. Activation functions that can be used in CNN models are shown in Figure 9.4.

In this study, the ReLu activation function is used in the hidden layers and the Sigmoid function is used in the last layer. ReLu is often preferred

| Name | Function |
|---|---|
| Sigmoid | $\sigma(x) = \frac{1}{1+e^{-x}}$ |
| Tanh | $tanh(x) = 2\sigma(2x) - 1$ |
| ReLU | $f(x) = max(0,x)$ |
| Leaky ReLU | $f(x) = \begin{cases} ax, & x < 0 \\ x, & x \geq 0 \end{cases}$ |
| ELU | $f(x) = \begin{cases} x, & if\ x > 0 \\ \alpha(e^x - 1), & if\ x \leq 0 \end{cases}$ |
| SELU | $selu(x) = \lambda \begin{cases} x, & x > 0 \\ \alpha e^x - \alpha, & x \leq 0 \end{cases}$ |
| PReLU | $f(x) = \begin{cases} x, & if\ x > 0 \\ \alpha x, & if\ x \leq 0 \end{cases}$ |
| Softmax | $f(x) = \frac{e^{z_j}}{\sum_k e^{z_k}}$ |

**Figure 9.4** Activation functions for CNN.

in hidden layers in CNN networks. The most important benefit of the ReLu function is that the deep network does not actively use all neurons in the same layer. If a neuron in the layer produces a negative value, its output value will be 0 and thus cannot be active. This makes ReLu work efficiently and fast and is more preferred in multilayer neural networks. The sigmoid function is one of the most used and nonlinear activation functions in deep learning applications. It is a probabilistic approach to decision-making and its value range is between [0, 1]. That is, it gives a probabilistic value of which class the output belongs to. Since the sigmoid function is a differentiable function, the learning process takes place. But Sigmoid is not perfect either because the derivative value converges to 0 at the extreme points.

In order to reduce the size of the model, a layer called pooling is passed. In the pooling layer, subsampling in the size of $p \times p$ ($p$ value is chosen between 2 and 5 according to the image size) is applied with the sliding window method [35]. In the pooling layer, a value is obtained by taking the maximum or average of the values in a specified area within each map produced in the convolution layer. Thanks to the pooling layers, the small parts of the previously mentioned input are reduced to a single fixed value according to the preferred method, thus improving the computational costs [36]. Max pooling and average pooling are the mostly used pooling functions in the literature. Pooling processes that can be used in CNN models are shown in Figure 9.5. In this study, max pooling function is used as a pooling function.

The loss function calculates the difference between the result value produced by the model and the actual value it should be. In other words, it can be defined as a function that measures the performance of the model. The

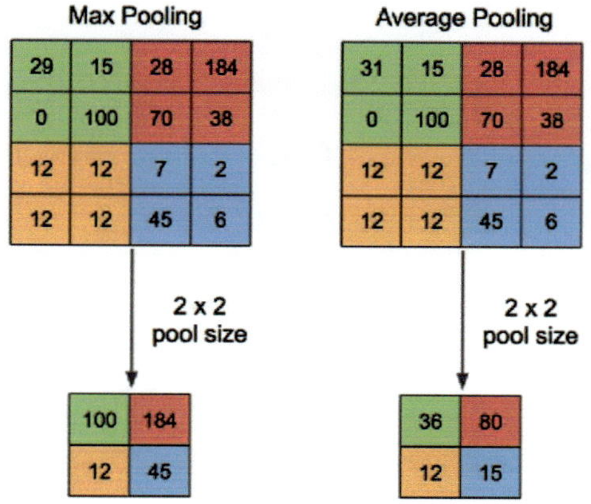


**Figure 9.5** Max pooling and average pooling [37].

| Name | Function |
|---|---|
| Mean Square Error | $Loss = \frac{1}{output\ size} \sum_{i=1}^{output\ size} (y_i - \hat{y}_i)^2$ |
| Categorical Cross Entropy | $\text{Loss} = -\sum_{i=1}^{\substack{\text{output}\\\text{size}}} y_i \cdot \log \hat{y}_i$ |
| Binary Cross Entropy | $\text{Loss} = -\frac{1}{\substack{\text{output}\\\text{size}}} \sum_{i=1}^{\substack{\text{output}\\\text{size}}} y_i \cdot \log \hat{y}_i + (1 - y_i) \cdot \log (1 - \hat{y}_i)$ |

**Figure 9.6** Loss functions for CNN.

loss function is defined in the last layer of deep networks. The loss function basically calculates the difference between the prediction made by the model and the true value. For this reason, the expected loss value from a good model is to be as close to 0 as possible. With the loss value obtained, the backpropagation process is started. By using the loss function, the weight values of all layers are recalculated and the error value is minimized. This process (forward and backpropagation) is repeated until the drop in loss stops or reaches a point where it will no longer matter. There are many loss functions used to calculate the loss value in the literature. The loss functions that can be used in CNN models are shown in Figure 9.6. In this study, binary cross-entropy function is used as loss function.

Learning rate is a coefficient used for error correction. It can also be called error correction coefficient. In simple terms, the learning rate defines how fast the weights will change in the neural network. The learning coefficient provides the convergence of the deep neural network. When the learning

| Name | Function |
|---|---|
| SGD | $\theta_{t+1} = \theta_t - \eta \cdot \nabla_\theta J(\theta_t; x^{(i)}; y^{(i)})$ |
| Adagrad | $\theta_{t+1,i} = \theta_{t,i} - \frac{\eta}{\sqrt{G_{t,ii} + \epsilon}} g_{t,i}$ |
| Adadelta | $\theta_{t+1} = \theta_t - \frac{\eta}{\sqrt{E[g^2]_t + \epsilon}} g_t$ |
| Adam | $\theta_{t+1} = \theta_t - \frac{\eta}{\sqrt{\frac{v_t}{1-\beta_2^t}} + \epsilon} \frac{m_t}{1-\beta_1^t}$ |
| Adamax | $\theta_{t+1} = \theta_t - \frac{\eta}{(1-\beta_1^t)} \frac{m_t}{u_t}$ |

**Figure 9.7** Optimizers for CNN.

coefficient is too large, it may be difficult to reach the target, and in cases where it is chosen too small, the convergence process will take quite a long time since very small steps will be taken in each iteration in the algorithm [38]. In this study, the learning coefficient was initially determined as 0.005.

The learning process in deep learning algorithms is basically an optimization problem. In the literature, optimization algorithms are generally used to find the most appropriate value in the solutions of nonlinear problems. Optimizers commonly used in deep neural networks are stochastic gradient descent (SGD), adagrad, adadelta, adam, and adamax. There are some differences between these optimizers in terms of speed and performance. In Figure 9.7, optimizers commonly used in deep learning are shown. In this study, the SGD function was used as the optimizer.

Dropout is a method that helps to prevent over-fitting by making the outputs of hidden neurons close to zero with a predetermined probability. In deep learning applications, this value is mostly determined as 0.5 or 0.7 [39]. On the other hand, dropout in convolutional layers is less effective due to fewer parameters. In this case, another method used to make the convolutional neural network more regular is the batch normalization process. Besides a regulatory effect, batch normalization also confers a resistance to the extinction gradient of the CNN network during training. This can reduce training time and make the model perform better. In this study, batch normalization was applied in the convolutional layer and 0.5 value dropout was applied in the fully connected layer.

### 9.2.2 Dataset

In this study, the ChestX-ray14 dataset, which was created with hospital-scale chest X-ray images extracted from the PACS system of the National

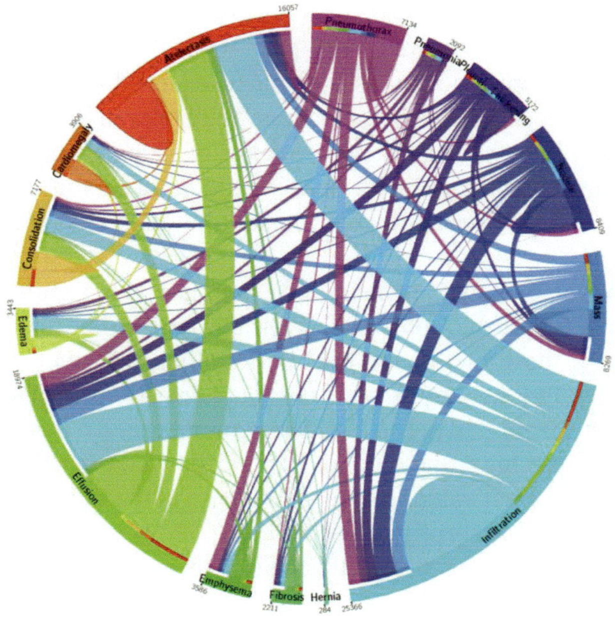


**Figure 9.8** Multi-label images in each of the 14 pathology classes [7].

Institutes of Health (NIH), was used [7]. This dataset contains 112,120 frontal chest X-ray images of 30,805 different patients. The images in the dataset are in high resolution .png format with 1024 × 1024 pixels. The images are labeled with 14 common chest diseases that are frequently observed and diagnosed, based on feedback from radiologists. Natural language processing techniques are adopted to generate image tags. The keywords used for the tags are completely taken from radiology reports. Many images in the dataset have multi-labels. A circular diagram showing the proportions and labels of the multi-label images in each of the 14 pathology classes is given in Figure 9.8.

Atelectasis is a disease that can be defined as the inability of all or part of the lungs to inflate sufficiently as a result of the inability to get air due to a physical obstruction [40]. After a detailed medical history and examination for the diagnosis of atelectasis, the first method doctors apply is a chest X-ray.

Cardiomegaly is a serious heart condition that can be defined by chest X-ray images, which can be expressed as enlargement or expansion seen in all or some parts of the heart [41].

Consolidation is solidification of the lungs for any reason, mostly filling of the lungs with liquid or gas. Lung consolidation is the irritation and destruction of the alveoli due to different reasons and thus the hardening of the soft tissue. Consolidation can affect only one lobe of the lung or spread to the entire lung surface [42].

Pulmonary edema occurs as a result of excess fluid collection in the lungs. This fluid accumulates in the numerous air sacs in the lungs, making it hard to breathe. If we have pulmonary edema, our lungs, which normally fill with air when we breathe, fill with fluid instead of air. In this case, our blood cannot get the oxygen it needs by our lungs. If left untreated, it can have fatal consequences.

Effusion, also known as pleural effusion, is the accumulation of water in the space between the outer surface of the lung called the pleura (lung membrane) and these two membranes surrounding the inner surface of the chest wall [43]. In a healthy person, there is normally a very small amount of fluid, about 20 mL, between these two membranes. Depending on any disease outside the lung, the amount of fluid between the two membranes increases above normal values due to an increase in the secretion of this fluid or a decrease in its reabsorption.

Emphysema is a lung disease that causes shortness of breath. In emphysema patients, the alveolar air sacs in the lungs are damaged. Emphysema occurs due to irreversible damage to the alveoli and the walls of the respiratory tract over time in the lungs exposed to smoking or some harmful gases. In emphysema patients, flexibility in the alveoli is lost. Small air sacs are replaced by large air sacs [44].

Fibrosis is a condition in which the spongy tissue of the lung thickens and hardens, and as a result, the diseased areas have a scar-like appearance. The word fibrosis is a medical term used to describe the hard tissue layer formed by wound healing [45].

Hernia is a health emergency and requires surgical intervention to be corrected. The diaphragm is a muscle barrier in the form of a dome between the thorax and the abdominal cavities. It separates the heart and lungs from the abdominal organs. A diaphragmatic hernia occurs when one or more of the abdominal organs move through an opening in the diaphragm into the chest cavity. Such a defect may be congenital or may occur later as a result of any injury [46].

Lung infiltration is generally caused by abnormal substances heavier than air, such as pus and blood, which gradually accumulate in the lung tissue [47].

Lung mass arises in the lung cells and is known as a tumor in the lung. A mass in the lung can also be associated with lung cancer. The uncontrolled and rapid proliferation of cells in the lung is called mass increase [48].

Lung nodules are masses less than 3 cm that appear as round, white dots (small tissues) that can be seen on chest X-ray images [49]. These nodules in the lung are usually benign. If the nodule is seen in the same size in radiological follow-ups at certain routine intervals, the probability of malignancy decreases. However, it should be followed meticulously and the size and shape of the nodules should be kept under observation with routine scans.

Pleural thickening is a thin, bilayer membrane that lines the chest cavity from the inside and surrounds the lungs. Normally, the pleura is an extremely thin membrane, like the onion skin. However, in some people, this membrane can reach the thickness of a paper or even a finger and harden. While this hardening can mostly be caused by an infection, in some cases, a tumor can also cause pleural thickening [50].

Pneumothorax is the condition of air filling between the lung membranes. Normally, air is trapped inside the lungs in the thorax. Due to a hole that may occur on the lungs, the air inside escapes out of the lungs and collects inside the rib cage, causing them to deflate by pressing on the lungs [51].

### 9.2.3 Experimental study

In this study, a CNN model was developed to perform multi-label classification on the ChestX-ray14 dataset. In the data pre-processing stage, each image with "1024 × 1024" pixels in the ChestX-ray14 dataset was resized to "224 × 224" pixels. The resizing of the images was done using the OpenCV library. In the next step, the dataset is divided into two parts as 80% training and 20% test set. In the developed model, ReLU is used as the activation function in the entire convolution network consisting of nine layers. In addition, batch normalization was applied at the end of each layer. At the end of the ninth layer, the data were transformed into a one-dimensional array by flattening. After this layer, the data continued to be processed in the fully connected layer. The fully connected layer consists of five layers and ReLU activation layer is used in each layer. The output layer consists of 15 neurons and the Sigmoid function is chosen as the activation function. SGD was chosen as the optimization algorithm. On the algorithm, 0.005 was chosen as the learning rate and binary_crossentropy was preferred as the loss function. In this way, learning is slow, but the probability of the algorithm missing the optimum value is reduced. The training process was carried out in 800 iterations. The model and architecture of the developed CNN are shown in Figures 9.9 and 9.10, respectively.

The performance criteria calculated using true positive, false positive, true negative, and false negative data to compare the performances of the experiments are shown in Figure 9.11.

The dataset obtained as a result of the pre-processing was trained for 800 epochs on the developed CNN model and 91.04% accuracy and 0.089

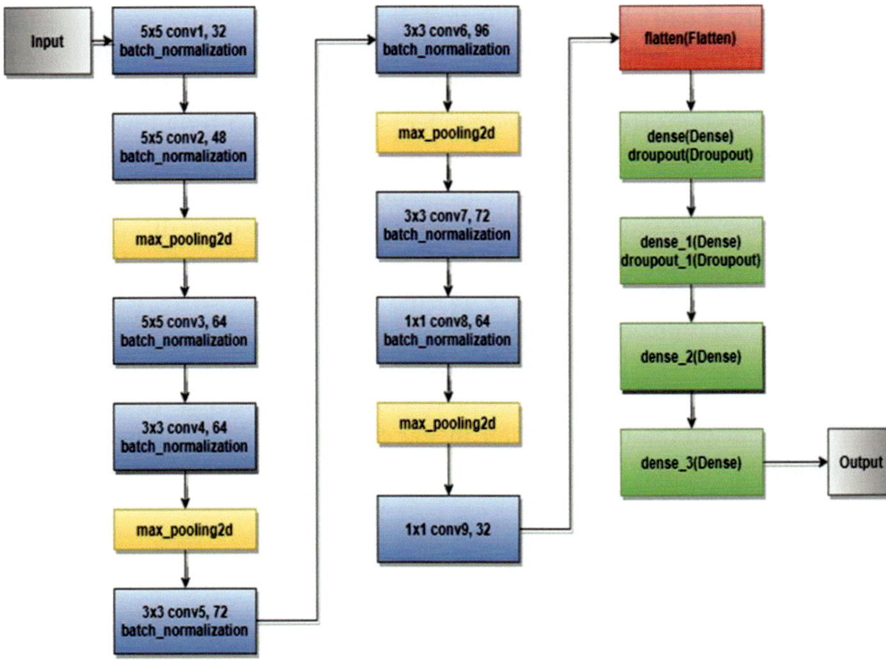


**Figure 9.9** The developed CNN model.

training loss were obtained. The convergence graph of accuracy and training loss values is shown in Figure 9.12.

The results of the developed CNN network on the basis of disease classes are shown in Figure 9.13.

In order to determine the performance of the CNN model developed in the study, it has been compared with the VGG-16 and ResNet-152 CNN models, which have achieved many successes in the field of image processing. The results of the comparisons on the basis of disease are shown in Figure 9.14. The developed CNN model has achieved a close accuracy with the VGG-16 and ResNet-152 models.

Finally, the developed CNN model was compared with the results of previous studies on the same dataset. The developed model achieved better results than previous studies. The results obtained from these comparisons made on the basis of diseases are shown in Figure 9.15.

## 9.3 Conclusion

Early diagnosis is the most fundamental problem facing the health systems of many countries in the world. In this study, multi-label classification was

| | Layer | Size | Filter Size | Feature Map | Activation Function |
|---|---|---|---|---|---|
| Input | İmage | 1024x1024x1 | - | 1 | |
| 1 | Convolution | 224x224 | 5x5 | 32 | ReLu |
| 2 | Convolution | 224x224 | 5x5 | 48 | ReLu |
| 3 | Max Pooling | 128x128 | 2x2 | 48 | ReLu |
| 4 | Convolution | 128x128 | 5x5 | 64 | ReLu |
| 5 | Convolution | 128x128 | 3x3 | 64 | ReLu |
| 6 | Max Pooling | 64x64 | 2x2 | 64 | ReLu |
| 7 | Convolution | 64x64 | 3x3 | 72 | ReLu |
| 8 | Convolution | 64x64 | 3x3 | 96 | ReLu |
| 9 | Max Pooling | 32x32 | 2x2 | 96 | ReLu |
| 10 | Convolution | 32x32 | 3x3 | 72 | ReLu |
| 11 | Convolution | 32x32 | 1x1 | 64 | ReLu |
| 12 | Max Pooling | 16x16 | 2x2 | 64 | ReLu |
| 13 | Convolution | 16x16 | 1x1 | 32 | ReLu |
| 14 | Dense | 2048 | - | - | ReLu |
| 15 | Dense | 512 | - | - | ReLu |
| 16 | Dense | 128 | - | - | ReLu |
| 17 | Dense | 32 | - | - | ReLu |
| Output | Dense | 15 | - | - | Sigmoid |

**Figure 9.10** The architecture of the developed CNN model.

| Performance Criteria | Formula |
|---|---|
| Accuracy | (TN + TP) / (TN + TP + FN + FP) |
| Error rate | (FN + FP) / (TN + TP + FN + FP) |
| Sensitivity | TP / (FN+TP) |
| False Positive Rate | FP / (TN+FP) |
| Specificity | TN / (TN+FP) |
| Precision | TP / (FP+TP) |

**Figure 9.11** Performance criteria.

performed on the ChestX-ray14 dataset using CNN models on chest X-ray images. It has been shown that a well-designed deep learning model can be successfully applied in the early diagnosis of diseases. In the test results obtained after the training of the CNN network, the training loss value was 0.0775 and the accuracy value was 84.74%. In the examinations made on the basis of class, the highest success was achieved for cardiomegaly with 89.86%, and the lowest success was obtained for hernia with 75.67%. These

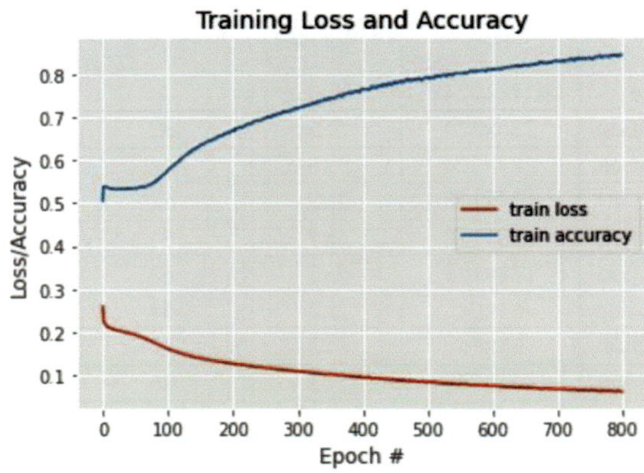


**Figure 9.12** Training loss and accuracy convergence graphic.

| Disease Name | Accuracy (%) | Error rate | Sensitivity | False Positive Rate | Specificity | Precision |
|---|---|---|---|---|---|---|
| Atelectasis | 82.61 | 0.1739 | 0.2232 | 0.1028 | 0.8972 | 0.2039 |
| Cardiomegaly | 97.57 | 0.0243 | 0.0000 | 0.0000 | 1.0000 | - |
| Consolidation | 95.28 | 0.0472 | 0.0090 | 0.0029 | 0.9971 | 0.1268 |
| Edema | 97.03 | 0.0297 | 0.0796 | 0.0125 | 0.9875 | 0.1104 |
| Effusion | 85.89 | 0.1411 | 0.2537 | 0.0598 | 0.9402 | 0.3631 |
| Emphysema | 97.65 | 0.0235 | 0.0020 | 0.0008 | 0.9992 | 0.0526 |
| Fibrosis | 98.45 | 0.0155 | 0.0000 | 0.0000 | 1.0000 | - |
| Hernia | 99.80 | 0.0020 | 0.0000 | 0.0000 | 1.0000 | - |
| Infiltration | 73.41 | 0.2659 | 0.2675 | 0.1657 | 0.8343 | 0.2573 |
| Mass | 94.66 | 0.0534 | 0.0035 | 0.0021 | 0.9979 | 0.0816 |
| Nodule | 91.73 | 0.0827 | 0.0510 | 0.0313 | 0.9687 | 0.0880 |
| Pleural Thickening | 96.93 | 0.0307 | 0.0000 | 0.0000 | 1.0000 | - |
| Pneumonia | 98.82 | 0.0118 | 0.0000 | 0.0000 | 1.0000 | - |
| Pneumothorax | 94.14 | 0.0586 | 0.0847 | 0.0154 | 0.9846 | 0.2167 |
| No Finding | 61.56 | 0.3844 | 0.5711 | 0.3330 | 0.6670 | 0.6642 |

**Figure 9.13** The results of developed CNN on the basis of disease classes.

| Disease Name | Developed CNN (%) | VGG-16 (%) | ResNet-152 (%) |
|---|---|---|---|
| Atelectasis | 82.61 | 87.36 | 88.40 |
| Cardiomegaly | 97.57 | 97.16 | 97.47 |
| Consolidation | 95.28 | 94.27 | 95.13 |
| Edema | 97.03 | 97.51 | 97.94 |
| Effusion | 85.89 | 87.62 | 88.61 |
| Emphysema | 97.65 | 97.36 | 97.64 |
| Fibrosis | 98.45 | 98.04 | 98.43 |
| Hernia | 99.80 | 99.79 | 99.80 |
| Infiltration | 73.41 | 78.25 | 80.11 |
| Mass | 94.66 | 94.06 | 94.58 |
| Nodule | 91.73 | 93.18 | 93.94 |
| Pleural Thickening | 96.93 | 96.15 | 96.70 |
| Pneumonia | 98.82 | 98.68 | 98.77 |
| Pneumothorax | 94.14 | 94.88 | 95.13 |
| No Finding | 61.56 | 65.81 | 66.71 |

**Figure 9.14** The comparison of the developed CNN with VGG-16 and ResNet-152.

| Disease Name | Developed CNN (%) | [7] (%) | 13 (%) | [52] (%) |
|---|---|---|---|---|
| Atelectasis | 82.61 | 70.03 | 73.23 | 76.71 |
| Cardiomegaly | 97.57 | 81.0 | 85.56 | 88.13 |
| Consolidation | 95.28 | 70.32 | 71.01 | 74.25 |
| Edema | 97.03 | 80.52 | 80.56 | 83.55 |
| Effusion | 85.89 | 75.85 | 80.56 | 82.78 |
| Emphysema | 97.65 | 83.3 | 84.12 | 89.45 |
| Fibrosis | 98.45 | 78.59 | 74.23 | 81.88 |
| Hernia | 99.80 | 87.17 | 77.55 | 89.76 |
| Infiltration | 73.41 | 66.14 | 67.33 | 70.89 |
| Mass | 94.66 | 69.33 | 71.88 | 82.01 |
| Nodule | 91.73 | 66.87 | 77.87 | 75.78 |
| Pleural Thickening | 96.93 | 68.35 | 72.44 | 76.01 |
| Pneumonia | 98.82 | 65.8 | 68.45 | 73.01 |
| Pneumothorax | 94.14 | 79.93 | 80.52 | 84.56 |

**Figure 9.15** The comparison of the developed CNN with studies in the literature.

results show that better rates can be achieved with more data and improved algorithms by using more advanced hardware in future studies.

## References

[1] Kulkarni, H. (2016). What is Pneumonia?. American Journal of Respiratory and Critical Care Medicine, 193(1), I.
[2] ATS (American Thoracic Society). Available at: https://www.cdc.gov/features/pneumonia/index.html [accessed July, 18, 2022]
[3] CDC. Available at: https://www.cdc.gov/features/pneumonia/index.html [accessed July, 18, 2022]
[4] Dadonaite B. and Roser M. (2018). Pneumonia. Available at: https://ourworldindata.org/pneumonia [accessed July, 18, 2022]
[5] Zar, H. J., Madhi, S. A., Aston, S. J., & Gordon, S. B. (2013). Pneumonia in low and middle income countries: progress and challenges. Thorax, 68(11), 1052–1056.
[6] Speets, A. M., van der Graaf, Y., Hoes, A. W., Kalmijn, S., Sachs, A. P., Rutten, M. J., ... & Mali, W. P. (2006). Chest radiography in general practice: indications, diagnostic yield and consequences for patient management. British Journal of General Practice, 56(529), 574–578.
[7] Wang, X., Peng, Y., Lu, L., Lu, Z., Bagheri, M., & Summers, R. M. (2017). Chestx-ray8: Hospital-scale chest x-ray database and benchmarks on weakly-supervised classification and localization of common thorax diseases. In Proceedings of the IEEE conference on computer vision and pattern recognition (pp. 2097–2106).
[8] World Health Organization. (2001). Standardization of interpretation of chest radiographs for the diagnosis of pneumonia in children / World Health Organization Pneumonia Vaccine Trial Investigators' Group. World Health Organization. Available at: https://apps.who.int/iris/handle/10665/66956 [accessed July, 18, 2022]
[9] Hardy, M., Snaith, B., & Scally, A. (2013). The impact of immediate reporting on interpretive discrepancies and patient referral pathways within the emergency department: a randomised controlled trial. The British journal of radiology, 86(1021), 20120112-20120112.
[10] NHS, 2019, Diagnostic Imaging Dataset Statistical Release, Available at: https://www.england.nhs.uk/ [accessed July, 18, 2022]
[11] Mardani, M., Gong, E., Cheng, J. Y., Vasanawala, S. S., Zaharchuk, G., Xing, L., & Pauly, J. M. (2018). Deep generative adversarial neural networks for compressive sensing MRI. IEEE transactions on medical imaging, 38(1), 167–179.

[12] Hassen, M., Toma, A., Tesfay, M., Degafu, E., Bekele, S., Ayalew, F., ... & Tadesse, B. T. (2019). Radiologic diagnosis and hospitalization among children with severe community acquired pneumonia: a prospective cohort study. BioMed Research International, 2019.

[13] Yao, L., Poblenz, E., Dagunts, D., Covington, B., Bernard, D., & Lyman, K. (2017). Learning to diagnose from scratch by exploiting dependencies among labels. arXiv preprint arXiv:1710.10501.

[14] Abdullah, A. B. M. (2020). Radiology in Medical Practice-E-book. Elsevier Health Sciences.

[15] Hopstaken, R. M., Witbraad, T., Van Engelshoven, J. M. A., & Dinant, G. J. (2004). Inter-observer variation in the interpretation of chest radiographs for pneumonia in community-acquired lower respiratory tract infections. Clinical radiology, 59(8), 743–752.

[16] Nodine, C. F., & Krupinski, E. A. (1998). Perceptual skill, radiology expertise, and visual test performance with NINA and WALDO. Academic radiology, 5(9), 603–612.

[17] Gatt, M. E., Spectre, G., Paltiel, O., Hiller, N., & Stalnikowicz, R. (2003). Chest radiographs in the emergency department: is the radiologist really necessary?. Postgraduate medical journal, 79(930), 214–217.

[18] Fabre, C., Proisy, M., Chapuis, C., Jouneau, S., Lentz, P. A., Meunier, C., ... & Lederlin, M. (2018). Radiology residents' skill level in chest x-ray reading. Diagnostic and interventional imaging, 99(6), 361–370.

[19] Gulshan, V., Peng, L., Coram, M., Stumpe, M. C., Wu, D., Narayanaswamy, A., ... & Webster, D. R. (2016). Development and validation of a deep learning algorithm for detection of diabetic retinopathy in retinal fundus photographs. Jama, 316(22), 2402–2410.

[20] Grewal, M., Srivastava, M. M., Kumar, P., & Varadarajan, S. (2018, April). Radnet: Radiologist level accuracy using deep learning for hemorrhage detection in ct scans. In 2018 IEEE 15th International Symposium on Biomedical Imaging (ISBI 2018) (pp. 281–284). IEEE.

[21] Esteva, A., Kuprel, B., Novoa, R. A., Ko, J., Swetter, S. M., Blau, H. M., & Thrun, S. (2017). Dermatologist-level classification of skin cancer with deep neural networks. nature, 542(7639), 115–118.

[22] Shalbaf, A., Bagherzadeh, S., & Maghsoudi, A. (2020). Transfer learning with deep convolutional neural network for automated detection of schizophrenia from EEG signals. Physical and Engineering Sciences in Medicine, 43(4), 1229–1239.

[23] Hashmi, M. F., Katiyar, S., Keskar, A. G., Bokde, N. D., & Geem, Z. W. (2020). Efficient pneumonia detection in chest xray images using deep transfer learning. Diagnostics, 10(6), 417.

[24] Khalifa, N. E. M., Taha, M. H. N., Hassanien, A. E., & Elghamrawy, S. (2020). Detection of coronavirus (covid-19) associated pneumonia based on generative adversarial networks and a fine-tuned deep transfer learning model using chest x-ray dataset. arXiv preprint arXiv:2004.01184.
[25] Uçar, M., & Uçar, E. (2019). Computer-aided detection of lung nodules in chest X-rays using deep convolutional neural networks.
[26] Yao, L., Poblenz, E., Dagunts, D., Covington, B., Bernard, D., & Lyman, K. (2017). Learning to diagnose from scratch by exploiting dependencies among labels. arXiv preprint arXiv:1710.10501.
[27] Rajpurkar, P., Irvin, J., Zhu, K., Yang, B., Mehta, H., Duan, T., ... & Ng, A. Y. (2017). Chexnet: Radiologist-level pneumonia detection on chest x-rays with deep learning. arXiv preprint arXiv:1711.05225.
[28] Deng, L., & Yu, D. (2014). Deep learning: methods and applications. Foundations and trends® in signal processing, 7(3–4), 197-387.
[29] Bengio, Y., Goodfellow, I., & Courville, A. (2017). Deep learning (Vol. 1). Cambridge, MA, USA: MIT press.
[30] Song, H. A., & Lee, S. Y. (2013, November). Hierarchical representation using NMF. In International conference on neural information processing (pp. 466-473). Springer, Berlin, Heidelberg.
[31] Bengio, Y. (2009). Learning deep architectures for AI. Foundations and trends® in Machine Learning, 2(1), 1–127.
[32] Le Cun, Y., Jackel, L. D., Boser, B., Denker, J. S., Graf, H. P., Guyon, I., ... & Hubbard, W. (1989). Handwritten digit recognition: Applications of neural network chips and automatic learning. IEEE Communications Magazine, 27(11), 41–46.
[33] Lu, J., Feng, J., Fan, Z., Huang, L., Zheng, C., & Li, W. (2019). Automated strabismus detection based on deep neural networks for telemedicine application. Knowledge-based systems, 13.
[34] Yang, R., Wang, S., Wu, X., Liu, T., & Liu, X. (2022). Using lightweight convolutional neural network to track vibration displacement in rotating body video. Mechanical Systems and Signal Processing, 177, 109137.
[35] Scherer, D., Müller, A., & Behnke, S. (2010, September). Evaluation of pooling operations in convolutional architectures for object recognition. In International conference on artificial neural networks (pp. 92–101). Springer, Berlin, Heidelberg.
[36] Dumoulin, V., & Visin, F. (2016). A guide to convolution arithmetic for deep learning. arXiv preprint arXiv:1603.07285.
[37] Yani, M. (2019, May). Application of transfer learning using convolutional neural network method for early detection of terry's nail. In

Journal of Physics: Conference Series (Vol. 1201, No. 1, p. 012052). IOP Publishing.

[38] Haykin, S. (2009). Neural networks and learning machines, 3/E. Pearson Education India.

[39] Krizhevsky, A., Sutskever, I., & Hinton, G. E. (2012). Imagenet classification with deep convolutional neural networks. Advances in neural information processing systems, 25.

[40] Atelectasis. Available at: https://www.acibadem.com.tr/ilgi-alani/atelektazi/ [accessed July, 18, 2022]

[41] Buchanan, J. W., & Bücheler, J. (1995). Vertebral scale system to measure canine heart size in radiographs. Journal-American Veterinary Medical Association, 206, 194–194.

[42] Consolidation, Available at: https://akciger.info/konsolidasyon-akciger.html [accessed July, 18, 2022]

[43] Effusion, Available at: http://www.tgcd.org.tr/3-soruda-akciger-zarlari-arasinda-su-birikmesi-plevralefuzyon/ [accessed July, 18, 2022]

[44] Emphysema, Available at: https://www.medikalakademi.com.tr/amfizem-tedavi/ [accessed July, 18, 2022]

[45] Fibrosis, Available at: https://www.acibadem.com.tr/ilgi-alani/pulmoner-fibrozis/ [accessed July, 18, 2022]

[46] Hernia, Available at: https://www.turkiyeklinikleri.com/article/tr-gogus-duvarindan-akciger-herniasyonu/ [accessed July, 18, 2022]

[47] Infiltration, Available at: https://akciger.info/akcigerde-infiltrasyon-nedir.html [accessed July, 18, 2022]

[48] Mass, Available at: https://www.milliyet.com.tr/pembenar/akcigerde-kitle-nedir-neden-olusur-akcigerde-kitle-tumor-nasil-tedavi-edilir/ [accessed July, 18, 2022]

[49] Nodule, Available at: https://www.acibadem.com.tr/ilgi-alani/akciger-nodulleri [accessed July, 18, 2022]

[50] Pleural Thickening, Available at: http://www.tgcd.org.tr/3-soruda-akciger-zarlari-arasinda-su-birikmesi-plevral-efuzyon/ [accessed July, 18, 2022]

[51] Pneumothorax, Available at: https://okanhastanesi.com.tr/akciger-sonmesi-hakkinda-her-sey/ [accessed July, 18, 2022]

[52] Gündel, S., Setio, A. A., Ghesu, F. C., Grbic, S., Georgescu, B., Maier, A., & Comaniciu, D. (2021). Robust classification from noisy labels: Integrating additional knowledge for chest radiography abnormality assessment. Medical Image Analysis, 72, 102087

# 10

# Explainable Artificial Intelligence Applications in Dentistry: A Theoretical Research

**B. Aksoy, M. Yücel, H. Sayın, O.K.M. Salman, M. Eylence, and M.M. Özmen**

Faculty of Technology, Department of Mechatronics Engineering, Isparta University of Applied Sciences, Turkey
Email: bekiraksoy@isparta.edu.tr; mehmetyucel9696@gmail.com; hsayin32@gmail.com; osamahkms1994@gmail.com; meylence@yandex.ru; cadet.2045@gmail.com

## Abstract

With the rapid development of technology, the use of artificial intelligence and related technologies in almost every field has increased significantly. Artificial intelligence applications are used in almost all areas, such as education, engineering, and the defense industry. One of the essential areas of artificial intelligence applications in the health sector. In this chapter of the book, artificial intelligence methods that are frequently used in dentistry and explainable artificial intelligence methods are examined, along with an overview of the dental field, which is one of the critical sectors in health. In addition, theoretical research was carried out by examining the academic studies published in the field of artificial intelligence and explainable artificial intelligence in dentistry.

## 10.1 Introduction

Today, with the rapid development in the health sector, the use of artificial intelligence applications in the health sector is increasing daily. Artificial intelligence applications have achieved high accuracy results in recent years. They are believed to significantly contribute to reducing human-induced errors in the diagnosis and treatment phase in the health sector. One of the critical areas of artificial intelligence applications in the dental field. In the introductory part of the study, basic information about dentistry, dental imaging techniques, and the use of artificial intelligence in dental images subtitles will be mentioned.

### 10.1.1 An overview of the dentistry

The appearance of the human face has significant social and psychological effects on the individual. The eyes and mouth are the most important essential elements that increase facial attractiveness [1]. In dentistry, the typical structure of the head, face, mouth, jaws, and teeth, the function of these structures, and their diseases are examined, and preventive and curative treatments of these diseases are made. Diseases that occur with the deterioration of oral and dental health affect general health negatively in the long term. This situation can lead to various problems such as the deterioration of the patient's nutrition, the restriction of his social life, and even the adverse alteration in psychological status. For these reasons, the protection of oral and dental health has great importance in terms of general health protection [2]. This clearly shows that oral and dental health is integral to general health [3]. Human teeth have essential functions for speaking, chewing, and esthetics. The loss or decrease of these functions negatively affects the life quality of a person [4]. In the world, and especially in our country, a large part of the population suffers from dental and gingival diseases [5]. Diagnosis of dental and gingival diseases can be achieved respectively by listening to the patient's history of pain or discomfort; learning about previous complaints such as trauma and previous treatments like restorative procedures; clinical examination; clinical and laboratory tests, and evaluation of the results; and radiographic examination of the teeth and surrounding tissues [6]. Diagnosis is based on a series of observations, and not a single finding. The clinical situation can be so complex that the appropriate diagnosis and treatment decision may require following a diagnostic process consisting of several steps [7]. Dentistry is an updated science with changing and developing technology and new treatment practices and techniques. Devices and dental materials used in this field are rapidly diversifying. With the advancement of digital technology, the use of assistive technologies is increasing in the stages of diagnosis of diseases, evaluation of the patient, and treatment planning. Due to the rapid developments in dental materials and dental technologies that have created new options in recent years, a new perspective needs to be brought to the previously used diagnostic and planning techniques in dentistry [8].

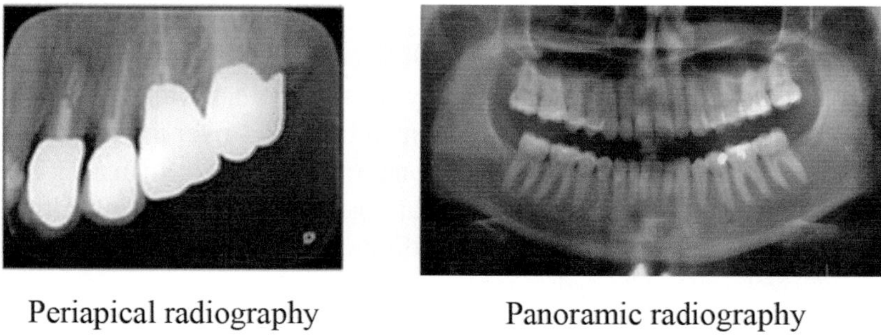


**Figure 10.1** Periapical and panographic radiography images [13, 14].

### 10.1.2 Imaging techniques in the dentistry

Radiographs are one of the most important tools used in the diagnosis and post-treatment evaluation of the patient in dentistry. The rapid technological development of imaging systems for dental practice requires continuous updates and justification of radiographic applications and guidelines. The main purpose of dental imaging is to demonstrate the three-dimensional anatomy and to completely visualize the target area in at least two planes, with minimal superposition, minimal distortion, and maximum detail. It is also needed to balance the diagnostic values of the imaging in terms of the risk and cost of the imaging process [9, 10]. There are many different imaging techniques to be used in the diagnosis and treatment of dental and gingival diseases. The most frequently used techniques are bitewing, periapical, and panoramic radiographs [11]. Bitewing radiographs are mostly used in dentistry for the detection of caries and the determination of alveolar bone levels [12]. Figure 10.1 shows the periapical and panoramic radiography image samples.

Periapical radiographs ("peri," "periphery," and apical "tip of the tooth root," "apex of the root") are used to determine teeth and surrounding tissues, their position, and tooth size [15]. The periapical radiography technique has the highest image quality among many imaging techniques [16].

The panoramic radiography technique, which displays the entire maxillomandibular region on a single film, has become a popular diagnostic tool since its introduction into the general dental practice and allows easy examination of all teeth, alveolar bone, temporomandibular joints, and adjacent structures [17].

Studies to improve image quality and reduce the amount of radiation in dental radiology continue to develop with the introduction of different digital systems [18]. With the developing radiographic technology, conventional beam receivers are replaced by digital sensors, and the radiation dose reaching the patient can be reduced by 80%–90% compared to conventional films with the use of sensors with greater X-ray sensitivity than films [19]. In addition, digital imaging techniques have many advantages over the conventional method. The image obtained in conventional radiography is an analog image. Here, the image is on an X-ray film and cannot be changed after it is obtained; it is difficult to transport and store. In digital radiography, these problems have been overcome. The radiographic image can be stored in the computer memory, and the obtained image can be modified, measured, and improved by using all the features and techniques of computer technology. Radiographic image quality and diagnostic capacity of the image can be increased, and dimensional measurements can be made easily with image processing techniques performed on digital images using various software [20].

While conventional methods only provide two-dimensional images, three-dimensional imaging has become possible in dentistry in the last 20 years [21]. Three-dimensional imaging systems, which have come to use as another important development in the field of dentomaxillofacial radiology, are called dental volumetric tomography (DVT) or cone beam computed tomography (CBCT) [22]. In this technique, images are obtained by processing the data obtained by rotating a circular rotational X-ray source and the sensor positioned opposite it by rotating around the patient, using a computer [23]. In the creation of CBCT images, first, volumetric 3D data of the facial skeleton, which is formed by rotating the conical X-ray around the patient's head, is obtained. The cylindrical volumetric data are then split into small voxels for analysis. In the last step, 2D images and 3D reconstruction images are prepared in sagittal, coronal, and axial anatomical planes from the data separated into voxels [24]. It is possible to prepare dental materials and models to be applied to the patient by using measurements on the images, digital analysis, and 3D printers.

### 10.1.3 Problem solving with artificial intelligence in dentistry images

Artificial intelligence, which is an area to develop various algorithms to mimic the cognitive abilities of the human brain, has also started to be used in dental and medical applications for purposes such as analyzing medical data, predicting disease, and prognosis, detecting abnormalities, classifying diseases, and determining the functional performance of tissues [25]. Artificial intelligence based virtual assistants were used in early applications to coordinate appointments, patient check-ups, and treatment planning.

Later, it evolved into artificial intelligence systems that can help in diagnosis from radiographic images by analyzing the symptoms that the human eye cannot easily perceive [26]. Over the years, the use of artificial intelligence applications in the evaluation and follow-up of the oral and surrounding soft tissues and the diagnosis and follow-up of oral cancers have been considered. In orthodontic applications, it is used for purposes such as artificial intelligence based systems that can be used to design the appropriate apparatus and prosthesis by using different variables such as the patient's face size and for treatment planning in orthodontic surgeries [27]. Another breakthrough in the field of restorative and prosthetic dentistry is the use of computer-aided design and computer-aided manufacturing technologies for the precise fit of the prosthesis. In addition, artificial intelligence systems are used to create dental restoration products developed automatically in laboratories, along with innovations in generative adversarial networks (GAN). These solutions are expected not only to assist dentistry but also to have great potential and impact on orofacial or craniofacial prostheses [28]. In addition, in dentistry, regular clinical records should be kept, and general health information such as the patient's systemic condition and medications and data that do not contain radiographic images, such as dental history data, should also be evaluated. Data are usually collected at multiple time points. Artificial intelligence is well suited to effectively integrating, cross-linking, and developing diagnostic, predictive, and decision support systems [29]. However, it is among the expectations of dentists to produce a device that includes software that combines both dental imaging and image analysis with artificial intelligence to facilitate the diagnosis and treatment processes of dentists [30].

## 10.2 Imaging Techniques using X-rays

X-rays were discovered by Wilhelm Conrad Rontgen in 1895. He aimed to obtain fluorescence using a Hittorf–Crookes tube made of deaerated X-ray glass containing positive and negative electrons and a barium platinocyanide plate. After covering the tube with opaque dark black cardboard, he applied a high voltage to the electrodes using a Ruhmkoff coil. Meanwhile, a green fluorescent emission was observed at a distance of 1–2 m from the tube [31–33]. The source of this glow was another plate coated with barium platinocyanide. Roentgen determined that a different form of radiation energy emitted from the tube, different from the cathode rays but produced by the cathode rays, hit the plate, producing radiation. He called these rays "X-rays" because of their unknown nature. Figure 10.2 shows the first X-ray images, which are of the fingers of Rontgen's wife [34, 35].

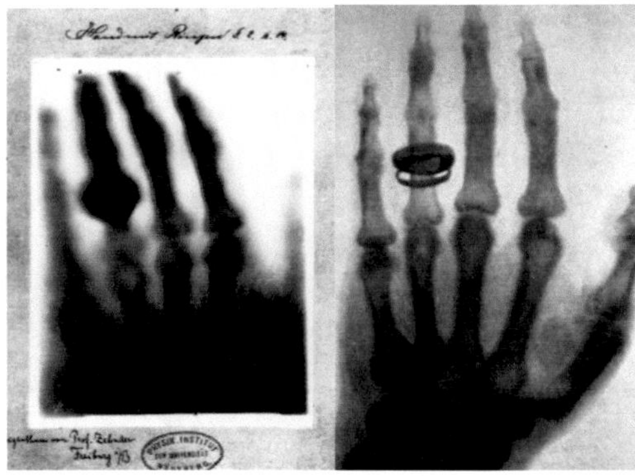

**Figure 10.2** X-ray image of the hand of Wilhelm Conrad Rontgen's wife, Anna Bertha, captured by himself [34, 35].

Since the discovery of X-rays by Rontgen, they have been used frequently in the field of health and have been continuously developed until today. The basis of the X-ray imaging technique is based on the different absorption properties of materials. X-rays are used to digitally visualize the structures of the hard tissues of living things. The X-rays thus obtained are used by radiologists and doctors in disease detection and disease follow-up. The rays produced by a source are directed to the patient. X-rays passing through the patient's body are detected by detectors. The main purpose of X-ray detectors is to collect the X-ray photons they detect. The image detector is a film in the conventional method, and the image is formed on the film after processing. Since the discovery of X-rays, there have been significant advances in X-ray film, image acquisition, and archiving of images taken. With the invention of computers in the early 1940s, the first steps of digitalization were taken in the field of radiology, as in many other fields. Digital radiography aims to capture X-rays with the help of sensors and convert and store data in electronic form [36]. Digital images are obtained from the converted electrical signal. The sensors used in digital systems are more sensitive to X-rays than conventional systems. Thus, less radiation is sufficient for imaging [36, 37]. While working time is reduced with digital radiography, disadvantages such as film cost and chemical processing are eliminated. It is more practical to make measurement and color adjustments on digital images and to enlarge the images in detail.

In the sample X-ray image shown in Figure 10.3, the light gray parts show the hard tissues, while the dark gray parts show the soft tissues of the head.

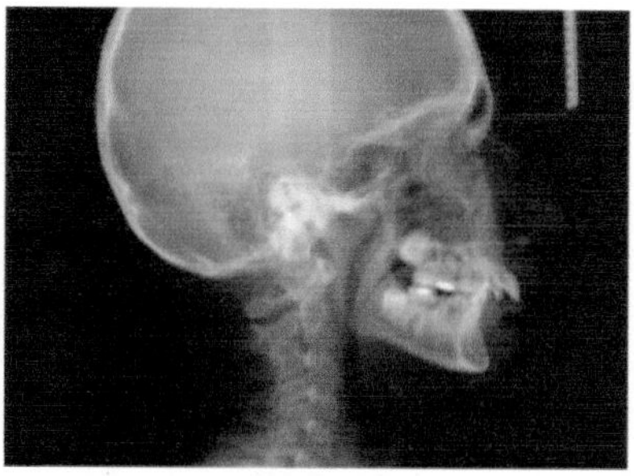

**Figure 10.3** Sample of a head X-ray [38].

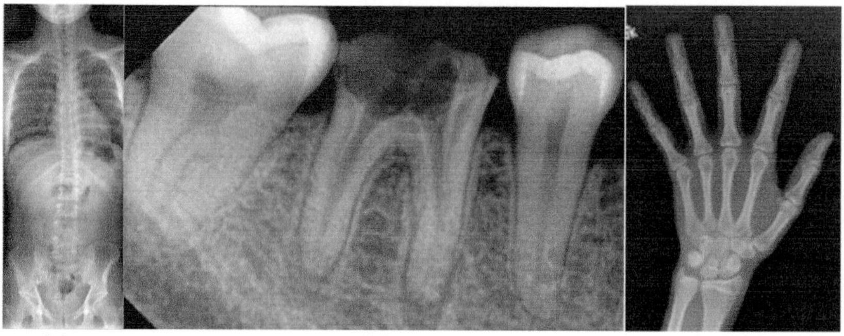

(a) (b) (c)

**Figure 10.4** Example X-ray images. (a) Spinal cord [39]. (b) Tooth [40]. (c) Hand [41].

Various diseases in living things can be detected easily by using the X-ray imaging method. Imaging of hard tissues such as bones and teeth is performed with imaging methods using X-ray. For example, in bones and teeth, fractures, changes due to infection, arthritis, dental caries, and cancers affecting bones can be viewed, and an evaluation of growth and development in bones can be made. Various X-ray diagnoses are shown in Figure 10.4.

In addition to all these advantages, X-rays cause the atoms of the material imaged to lose electrons. Thus, atoms that lose electrons become ionized. Depending on the dose of X-rays, imaging procedures should be completed in the cells of living things when necessary and with the lowest possible dose, and patients and personnel who take X-rays should be protected [42].

## 10.3 CBCT Imaging

Today, with the rapid development of imaging techniques, three-dimensional imaging is frequently used in the health sector [43]. Computed tomography (CT) is used for three-dimensional imaging in the head and neck regions in medical evaluation [44, 45]. The high cost of CT devices, large area coverage, and high amount of radiation dose given to the patient are among the disadvantages. However, with the latest developments in medical technology, machines that obtain images using lower doses and occupy less space are designed [44]. In recent years, cone beam computed tomography (CBCT) has replaced conventional tomography and CT for head and neck imaging in some cases in dentistry.

Cone beam computed tomography (CBCT), also known as dental volumetric tomography (DVT), is a digital radiographic technique in which three-dimensional isometric images of the bone structure of the head and neck regions are obtained in dentistry, maxillofacial surgery, and ear–nose–throat (ENT) areas. CBCT is an imaging method that works with the principle of directing a conical X-ray beam on a two-dimensional flat panel detector [46]. CBCT was first developed for angiography in 1982; it has also been used for radiotherapy guidance and for mammography [47, 48]. The first device of CBCT developed for dentistry is the "NewTom" (Quantitative Radiology, Italy) device produced in 1998 [33].

In conical beam computed tomography, a conical X-ray instead of a fan-shaped beam with a two-dimensional sensor can be used to obtain a volumetric image of the head and neck regions with a simple rotation of the beam and the sensor [45]. In CBCT, a conical X-ray beam is used instead of a fan-shaped beam and multiple rotations, and a single 360° rotation takes place around the area to be imaged [21].

CBCT scanners are systems that can create three-dimensional reconstructions that allow two-dimensional images to be reformatted. The scan is performed in a single 360° scan, in which the X-ray source and a reciprocating field detector move synchronously around the patient's head [49]. The data created by the projections as a result of this scan are reconstructed, and axial, coronal, and sagittal sections are created. Parasagittal cross-sectional images can be created from the desired area on these cross-sectional images. As a result of a single scan, the amount of radiation dose received by the patient can be reduced by reducing the irradiation time [45].

A display area, namely FOV (field of view), can be selected in accordance with the size of the region to be examined.

All CT scanners consist of an X-ray source and a detector mounted on a rotating gantry. As the gantry rotates, the X-ray source generates radiation, and the receptor records the X-ray data that arrive past the imaged area. These data constitute the raw data, which is reconstructed by a computer algorithm to create the cross-sectional images. Pixel values are the basic components of grayscale images, and the grayscale value of each pixel is related to the photon intensities reaching the detector [50]. Voxels are the smallest unit of digital volumetric data. Voxel sizes, which are isotropic in CBCT, range from 125 to 400 μm [33].

CBCT is used in the following areas of dentistry: diseases and imaging of the jaw joint, pre-surgical planning of the head and neck region, determination of the size of pathological lesions such as cysts and tumors and their relationship with the surrounding anatomical structures and pre-surgical planning, post-surgical follow-up imaging, implant planning, examination of the position and localization of impacted teeth, sinus lift operation evaluation, determination of the localization of impacted teeth in orthodontics, evaluation of patients with cleft lip and palate, orthodontic and orthognathic surgery planning, examination of root canal morphology, evaluation of periapical lesions, fracture instrument localization, tooth root resorptions, examination of tooth root fractures, and examination of bone defects and tooth in gum diseases. It is used in many areas such as the evaluation of the surrounding bone structure [51–53].

One of the important disadvantages of CBCT images is the generation of noise due to factors such as digital rounding errors of voxels and the number of photons. The resulting noises often occur during the acquisition of images. In addition, errors may occur in different situations, such as combining the voxel values of the image and transferring the data. When academic studies are examined, image filtering methods are used to reduce noise in the image and increase the image quality. Among these methods, linear and non-linear filters such as linear filters, nonlocal means, mean, anisotropic diffusion, and Gaussian and median filters are used [45–47].

## 10.4 Artificial Intelligence Techniques in Dental Applications

Although there are very broad definitions of artificial intelligence, it can be explained as a set of hardware and software systems that have the ability to think and make decisions like humans. Samuel [54] defined artificial intelligence as a field of study that develops computers that can learn without reprogramming. According to this definition, artificial intelligence can also be defined as systems that find solutions by self-inferring repetitive models and patterns on given problems [55]. The sub-branches of artificial intelligence are given in Figure 10.5.

As seen in Figure 10.5, artificial intelligence includes sub-branches such as neural networks, machine learning, and deep learning. Neural networks are a structure consisting of an input layer, hidden layer, and output

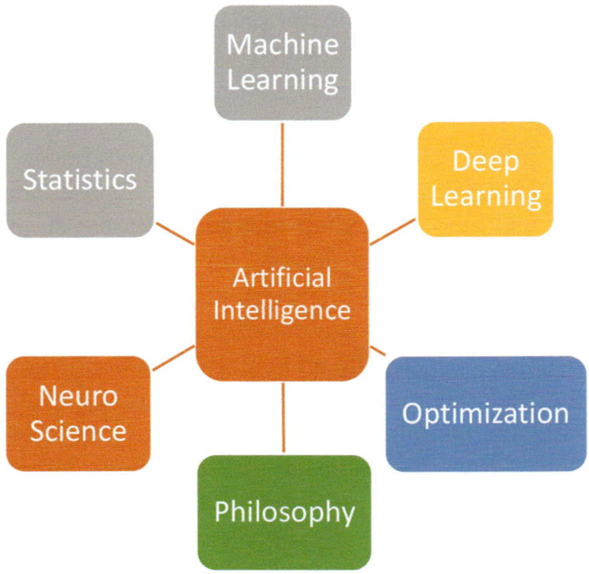


**Figure 10.5** Artificial intelligence sub-branches.

layer, which is modeled on the human brain [56]. These structures enable learning and adapting the system according to the inputs, which are the most important features of artificial intelligence. Neural networks form the basis of machine learning and deep learning structures. Machine learning is a structure that enables the extraction of meaningful patterns from structured data without detailed programming and making predictions by learning from data [57, 58]. Deep learning, on the other hand, is a type of machine learning based on big data and parallel and distributed computing that can handle larger data sources [59, 60]. With deep learning, the information is made hierarchical and multi-layered, and the learning process is carried out more easily [61]. Artificial intelligence and its subcategories are implemented along with the developments in technology, which are health [62, 63], energy [64], cyber security [65], job security [66, 67], entrepreneurship/business world [68], education [69], robotics [70], and agriculture [71], especially in many different areas.

### 10.4.1 Explainable artificial intelligence

Explainable artificial intelligence (XAI) is defined as the methods and techniques that translate the results of a solution reached by artificial intelligence in a way that can be understood by humans. In order to bring image-based deep learning models to an explainable level, various integrations are basically added to the target technique. XAI is a method that emerged with the use of traditional machine learning techniques, which are known to be interpretable, in a hybrid formation. In addition, it is tried to obtain meaningful visuals on the input data by supporting some mathematical processes in the existing artificial neural network model with additional solutions [72, 73]. The second solution process is class activation mapping (CAM), which is one of the frequently preferred techniques. It is the creation of activation maps by gathering weighted feature maps with the CAM technique in line with different class results and by showing the visual regions of these maps on the input data with heat maps [74–76].

Class activation map (CAM) is an image visualization used as a result of classification. It can also be used to determine the position of objects in images in different applications such as image segmentation and object recognition using the CAM technique [76]. In addition, the GRAD-CAM method can be applied to different CNN architectures. The GRAD-CAM method is a visualization technique using gradient information flowing into the last convolution layer in a CNN architect [77]. The mathematical equation of the GRAD-CAM structure is given in the following equation:

$$\alpha_k^c = \frac{1}{z}\sum_i \sum_j \frac{\partial y^c}{\partial A_{ij}^k}. \tag{10.1}$$

To obtain the class-differential localization map in eqn (10.1), GRAD-CAM calculates the gradient (score for class $c$) relative to the feature map $A$ of a convolution layer. These backflowing gradients are pooled into the global mean to obtain significant weights. GRAD-CAM heatmap is a weighted combination of feature maps. A ReLU function needs to be added using eqn (10.2) to perform the classification after the calculation.

$$L_{\text{GRAD-CAM}}^c = \mathrm{Re}\,LU\left(\sum_k \alpha_k^c A^k\right). \tag{10.2}$$

An example of GRAD-CAM structure is shown in Figure 10.6. When Figure 10.6 is examined, GRAD-CAM. When an image or a related class is given as input, the class of the image is determined by special calculations. By propagating back to the rectified convolutional feature maps (blue heatmap), which are combined to calculate the GRAD-CAM localization, the model explains which region should be examined to make a particular decision. Finally, point multiplication with guided backpropagation is performed on the heatmap to obtain both high-resolution and GRAD-CAM-specific visualizations [78–81].

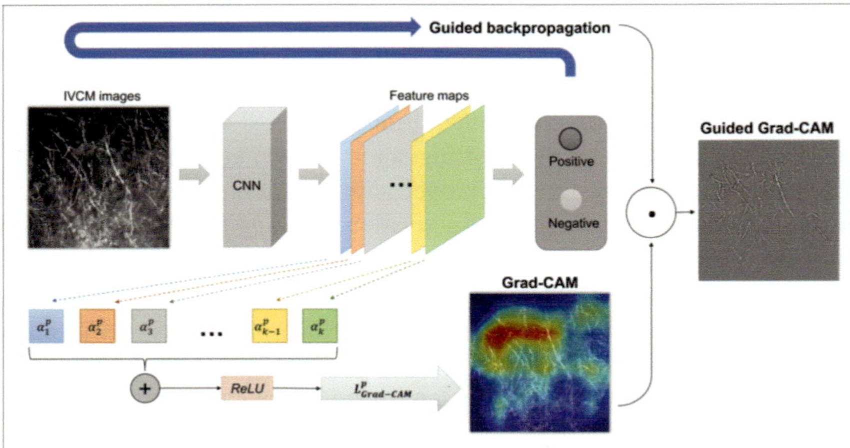


**Figure 10.6** Example of GRAD-CAM model [82].

### 10.4.2 The importance of artificial intelligence and explainable artificial intelligence in dental practices

Artificial intelligence applications in the field of general health services appear in two categories, physical and virtual. Physical applications are represented by complex robots or automated robotic arms, while virtual components are software-type algorithms that support clinical decision-making [83]. A growing link between genes and susceptibility to dental disease can be identified, thanks to the vast amounts of medical and genetic data possessed by nearly everyone born in our time. The process of finding any genetic information and correlation related to the disease in dental diseases are accepted as an irreplaceable prediction regarding the correct diagnosis and treatment. For this reason, it has become a necessity to include computer and artificial intelligence applications in medicine and dentistry [84]. In Table 10.1, research trends prepared in the field of artificial intelligence in the dental field between 2008 and 2019 are given.

Examining Table 10.1, it can be seen that artificial intelligence applications prepared in the field of dentistry increase with a high acceleration value. Because of its powerful capabilities in data analysis, artificial intelligence, a technology that uses machines to mimic intelligent human behavior, has improved the accuracy and effectiveness of dental diagnosis in the clinical setting, providing visualized anatomical guidance for treatment, and post-evaluation by simulating prospective outcomes, and reflecting the occurrence and prognosis of oral diseases. It has an important area of use in medicine [86].

**Table 10.1** Research trends on artificial intelligence in dentistry by years [85].

| **Year** | **2008** | **2010** | **2012** | **2016** | **2017** | **2018** | **2019** |
|---|---|---|---|---|---|---|---|
| Number of studies done | 1 | 1 | 2 | 1 | 5 | 7 | 20 |

While data-driven AI applications analyze the output in a purely computational way, they cannot represent the decision-making process in a medically acceptable way. The lack of interpretability and transparency reflects the black box nature of many machine learning approaches that are not amenable to validation [87]. In medical AI studies, interpretability is important for two reasons. First, ensuring that the algorithm has a reasonable interpretation of medical events is critical to the relationship between technology and humans. Failure to explain the system's internal working structure inevitably undermines practitioners' confidence in the clinical value of AI. Second, the lack of transparency and interpretability makes it difficult to predict errors and generalize specific algorithms for similar cases [88]. As new explainable AI models emerge and are used for dental radiography analysis, it has become more difficult to interpret results and extract broader principles from existing studies. One possible solution to this problem is to adopt an evidence-based paradigm. To understand the role of evidence, there appears to be a need for methods that allow the objective and consistent collection of results across multiple experimental studies in different study disciplines [29]. Experts from different disciplines and scientific fields need to work together to ensure the reliability of artificial intelligence. Only then can meaningful and acceptable standards that ensure the quality of medical AI applications be developed. Also, the need for high-quality tools such as XAI that provides insight into individual predictions, as well as general reasoning of a model, is evident [89].

## 10.5 Academic Studies in the Dentistry

Academic studies in the field of artificial intelligence and explainable artificial intelligence in the dental field are discussed in detail below.

Academic studies in the field of artificial intelligence and explainable artificial intelligence in the dental field are discussed in detail below.

Figueroa et al. used Selvaraju et al.'s GRAD-CAM to integrate explainability into a CNN network for oral cancer diagnosis. In the study, GAIN and a two-stage training process were carried out with data augmentation techniques. The dataset used includes oral images from volunteer patients. Before the data were trained on the GAIN architecture, it was used for transfer learning on VGG19. Then, CNN was trained using GAIN training architecture and classified with attention maps obtained by GRAD-CAM. A success rate of 86.38% was achieved in the validation dataset and 84.84% in the test dataset. As a result, explainability is provided by showing where a CNN focuses most in the input image [90].

Asci et al., in their study, detected and classified dental restorations in panoramic radiographs with artificial intelligence. In the study, 789 panoramic radiographs taken from children aged 12–15 were used for the training of the model. The images used are divided into two groups: filling and root canal treatment. Thanks to the U-Net model used with the PyTorch library, the detection and segmentation of restorative materials are provided. The artificial intelligence performance of the filler group was evaluated with the complex matrix, and the sensitivity, precision, and $F1$ score values were 0.9569, 0.9888, and 0.9726, respectively. When the performance test of the root canal treatment group was performed, the sensitivity, precision, and $F1$ score values were obtained as 0.8450, 1, and 0.9160, respectively [91].

Miki et al., in their study, used the deep convolutional neural network (DCNN) model to classify tooth types in CBCT images. In the study, they trained the DCNN model by randomly separating 42 as training images and 10 as test images from 52 CBCT images to divide the teeth into seven different classes. AlexNet architecture consisting of five convolution layers, three pool layers, and two full link layers is used in the training model. They determined the classification process with an accuracy rate of 88.8% using the training data augmented by image rotation and intensity transformation [92].

Lee et al. used deep CNN algorithms for the detection and diagnosis of dental caries on periapical radiographs. In the study, a pre-trained GoogLeNet Inception v3 CNN network model was used for preprocessing and learning transfer, divided into 3000 periapical radiographic images, 80% (2400) training, and 20% (600) test datasets. According to the evaluations made at the end of the study, the diagnostic accuracy of the models was determined as 89.0% premolar, 88.0% molar, and 82.0% both premolar and molar, respectively. It has been observed that the CNN model used in the study provides a very successful performance in detecting dental caries in periapical radiographs [93].

Ekert et al., in their study, proposed a model that uses deep convolutional neural networks to detect apical lesions on panoramic dental radiographs. The model was trained and validated by using a synthesized dataset of 2001 tooth segments from panoramic radiographs, the prepared seven-layer deep mesh, and group shuffling repeated 10 times. In the evaluation, it was seen that the model successfully detected apical lesions on dental radiographs with an accuracy of 85% [94].

Jaskari et al. tried to detect the mandibular canals on CBCT images in their studies. In the study, a deep learning model that automatically detects the mandibular canals using the fully convolutional network (FCN) model on the dataset containing 637 different CBCT images labeled by radiologists is proposed. As a result of the evaluation of the model, it was observed that the mean curve distance and the mean symmetrical surface distance were successfully obtained as 0.56 and 0.45 mm, respectively [95].

Cejudo et al., in their study, used three different deep learning architectures, namely ResNet, baseline CNN, and CapsNet, to evaluate and classify radiographic images used in dentistry such as panoramic, namely periapical, bitewing, and cephalometric. *K*-fold cross-validation was used to evaluate the performance of deep learning models. They used the GRAD-CAM explainable artificial intelligence (XAI) method to visualize the areas most relevant to classification, helping to understand and interpret the output of the models. Among the models used, the ResNet model showed the best performance. Misclassification results were mostly found in bitewings and periapical classes [96].

Glick et al., in their study, evaluated dental students' performance, competence, and confidence levels in radiographically determining furcation involvement (FI) with and without explainable AI. When the performance between the groups with and without explainable artificial intelligence assistance was evaluated, they determined that there was no statistical difference between the two groups. However, it has been observed that there is a tendency to be wrong ($P < 0.05$) in the answer produced by artificial intelligence for a single question. However, both groups with and without AI predicted that the use of AI would improve clinical decision-making [97].

## 10.6 Conclusion

With the introduction of artificial intelligence applications into our lives, it has started to be used in many applications such as education, health, and defense industry. One of the important areas of use of artificial intelligence applications has been the field of health. In particular, the use of artificial intelligence applications in minimizing human-induced errors has provided great convenience to physicians in the diagnosis and treatment of diseases.

Artificial intelligence applications have been applied in a way to help physicians in many applications, such as identifying diseases in dentistry and implant treatment. In the first stage of the study, brief information about the imaging methods used in dentistry is presented. In the second stage, explanatory information about artificial intelligence and explainable artificial intelligence methods that are frequently used in dental applications are presented. In the last stage of the study, academic studies carried out with artificial intelligence and explainable artificial intelligence applications in dentistry were examined.

In further academic studies, it is aimed to develop software that will guide physicians in diagnosis and treatment by using imaging techniques used in dentistry and artificial intelligence methods that can be explained.

## References

[1] Lin, M.T., Munoz J., Munuz, C.A., Goodacre, C.J., Naylor W.P. (1998) The effect of tooth preparation form on the fit of Procera copings. Int J Prosthodont, 11, 580–590.

[2] Aydıntuğ, Y. S., Şençimen, M., Bayar, G. R., Mutlu, İ. & Bayar A. (2010) Ağız, diş, çene hastalıkları ve cerrahisi polikliniğine başvuran erişkin hastalarda çeşitli sistemik hastalıkların görülme sıklıkları. Gülhane Tıp Dergisi, 52, 7–10.

[3] İçtin E. G. (2013) Dünya Sağlık Örgütü 2003 Dünya Ağız Diş Sağlığı Raporunun Değerlendirilmesi. PhD thesis, Ege Üniversitesi, Diş hekimliği Fakültesi, İzmir.

[4] Marakoğlu, İ., Demirer, A. G. S., Özdemir, U. P. D. & Sezer, H. (2003) Periodontal tedavi öncesi durumluk ve süreklik kaygi düzeyi. Cumhuriyet Üniversitesi Diş Hekimliği Fakültesi Dergisi, 6, 74–9

[5] Kozacıoğlu, G. and Gördürür, H. E. (1995) Bireyden Topluma Ruh Sağlığı. Alfa Basım Yayım Dağıtım

[6] Momeni-Moghaddam, M., Hashemi, C., Fathi, A., and Khamesipour, F. (2022) Diagnostic accuracy, available treatment, and diagnostic methods of dental caries in practice: a meta-analysis. Beni-Suef University Journal of Basic and Applied Sciences, 11(1), 1–11.

[7] Mejàre, I. A., Axelsson, S., Davidson, T., Frisk, F., Hakeberg, M., Kvist, T., and Bergenholtz, G. (2012) Diagnosis of the condition of the dental pulp: a systematic review. International Endodontic Journal, 45(7), 597–613.

[8] Greven, M., Landry, A., & Carmignani, A. (2016) Comprehensive dental diagnosis and treatment planning for occlusal rehabilitation: a perspective. Cranio, 34, 215–217.

[9] Harrel S.K., Nunn M.E. (2001) The Effect of Occlusal Discrepancies on Periodontitis. II. Relationship of Occlusal Treatment to the Progression of Periodontal Disease. J Period, 7, 495–505.

[10] T.M. Graber, R.L. Vanarsdall,(1994) Diagnosis and Treatment Planning in Orthodontics, Orthodontics-Current Principles and Techniques, Mosby-Year Book.

[11] Tugnait, A., and Carmichael, F. (2005) Use of radiographs in the diagnosis of periodontal disease. Dental update, 32(9), 536–542.B.M.

[12] Eley, B.M., and Cox, S.W. (1998) Advances in periodontal diagnosis. 1. Traditional clinical methods of diagnosis. British dental journal, 184(1), 12–16.

[13] Kruse, C., Spin-Neto, R., Reibel, J., Wenzel, A., Kirkevang, L. L. (2017) Diagnostic validity of periapical radiography and CBCT for assessing periapical lesions that persist after endodontic surgery. Dentomaxillofacial Radiology, 46(7), 20170210.

[14] Crow, H. C., Parks, E., Campbell, J. H., Stucki, D. S., Daggy, J. (2005) The utility of panoramic radiography in temporomandibular joint assessment. Dentomaxillofacial Radiology, 34(2), 91–95.

[15] Gupta, A., Devi, P., Srivastava, R., and Jyoti, B. (2014) Intra oral periapical radiography-basics yet intrigue: A review. Bangladesh Journal of Dental Research and Education, 4(2), 83–87.

[16] White, S.C., Heslop, E.W., Hollender, L.G., Mosier, K.M., Ruprecht, A., & Shrout, M.K. (2001) Parameters of radiologic care: An official report of the American Academy of Oral and Maxillofacial Radiology. Oral Surgery, Oral Medicine, Oral Pathology, Oral Radiology, and Endodontology, 91(5), 498–511.

[17] Choi, J.W. (2011) Assessment of panoramic radiography as a national oral examination tool: review of the literature. Imaging science in dentistry. 41(1), 1–6.

[18] Soğur, E., and Baksı, B.G. (2014) Imaging systems used for diagnosis of periodontal pathology Part 2: Alternative Imaging Systems and Image Processing Methods. Ege Universitesi Dis Hekimligi Fakültesi Dergisi, 35(1), 10–18.

[19] Brettle, D.S., Workman, A., Ellwood, R.P., Launders, J.H., Horner, K., and Davies, R.M. (1996) The imaging performance of a storage phosphor system for dental radiography. The British Journal of Radiology, 69(819), 256–261.H.J.

[20] Naoum, H.J., Chandler, N.P., and Love, R.M. (2003) Conventional versus storage phosphor-plate digital images to visualize the root canal system contrasted with a radiopaque medium. Journal of endodontics, 29(5), 349–352.

[21] Ergün, S., and Güneri, P. (2019) Dental dijital görüntülemede üçüncü boyut. Atatürk Üniversitesi Diş Hekimliği Fakültesi Dergisi, 29(1), 133–142.

[22] Evlice, B.K., and Öztunç, H. (2013) Dijital Radyografi ve Diş hekimliğinde İleri Görüntüleme Yöntemleri. Arşiv Kaynak Tarama Dergisi, 22(2), 230–238.
[23] Ludlow, J.B., Timothy, R., Walker, C., Hunter, R., Benavides, E., Samuelson, D. B., and Scheske, M. J. (2015) Effective dose of dental CBCT—a meta analysis of published data and additional data for nine CBCT units. Dentomaxillofacial Radiology, 44(1).
[24] H. Sayın, (2021) Dental implant planlamasında konik ışınlı bilgisayar tomografi verilerini görüntü işleme yöntemleri kullanılarak optimizasyonu ve üç boyutlu yazıcı ile üretimi. PhD thesis, Isparta Uygulamalı Bilimler Üniversitesi, Lisansüstü Eğitim Enstitüsü,Isparta.
[25] Nagi, R., Aravinda, K., Rakesh, N., Gupta, R., Pal, A., and Mann, A. K. (2020) Clinical applications and performance of intelligent systems in dental and maxillofacial radiology: A review. Imaging Science in Dentistry, 50(2), 81..
[26] Khanna, S.S., andDhaimade, P.A. (2017) Artificial intelligence: transforming dentistry today. Indian J Basic Appl Med Res, 6(3), 161–167.
[27] Grischke, J., Johannsmeier, L., Eich, L., Griga, L., and Haddadin, S. (2020) Dentronics: Towards robotics and artificial intelligence in dentistry. Dental Materials, 36(6), 765–778.
[28] Hwang, J.J., Azernikov, S., Efros, A.A., and Yu, S.X. (2018) Learning beyond human expertise with generative models for dental restorations. arXiv preprint arXiv:1804.00064.
[29] Schwendicke, F.A., Samek, W., and Krois, J. (2020) Artificial intelligence in dentistry: chances and challenges. Journal of dental research, 99(7), 769–774.
[30] Egeli, S.S., İşler, Y., (2020) Mini Review on Dental Imaging Devices and Use of Artificial Intelligence in Dentistry. Akıllı Sistemler ve Uygulamaları Dergisi, 3(2), 114–117.
[31] Ambika, D., Narender, S., Rishabh, K., & Rajan, R. J. A. o. D. R. (2012). History of X-Rays in Dentistry. 2(1), 21–25.
[32] Forrai, J. (2007). History of x-ray in dentistry. 3(3), 205–211.
[33] Harorlı, A. (2014). Ağız, Diş Ve Çene Radyolojisi, Nobel Tıp Kitapevi.
[34] 1896'da Wilhelm Rontgen tarafından oluşturulan, eşi Anna Bertha'nın elinin X ışını görüntüsü: Available at: https://www.hekim.net/doktor/page.php?i=view-photo&id=233 [accessed July 13, 2022].
[35] Aslan, N. (2022) Nükleer kimya, Bölüm 1: Radyoaktif elementler. Ankara: İksadyayinevi.
[36] Kurt, H., (2016) Direkt Sistemler, CCD, CMOS, Düz Panel Dedektörler, İndirekt Sistemler, Yarı Direkt Dijital Görüntüleme, Fosfor Plak

Taramaları. *Türkiye Klinikleri J Oral Maxillofac Radiol-Special Topics*, 2, 4–9.

[37] Jayachandran, S. (2017). Digital imaging in dentistry: A review. Contemporary clinical dentistry, 8(2), 193.

[38] Günaydın, Ç., Köklü, A., Cesur, E., Özdiler, O. (2014) Angle Sınıflı Divizyon 1 Tedavisinde Farklı Bir Yaklaşım: Olgu Sunumu. *European Annals of Dental Sciences*, 41(2), 107–114.

[39] Fatima, J., Akram, M. U., Jameel, A., &Syed, A. M. (2021) Spinal vertebrae localization and analysis on disproportionality in curvature using radiography—a comprehensive review. *EURASIP Journal on Image and Video Processing*, 2021(1), 1–23.

[40] Restrepo-Restrepo, F. A., Cañas-Jiménez, S. J., Romero-Albarracín, R. D., Villa-Machado, P. A., Pérez-Cano, M. I., Tobón-Arroyave, S. I. (2019) Prognosis of root canal treatment in teeth with preoperative apical periodontitis: a study with cone-beam computed tomography and digital periapical radiography. *International Endodontic Journal*, 52(11), 1533–1546.

[41] Pan, X., Zhao, Y., Chen, H., Wei, D., Zhao, C., Wei, Z. (2020) Fully automated bone age assessment on large-scale hand X-ray dataset. *International Journal Of Biomedical Imaging*, 2020.

[42] Röntgen Çekiminin Zararı Var mıdır?: Available at:https://www.lifemed.com.tr/blog/rontgen-cekiminin-zarari-var-midir/ [accessed July 13, 2022].

[43] Schendel, S.A., and Lane, C. (2009) 3D orthognathic surgery simulation using image fusion. In Seminars in Orthodontics, 15( 1), 48–56.

[44] Arai Y., Tammisalo E., Iwai, K., Hashimoto, K., Shinoda, K., (1999) Development of a compact computed tomographic apparatus for dental use. Dentomaxillofacial Radiology, 28(4), 245–8.

[45] Orhan, K., Eren H, 2017. *Diş Hekimliğinde Radyolojinin Esasları Konvansiyonelden-Dijitale.* İstanbul Medikal Sağlık ve Yayıncılık Hiz. Tic. Ltd. Şti., 228–230.

[46] Özdede, M, Paksoy C.S. (2019) Konik Işınlı Bilgisayarlı Tomografi: Teknik, Çalışma İlkeleri ve Görüntü Oluşumu. Turkiye Klinikleri Oral and Maxillofacial RadiologySpecial Topics. 5(1),1–6.

[47] Robb, R.A. (1982) Dynamic Spatial Reconstructor: An X-ray Video Fluoroscopic CT scanner for dynamic volume imaging of moving organs. IEEE Trans Med Imaging. 1, 22–3.

[48] Jaffray, D.A., Siewerdsen, J.H. (2000) Cone-beam computed tomography with a flat-panel imager: initial perforamnce characterization. Med Phys. 27,1311–1323.

[49] Luminati, T., and Tagliafico, E. (2014). CBCT systems and imaging technology. In Cone Beam CT and 3D imaging, 1–12.

[50] White, S. C., and Pharoah, M. J. (2018). White and Pharoah's Oral Radiology: Principles and Interpretation. Elsevier Health Sciences.

[51] Harorlı, A. A.M., Dağıstan,(2014) S. Diş Hekimliği Radyolojisi Kitabı. Eser Ofset Matbaacılık.

[52] White, S.C. P.M. (2014)Principles and interpretation. Elsevier Health Sciences.

[53] Scarfe, W.C., Farman, A.G., Sukovic, P.J.J. (2006) Clinical applications of cone-beam computed tomography in dental practice. 72(1), 75.

[54] Samuel, A. L. (1959) Some studies in machine learning using the game of checkers. *IBM Journal of research and development.* 3(3), 210–229.

[55] Langerhuizen, D. W., Janssen, S. J., Mallee, W. H., van den Bekerom, M. P., Ring, D., Kerkhoffs, G. M., and Doornberg, J. N. (2019) What are the applications and limitations of artificial intelligence for fracture detection and classification in orthopaedic trauma imaging? A Systematic Review. *Clinical Orthopaedics and Related Research.* 477(11), 2482–2491. DOI: 10.1097/CORR.0000000000000848.

[56] Shanmuganathan S. (2016) Artificial Neural Network Modelling: An Introduction. *Artificial Neural Network Modelling. Studies in Computational Intelligence.* 628, 1–14. DOI: 10.1007/978-3-319-28495-8_1.

[57] Sen, P. C., Hajra, M., and Ghosh, M. (2020) Supervised Classification Algorithms in Machine Learning: A Survey and Review. *Emerging Technology in Modelling and Graphics.* Singapore: Springer, 99–111. DOI: 10.1007/978-981-13-7403-6_11.

[58] Erickson, B. J., Korfiatis, P., Akkus, Z., and Kline, T. L. (2017) Machine learning for medical imaging. *Radiographics.* 37(2), 505–515. DOI: 10.1148/rg.2017160130.

[59] Kreutzer, R. T., and Sirrenberg, M. (2020) *Understanding Artificial Intelligence.* Springer International Publishing. Switzerland: Springer, DOI: 10.1007/978-3-030-25271-7

[60] Min, S., Lee, B., and Yoon, S. (2017) Deep learning in bioinformatics. *Briefings in bioinformatics.* 18(5), 851–869. DOI: 10.1093/bib/bbw068.

[61] Bronstein, M. M., Bruna, J., LeCun, Y., Szlam, A., and Vandergheynst, P. (2017) Geometric deep learning: going beyond euclidean data. *IEEE Signal Processing Magazine.* 34(4), 18–42. DOI: 10.1109/MSP.2017.2693418.

[62] Doupis, J., Papandreopoulou, V., Glykofridi, S., and Andrianesis, V. (2018) Mobile-Based Artificial Intelligence Significantly Improves

# 11

# Application of Explainable Artificial Intelligence in Drug Discovery and Drug Design

**Najam-ul-Lail[1], Iqra Muzammil[2,*], Muhammad Aamir Naseer[3], Iqra Tabussam[4], Sidra Muzmmal[5] and Aqsa Muzammil[6]**

[1]Department of Pharmacology and Toxicology, University of Veterinary and Animal Sciences, Pakistan
[2]Department of Veterinary Medicine, University of Veterinary and Animal Sciences, Pakistan
[3]Department of Clinical Medicine and Surgery, University of Agriculture, Pakistan
[4]Department of Pathology, University of Agriculture, Pakistan
[5]Department of Biochemistry and Biotechnology, Islamia University, Pakistan
[6]Department of Computer Science, Islamia University, Pakistan
***Corresponding author: Iqra Muzammil**

## Abstract

Drug discovery is the process of introducing a novel drug molecule into medical practice. Drug discovery is a very costly and time-consuming process, and that is why initiatives that contribute to facilitating and accelerating the drug discovery process are of major interest. Artificial intelligence is the investigation of complicated medical data utilizing powerful algorithms and software to replicate human cognition and investigate the relationships between preventive or curative interventions and health outcomes. In recent years, several artificial intelligence (AI) approaches have been effectively used for computer-assisted drug discovery like deep learning (DL), machine learning (ML), and neural networks (NNs). Explainable artificial intelligence (XAI) makes an effort to help researchers comprehend how the model came to a certain conclusion and provide reasons for why the model's response is reasonable. To make the decision-making process transparent,

XAI also offers thorough explanations in addition to the mathematical models. In this chapter, we have outlined the most important artificial intelligence approaches that aid in drug discovery. We have discussed the uses, prospects, and limitations of XAI.

## 11.1 Introduction

### 11.1.1 Drug discovery

Drug development refers to the process of introducing a novel drug molecule into medical practice. It encompasses all phases, from preliminary studies to identifying a promising therapeutic target to extensive phase 3 clinical trials that promote the commercial launch of the drug to studies on pharmaco-surveillance and drug repurposing after the drug has been released [1, 2]. Pharmacological compounds that may evolve into chemotherapeutic drugs are found and put through an extensive testing process as part of the long and expensive drug discovery process. According to estimates, each new treatment that is launched in the market often requires billions of dollars and more than 10 years of labor. While incredible proportions of them fail phase 2, studies account for the greatest number of clinical failures. As a result, initiatives that help facilitate and speed up the drug discovery process are of great interest [3, 4].

The main factors raising the price of drug invention include waste of funding due to failure of the drug in the end phase of the clinical trial, more strict regulations that put a high standard for authorization, and increased cost of tests in clinics, particularly for essential studies. Considering these facts, businesses in the pharmaceutical and biotechnology industries are encouraged to develop and use novel technology to increase production, reduce expenses, and guarantee sustainable development [5, 6].

Considering this, it is not surprising that scientists are looking forward to AI's unmatched data processing ability as a method to speed up and lower the cost of developing new medicines. AI technologies can accelerate the development of new drugs, promote innovation, increase the effectiveness of clinical studies, and regulate the dosage of medications.

### 11.1.2 Explainable artificial intelligence

Explainable artificial intelligence is a set of complex medical data using advanced algorithms and software to simulate human cognition and examine the connections between preventive or curative measures and health outcomes [7].

In many fields, artificial intelligence (AI) is recognized as a successful solution to many problems. But sometimes the method is not well comprehended. There is frequently an atmosphere of mystery – and even anxiety – established about AI. For instance, it is science fiction to predict that computers would "think" autonomously and make judgments that go beyond human logic. Depending on the circumstance, these decisions may be dangerous. Artificial intelligence in computer science refers to several fields [8]. Among them, recent advancements in object recognition and natural language processing have been attributed to deep learning (DL) employing neural networks (NNs), a subfield of machine learning (ML). These developments have significantly increased interest in AI among scientists. Another branch of AI called robotics is a cornerstone of the business and is crucial to scientific lab automation. Furthermore, the natural sciences are starting to investigate professional and ranking algorithms, which are also a component of artificial intelligence. The term AI is typically used interchangeably with deep learning. Deep learning predominates in biological science, particularly in the field of medicinal chemistry and early-stage medicine development [9–11]. In medicine, deep learning is seen to predominate in a variety of therapeutic fields, including radiography and cancer [12–14]. Medical image analysis is a promising growth area for deep learning in medical practice [15].

With Google's Deep Mind Health and IBM Watson Health, AI is influencing the development of whole sectors, including the healthcare sector. It should come as no surprise that the pharmaceutical and biotechnology sector is also aware of the potential benefits of AI and has expressed a strong intention to adopt discovery platforms based on artificial intelligence to optimize real data activities, lowering expenses and timelines for discovery, and enhancing effectiveness [16, 17]. Several pharmaceutical corporations have invested a lot of money in AI technology, whether through stock investments, collaborations with or purchase of AI-focused businesses, internal capacity creation, or a mix of these strategies. Collaborations seem to be centered on accelerating the discovery of new medicines, extending the target universe by identifying new targets, and improving clinical efficacy [18]. Big-tech firms with AI competencies and knowledge, including IBM, Microsoft, Amazon, and Google, are also entering the drug development industry [19]. Public-private projects to revolutionize drug development through data-driven modeling have also been formed, such as the ATOM collaboration (https://atomscience.org). The machine learning and chemo-informatics principles of the past have given rise to the AI technologies employed in drug development today. For instance, there is a long history of using ML to create efficient systems for toxin detection and developing QSAR models (quantitative structure–activity relationship) models [20, 21]. Recent developments in big data, analytic tools, Cloud technology, computational methods development, GPU acceleration, and the democratization of AI toolkits have all contributed to the massive use of these technologies [16].

In recent years, several "artificial intelligence" (AI) approaches have been effectively used for computer-assisted drug discovery [22–24]. Deep learning algorithms, or artificial neural networks with variou processing layers, are largely responsible for this advancement because they can model complicated non-linear input–output interactions and conduct pattern recognition and feature extraction from basic data representations. Certain deep learning models have been found to match or even outperform conventional machine learning and quantitative structure–activity relationship (QSAR) approaches for drug discovery [25, 26]. Deep learning has also increased the potential and widened the use of computer-aided discovery, for instance in protein structure prediction [27], molecular design [28, 29], chemical synthesis planning [30, 31], and macromolecular target identification [32, 33].

Thanks to both the exponential rise in computer power and the advancements in AI techniques, the area of AI, including ML/DL, has shifted from primarily theoretical research to practical applications [34]. Numerous phases of the drug development process have made extensive use of AI to find new targets [35], better understand disease processes [36], and create new biomarkers [37]. To promote research in AI and ML/DL, several pharmaceutical firms have started to invest in tools, technologies, and services, particularly in creating and combining datasets. Many of these datasets come from real-world data (RWD) sources.

The demand for approaches that aid in understanding and interpreting the models will rise, given the rate at which AI is being used in drug development and related domains. To reduce the inability of certain machine learning models to be interpreted, and to improve human thinking and decision-making [38], XAI techniques have gained attention [39, 40].

Explainable artificial intelligence (XAI) attempts to assist researchers in understanding how the model arrived at a certain answer and justification for why the model's response is appropriate [41, 42]. Along with the mathematical models, XAI provides detailed explanations to make the decision-making process visible ("comprehensible") [43], to prevent making accurate forecasts for the wrong motives [43], to prevent unjust prejudice or unethical discrimination [44], and to bridge the gap between the machine learning community and other scientific fields. Effective XAI can also aid researchers in navigating "cognitive valleys" [38], enhancing their understanding and convictions on the process under investigation [45].

There are numerous domain-specific difficulties for future AI-aided drug development, such as the data format provided by such techniques. The selection of the chemical "representation model" limits the amount of chemical information that can be maintained, including pharmacophores, physicochemical characteristics, and functional groups, as well as the amount of information that can be explained and how well the resulting AI model performs [46].

In designing new drugs, we must admit that our knowledge of molecular pathology is limited and that we are unable to create mathematical models of medication action and associated justifications that are accurate. In this situation, XAI has the promise of enhancing human creativity and aptitude for creating innovative bioactive substances with desired qualities [47].

The dilemma of whether the therapeutic activity can be derived from molecular structure, and which components of that structure are significant, characterizes the process of developing novel medications. The added difficulties and occasionally poorly presented issues brought on by multi-objective design lead to frequently compromised molecular structures. The practical strategy is to reduce the number of syntheses and screenings required to discover and improve novel drug candidates, particularly when complex and costly experiments are conducted. Some of these challenges are likely to be addressed by XAI-assisted drug design, which allows for informed action while also taking medicinal chemistry information, model reasoning, and understanding of the system's limitations [48]. XAI will promote communication between medicinal chemists, chemo-informaticians, and data scientists [49, 50].

XAI already makes it possible to mechanistically interpret how drugs work [51, 52], and it helps improve drug safety while also aiding in the planning of organic synthesis [53]. If effective in the long run, explainable artificial intelligence will give critical assistance in the processing and understanding of extremely complicated chemical data, as well as in the creation of new therapeutic hypotheses [54, 55].

In this chapter, we intend to discuss the role of XAI in drug discovery, current research on XAI, and different XAI models used in drug discovery, emphasizing its advantages, limitations, and potential for future drug development (Figures 11.1 and 11.2).

## 11.2 Deep Learning and Machine Learning

AI is influenced by a wide range of fields and combines several technologies, including machine learning (ML), deep learning (DL), and data analytics.

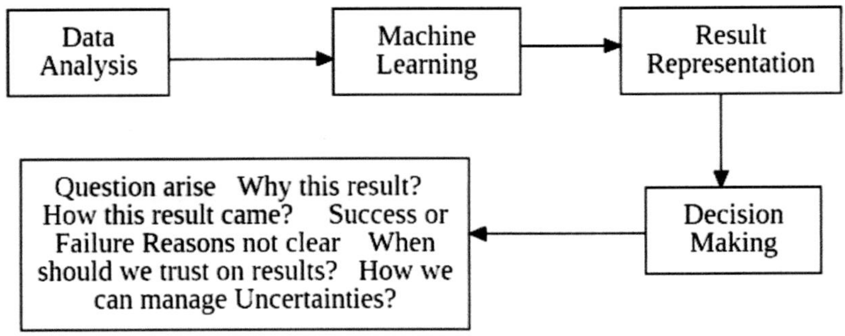


**Figure 11.1** Drug discovery without explainable artificial intelligence.

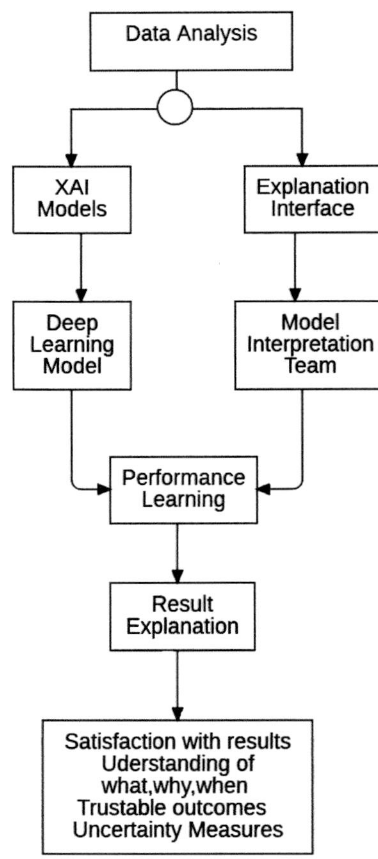


**Figure 11.2** Drug discovery with explainable artificial intelligence.

functioning. Neurosymbolic models integrate statistical and symbolic learning. This combination enables neural networks to make strong predictions, which are reinforced by the transparency offered by the application of logical principles that are comprehensible to people. One of the numerous benefits of employing these neurosymbolic models is the potential for interaction between users and the model throughout the learning process. Moreover, models that explain how things operate are more easily changed if some bias is identified. To find new drugs, these models are currently being applied to knowledge graphs (KGs) [83].

According to Paulheim [84], a KG possesses the qualities of combining data from several areas and specifying real-world entities and their interactions inside a graph, defining classes and relationships between these things in the form of a schema, and allowing entities to be freely connected. Because they are typically obtained from several databases, these data structures are ideally suited for expressing biological information, and KGs are ideal for retaining the semantic link between things. The application of AI models and algorithms to anticipate new relationships between existing entities in KGs has recently shown promising results [85, 86].

#### 11.2.10.1 Neural network characteristics

During the early phases of machine learning, shallow neural networks (NNs) were widely used in drug development. However, over time, alternative techniques like support vector machines, Bayesian modeling, and decision tree methods (random forest, gradient boosting, etc.), as well as other approaches mainly superseded them. This was due to shallow NNs' typical tendency to overfit algorithms to input data as well as their great sensitivity to altering input variables. Then, during the previous 10 years, deep neural networks (DNNs) – second-generation NNs – have drawn more and more attention. DNNs are appealing because they are very flexible computer frameworks [87]. Therefore, alternative DNNs may be explored for various applications, although selecting the best ones is not always simple.

Deep neural networks are very rich in hyperparameters when compared to other ML techniques, and constructing DNN models necessitates a significant amount of expertise, training, and experience. DNNs have not yet been studied as thoroughly as other ML strategies due to the diversity of DNN structures and their numerous parameters. In light of this, DL is not a strategy that is easily understandable by non-experts even if public domain software is accessible for building DNNs. There is a significant gap between the technicalities of the proposed model, which may be managed by less skilled users, and analysis of outcomes and the identification of possible cautions or model flaws, which take considerably more skills. Furthermore, DNNs have the famous "black box" aspect, which means that it is not clear how these models arrive at their judgments, comparable to other ML approaches, though not all of them [88].

#### 11.2.10.2 Graph neural networks

Graph neural network (GNN) principles such as estimation of structural features and de novo molecular production have been effectively used for drug discovery tasks in recent years [89, 90]. In comparison to current ML and quantitative structure–activity relationship (QSAR) approaches for therapeutic development, many graph neural network models have been found to produce more encouraging outcomes [91, 92]. This development is largely attributable to graph neural networks' capability to accurately simulate molecular graph data. With high-quality labeled data, GNN can develop improved molecular representations, which might eventually replace the depictions of handmade molecular fingerprints made 10 years ago. Despite their potential, graph neural networks have seen little success in drug development, in part because these models are sometimes referred to as "black boxes" [93].

There have been attempts to increase model comprehensibility based on model simplifications, feature sub-selection, or awareness [94, 95]; however, this problem is made worse by the fact that these models frequently produce the right answers for the wrong reasons [96]. Given the speed at which AI drugs are being discovered, there will be a greater need for interpretability techniques that enable humans to comprehend and interpret GNN models. So, the secret to accelerating drug discovery with graph neural networks may be a highly accurate and mechanically interpretable model. XAI methods might aid in the creation of graph neural networks in drug discovery applications, particularly for property prediction tasks, by quantifying the chemical substructures that are crucial for a specific prediction and describing how reliable a prediction is [93].

One method for measuring interpretability is feature attribution, which quantifies the significance of a feature concerning a model's ability to predict a target trait. Drug development is one area where attribution methods have been researched. For instance, McCloskey [97] created an attribution approach to check whether each model trained on protein–ligand binding data accurately learns the related binding logic. To evaluate the interpretability of GNN models in molecular property predictions, Jiménez-Luna [98] developed an integrated gradient (IG) feature attribution approach. Additionally, the exploration of the interpretability of models trained using graph convolution architecture in the domains of drug discovery is not surprising, given the development of graph neural networks. For example, Jin [99] used a Monte Carlo tree search with a property predictor to identify molecular substructures that are primarily accountable for each feature of interest.

Yu [100] introduced a framework of graph information bottleneck (GIB) for subgraph identification, which could identify a compressed subgraph with little information loss in terms of predicting chemical attributes. These techniques, which may be thought of as subgraph identification techniques, are interested in discovering the substructures that primarily reflect specific molecular features indirectly. As previously stated, various attempts have been made to overcome the basic shortcoming of deep learning systems, which is a lack of causal comprehension. Unfortunately, the quality and assessment of model interpretations are difficult to assess since obtaining ground truth sub-structures or attributes necessitates costly wet experimentation and subjective expert opinion.

Although Sanchez-Lengeling et al. [101] created an open-source synthetic benchmarking suite for attribution techniques using GNNs, the synthetic tasks were designed to distinguish basic subgraphs such as benzene from chemicals. Good XAI should expose more sophisticated facts to scientists and help them make decisions. In the case of toxicity prediction, for instance, there are sometimes hundreds of pieces responsible for certain toxicity, and some even need to be addressed in the context of many situations. Additionally, there is a class of molecular pairings known as "property cliffs" that have identical structures but very different properties. Such complex and realistic circumstances will present XAI with additional difficulties and opportunities [102].

### 11.2.11 Advances in XAI

Practical uses of DL in medicinal chemistry and drug development are still uncommon at the moment. Ultimately, the inclusion of DL in transdisciplinary research will depend on how significantly it affects experimental programs. This can be done by drastically lowering the design-test-make-analyze (DMTA) cycle times or by significantly advancing the discovery or production of molecules or biological agents with newer and better bioactivities, more controlled chemical probes, or innovative pharmaceutical candidates. Importantly, demonstrable progress in establishing DL in transdisciplinary contexts is only achievable if drug development practitioners agree to use predictions for experimental design. This will require much more model adoption in transdisciplinary contexts compared to the existing state. As with any new technology, it will take some time for DL to reach its maximum

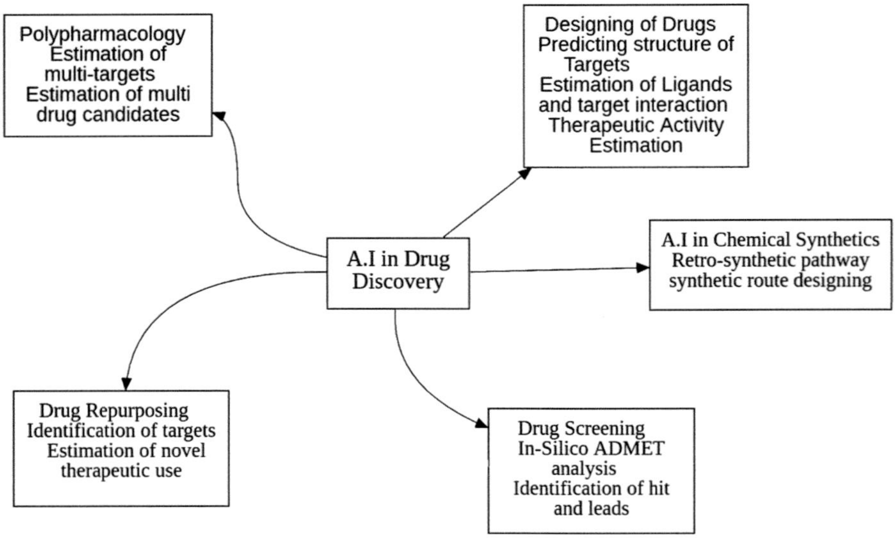


**Figure 11.4** Uses of explainable artificial intelligence in drug discovery.

potential in this regard. To further boost the trust of experimentalists in prediction models, several prerequisites must be addressed [103].

Naturally, researchers are hesitant to rely on hypotheses that are obscure or illogical. This poses a significant obstacle to the acceptability of advanced deep learning models for experiments considering the black box aspect of DNNs. To create predictions that can be rationalized and understood in terms of chemistry or biology, model-agnostic techniques for XAI are receiving more and more attention [104]. These techniques are feature weighting or specific methods to find representation characteristics that are most important for each specific estimation or other methods that establish feature subsets that are necessary to make valid (or incorrect) estimations (Figure 11.4). Such feature subsets may define structural patterns in medicinal chemistry that may be understood when mapped to test molecules [105].

### 11.2.12 Different XAI approaches that aid in drug discovery

#### 11.2.12.1 Instance-based methods

Instance-based techniques calculate a subgroup of pertinent attributes that should exist to keep (or alter) a given model's prediction. Instance-based techniques might be helpful in drug development to improve model transparency by identifying which chemical properties must be present or missing to ensure or alter the model prediction. For chemists, hypothetical reasoning also fosters informativeness by presenting possible new knowledge about the model and the data.

Instance-based methods can show promising results in various aspects of de novo drug design, according to the authors, including activity cliff prediction, which can better locate minute structural alterations that lead to huge biochemical alterations, fragment-based virtual screening, which highlights the smallest subcategory of atoms held to account for a given action, and hit-to-lead optimization, which can quickly find the very little structural change necessary to improve one molecule [93].

#### 11.2.12.2 Feature attribution methods

In recent years, feature attribution approaches including (gradient-based, perturbation-based, and surrogate model) have become the most widely employed XAI family of tools for ligand- and structure-based drug development. McCloskey [97] used gradient-based attribution to identify ligand pharmacophores necessary for affinity. Pope et al. [106] used gradient-based feature attribution to identify key functional groupings for adverse impact prediction [107]. SHAP was recently utilized to assess important aspects for the prediction of chemical strength and activities of combination therapy[108, 109].

It is advised to use understandable molecular markers or presentations for model development when using feature attribution methodologies. Simplified molecular input line entry systems (SMILES) [110] strings have recently been broken down into parts that are important for therapeutic potential or chemical and physical properties [111] using configurations taken from the field of natural language processing, such as long short-term memory networks and transformers [95, 112]. Depending on characterizations (atom and bond types, and molecular connectivity), these methods represent an initial effort to make the connection between the deep learning and medicinal chemistry communities. These depictions have direct chemical meaning and do not require subsequent descriptor-to-molecule decoding [110].

#### 11.2.12.3 Graph convolution networks

Molecular graphs are a natural mathematical depiction of molecular topology, with nodes representing atoms and edges reflecting chemical bonds. The structural information may be encoded to describe the relationships between entities and provide more insightful models of the data by presenting the data as graphs. Since the late 1970s [112], their use in mathematical chemistry and chemo-informatics has become widespread. Graph convolutions have been used in drug discovery to predict chemical properties [113] and in creating models for de novo drug design [99]. Currently, one of the most prominent research areas is investigating the interpretability of models trained using graph convolution architectures.

- Subgraph identification techniques seek to identify one or more portions of a graph that are accountable for a particular prediction.
- Attention mechanisms, which are taken from the field of natural language processing, can help with the interpretation of graph convolutional neural networks [114].

Graph convolution-based approaches are a significant tool in drug discovery because of their quick and natural relationship with chemists' intuitive representations (that is, chemical graphs and subgraphs). Additionally, when paired with mechanistic information, the ability to highlight atoms that are pertinent to a certain prediction can enhance a model's justification (i.e., clarify if an answer is acceptable) and its comprehensibility in the biochemical processes. Furthermore, solubility, polarity, synthetic accessibility, and photovoltaic efficiency have all been predicted using attention-based graph convolutional neural networks, among other attributes, which led to the discovery of pertinent chemical substructures for the desired attributes [115, 116]. In addition, attention-based graph approaches have been applied for the prediction of chemical reactivity, highlighting structural patterns that are in line with a chemist's intuition in the selection of appropriate reaction partners and activating agents [117].

#### 11.2.12.4 Ligand-based approaches

Ligand-based methods employ data obtained from samples and compounds whose bioactivity and relevant physical and chemical properties have to be estimated. Structural identifiers are typically utilized as signals to build models that connect chemical structure with bioactivity. In deep learning, graph neural networks are used for the graphical presentation of molecules [57].

Unterthiner et al. [118] used Tox21 Data Challenge to train a DNN to estimate various distinct binary hazardous effects associated with nuclear sensors and routes for responding to stress. Xu et al. [119] utilized undirected graph recursive neural networks to predict drug-induced liver damage. Individual models and database combinations were created using the datasets. The combined model performed better than the individual models, and the model created using a benchmark dataset forecasted more accurately than the original model. Moreover, the scientists compared DL to a typical neural network (NN), and the first strategy outperformed NN.

#### 11.2.12.5 Structure-based approaches

Structure-based procedures take data from the specimens and their molecular targets (such as receptors, enzymes, and other structural or functional proteins). Structure-based techniques can employ communication patterns (atomic pairings of ligand–target interactions) and/or ML scoring systems to classify the data as active or inactive [57].

This method was demonstrated by Wallach et al. [79], who built DL algorithms utilizing DUD-E, ChEMBL-20, and an internal variant of ChEMBL-20 that uses empirically inert chemicals. These algorithms were created by inserting characteristics from ligand–target interactions, like the presence of specific kinds of atoms and chemical bonds, into nodes of a 20 Å cubic box with its center at the binding site for the target. These networks were created using a convolution 3D layer approach that performed better in enrichment validations than the Smina scoring function (AutoDock Vina's optimized scoring version).

#### 11.2.12.6 Ligand–target interaction estimation

The main goal of this estimation is to determine the samples' (ligands') degree of affinity for a certain target molecule.

DBN models were created by [80] to estimate drug–target interactions. The extended connectivity fingerprints (ECFP) and protein sequence composition descriptors (PSC) were utilized as input characteristics to define compounds and targets, respectively.

#### 11.2.12.7 In silico ADMET analysis

The pharmaceutical industry underwent a paradigm change once it was discovered that the bad pharmacological activities of potential therapeutic agents were a significant factor in clinical failure in the late 1990s [120].

The goal of in silico ADMET modeling is to aid working groups in the choice and design of new molecules with better ADMET (absorption, distribution, metabolism, excretion, toxicity) properties and the allocation of experimental resources to the most beneficial compounds, thereby minimizing the total amount of substances that must be produced and recognized [121, 122]. In silico ADMET modeling changed from employing Bayesian neural networks, RFs, and SVMs to ML-based prediction models due to the development of ML algorithms and the accessibility of huge homogeneous ADMET data. These machine learning systems can accurately forecast endpoints with complicated non-linear relationships. After the 2012 Kaggle "Merck Molecular Activity Challenge," DNN techniques have become increasingly popular for simulating ADMET endpoints. The objective of the

Kaggle competition was to test the accuracy of ML algorithms in predicting 18 distinct ADMET endpoints using Merck proprietary datasets with a range of sizes (2000–50,000 molecules). The winning submission made use of an ensemble strategy that included the Gaussian process (GP), gradient-boosting machine (GBM), and DNN regression techniques [123].

DNNs have the unique capability to concurrently train neural networks that incorporate many endpoints into a single model. Multitask deep neural networks train datasets relevant to several ADMET endpoints and merge those in one model using an inductive transfer learning method. Multitask DNNs are designed to share their representation internally, which enables quicker learning and increased model accuracy [124]. The majority of multitask DNNs used to model ADMET endpoints employ a "Hard" parameter-sharing strategy, which denotes that all of the activities share the invisible layer [125].

Matched molecular pair (MMP) analysis is described as comparing two molecules that vary solely by a properly specified interference that corresponds to a difference in a property value [126]. In the past, one-to-one structural transformation frequency was examined in MMP analysis. It is now possible to do automated MMP analysis on big datasets because of developments in AI and molecular fragmentation algorithms. MCPairs is a remarkable application that employs an unsupervised ML technique to collect in vitro ADMET data from three distinct pharmaceutical firms (AstraZeneca, Genentech, and Roche). The application of artificial intelligence and the accessibility of enormous data aid in the development of next-generation MMP technologies that provide real answers to ADMET difficulties through explainable AI [127].

#### 11.2.12.8 Computer-aided synthesis planning

The invention of computer-aided synthetic planning (CASP) may be traced to the ground-breaking work of Corey [128], who, in the late 1960s, defined the idea of "retrosynthetic analysis." Retrosynthetic analysis is a method that includes consecutive disconnections and functional group interconversions to break down a target molecule into its basic, easily accessible basic components [128]. CASP software helps synthetic organic chemists choose the most effective and economical synthesis method by using the concept of retrosynthetic analysis [31, 129]. The discipline of computer-aided synthesis planning and technical advancements has been revived by the usage of AI [31, 130]. By suggesting workable synthetic pathways, AI-assisted synthesis planning tools aid chemists in enhancing their understanding of synthetic chemistry. Additionally, they aid chemists in making wiser choices, increasing productivity and efficiency by lowering synthesis failures. In the end, this speeds up the DMTA cycle's "create" step of the drug development process [131].

The two main kinds of computer-aided synthetic route-planning strategies are template-free approaches and rule- or template-based methods. Rule-based approaches offer synthetic pathways by using expert-coded rules and assumptions collected from response databases and literature. The response rules are manually retrieved and defined in rule-based methodologies. Synthia is one such example of retrosynthetic software that employs a database of expert-encoded rules for the planning of chemical synthesis (formerly Chematica). Such rule-based approaches have many drawbacks, including a knowledge base that is not fully covered and an inability to scale with the exponential increase of the chemical literature.

Template-free approaches are inspired by natural language processing (NLP) and treat forward or retrosynthetic prediction as a neural machine translation issue [132]. The sequence-to-sequence (Seq-2-Seq) model was the first template-free model for retrosynthetic analysis suggested by Liu and colleagues [133]. The usage of a graph, chemical reaction networks, and similarity-based algorithms are some other template-free techniques that have reportedly also shown promising outcomes [134]. Although artificial intelligence has shown considerable promise in expediting synthetic organic chemistry, there is still a need for advancements in different aspects [135].

#### 11.2.12.9 Self-explanation based approaches

The XAI techniques that have been discovered so far help in the interpretation of deep learning models. Although it has been demonstrated that such post hoc interpretations are helpful, some contend that ideal XAI systems should automatically provide a human-interpretable explanation in addition to their predictions [136]. Self-explanatory techniques would encourage verification and error analysis while also being directly linked to domain knowledge. Natural language explanation, prototype-based reasoning, self-explaining neural networks, human interpretable ideas, and concept activation vectors are examples of self-explanatory methodologies [137].

Interpretability by design might aid in bridging the gap between computer representation and human comprehension of certain drug development difficulties. For example, prototype reasoning has potential in the modeling of diverse collections of compounds with distinct modes of action, allowing both mechanistic interpretability and prediction accuracy to be preserved. Explanation-generation methodologies may be useful in some decision-making processes, such as the substitution of animal experimentation and in vitro to in vivo propagation, where explanations that human can understand are critical [93].

#### 11.2.12.10 Uncertainty predictions

These XAI methodologies are closely connected to techniques that measure the uncertainty of predictions. Getting uncertainty estimates increases model acceptability for planning experiments and increases trust in predictive modeling. However, certain ML techniques, such as Gaussian process modeling [138], give intrinsic prediction limitations, but most ML/DL techniques, including DNNs, give the predictions without any estimation of uncertainty. Probabilistic and ensemble approaches are methods for estimating prediction error that complements ML/DL [139, 140]. The latter techniques calculate prediction variability using different trained models produced by the same algorithm. The Bayesian DNNs offer an excellent illustration of probabilistic techniques. But Bayesian DNNs can only be used with big datasets if approximations are used because of their computing costs [139].

### 11.2.13 Limitations of XAI in drug discovery

Artificial intelligence technology encounters many difficulties especially in justifications and techniques to complete a task [141]. The majority of methods cannot be used immediately but need to be customized for each unique application. A thorough understanding of the issue is also essential for determining which model outcomes require further reasoning, and which sort of outputs are beneficial to the user [142]. In drug development, deep learning models are difficult to understand completely; however, the given insights can be helpful to the researcher [47]. It will be necessary to carefully plan a series of control studies to evaluate the hypothesis given by computer systems and strengthen their dependability and objectivity while aiming for interpretations that mimic human intuition [49].

## 11.3 Conclusion

The use of artificial intelligence offers significant potential for reducing the expense and time of therapeutic research. Even though artificial intelligence is not a fix-all for all issues in pharmaceutical research, it is undeniably a useful tool when used appropriately with correct knowledge. Artificial intelligence technology encounters many difficulties especially in justifications and techniques to complete a task. To improve the process in terms of clinical significance and cost reduction, it will be necessary to investigate how computational and reasoning techniques might be used. Achieving these objectives, artificial intelligence techniques have a lot of potential, but their effectiveness will rely on matching the correct technology with the relevant issue.

## References

[1] S. Decker and E. A. Sausville, "Drug Discovery," *Princ. Clin. Pharmacol.*, pp. 439–447, 2007, doi: 10.1016/B978-012369417-1/50068-7.
[2] L. McLean, "Drug development," *Rheumatol. Sixth Ed.*, vol. 1–2, pp. 395–400, 2015, doi: 10.1016/B978-0-323-09138-1.00049-8.
[3] S. M. Paul *et al.*, "How to improve R&D productivity: the pharmaceutical industry's grand challenge," *Nat. Rev. Drug Discov.*, vol. 9, no. 3, pp. 203–214, 2010, doi: 10.1038/nrd3078.
[4] T. J. Moore, H. Zhang, G. Anderson, and G. C. Alexander, "Estimated Costs of Pivotal Trials for Novel Therapeutic Agents Approved by the US Food and Drug Administration, 2015-2016," *JAMA Intern. Med.*, vol. 178, no. 11, pp. 1451–1457, Nov. 2018, doi: 10.1001/jamainternmed.2018.3931.
[5] O. J. Wouters, M. McKee, and J. Luyten, "Research and Development Costs of New Drugs—Reply," *JAMA*, vol. 324, no. 5, p. 518, 2020.
[6] A. Mullard, "2020 FDA drug approvals.," *Nat. Rev. Drug Discov.*, vol. 20, no. 2, pp. 85–91, 2021.
[7] F. Jiang *et al.*, "Artificial intelligence in healthcare: Past, present and future," *Stroke Vasc. Neurol.*, vol. 2, no. 4, pp. 230–243, 2017, doi: 10.1136/svn-2017-000101.
[8] W. J. Rapaport, "What is artificial intelligence?," *J. Artif. Gen. Intell.*, vol. 11, no. 2, pp. 52–56, 2020.
[9] S. Yu and J. Ma, "Deep learning for denoising," *Nature*, vol. 554, no. 7690, pp. 461–464, 2018, doi: 10.1190/igc2018-113.
[10] M. L. Leite *et al.*, "Artificial intelligence and the future of life sciences," *Drug Discov. Today*, vol. 26, no. 11, pp. 2515–2526, 2021.
[11] J. Bajorath, "State-of-the-art of artificial intelligence in medicinal chemistry," *Future Science OA*, vol. 7, no. 6. Future Science, p. FSO702, 2021. doi: 10.2144/fsoa-2021-0030.
[12] F. Wang, L. P. Casalino, and D. Khullar, "Deep Learning in Medicine - Promise, Progress, and Challenges," *JAMA Intern. Med.*, vol. 179, no. 3, pp. 293–294, 2019, doi: 10.1001/jamainternmed.2018.7117.
[13] A. Hosny, C. Parmar, J. Quackenbush, L. H. Schwartz, and H. J. W. L. Aerts, "Artificial intelligence in radiology," *Nat. Rev. Cancer*, vol. 18, no. 8, pp. 500–510, 2018.

[14] E. Farina, J. J. Nabhen, M. I. Dacoregio, F. Batalini, and F. Y. Moraes, "An overview of artificial intelligence in oncology," *Futur. Sci. OA*, vol. 8, no. 4, p. FSO787, 2022, doi: 10.2144/fsoa-2021-0074.
[15] D. Shen, G. Wu, and H.-I. Suk, "Deep learning in medical image analysis," *Annu. Rev. Biomed. Eng.*, vol. 19, p. 221, 2017.
[16] N. Fleming, "How artificial intelligence is changing drug discovery," *Nature*, vol. 557, no. 7706, pp. S55–S55, 2018.
[17] P. Schneider *et al.*, "Rethinking drug design in the artificial intelligence era," *Nat. Rev. Drug Discov.*, vol. 19, no. 5, pp. 353–364, 2020.
[18] F. Properzi, M. Steedman, K. Taylor, H. Ronte, and J. Haughey, "Intelligent drug discovery powered by AI," *Deloitte Insights*, pp. 1–38, 2019.
[19] A. Schuhmacher, A. Gatto, M. Kuss, O. Gassmann, and M. Hinder, "Big Techs and startups in pharmaceutical R&D–A 2020 perspective on artificial intelligence," *Drug Discov. Today*, vol. 26, no. 10, pp. 2226–2231, 2021.
[20] T. Aoyama, Y. Suzuki, and H. Ichikawa, "Neural networks applied to pharmaceutical problems. III. Neural networks applied to quantitative structure-activity relationship (QSAR) analysis," *J. Med. Chem.*, vol. 33, no. 9, pp. 2583–2590, 1990.
[21] D. E. Klingler, "Expert systems in the pharmaceutical industry," *Drug Inf. J.*, vol. 22, no. 2, pp. 249–258, 1988.
[22] E. Gawehn, J. A. Hiss, and G. Schneider, "Deep learning in drug discovery," *Mol. Inform.*, vol. 35, no. 1, pp. 3–14, 2016.
[23] E. A. Ashour *et al.*, "Impacts of green coffee powder supplementation on growth performance, carcass characteristics, blood indices, meat quality and gut microbial load in broilers," *Agric.*, vol. 10, no. 10, pp. 1–19, 2020, doi: 10.3390/agriculture10100457.
[24] E. N. Muratov *et al.*, "QSAR without borders," *Chem. Soc. Rev.*, vol. 49, no. 11, pp. 3525–3564, 2020.
[25] E. B. Lenselink *et al.*, "Beyond the hype: deep neural networks outperform established methods using a ChEMBL bioactivity benchmark set," *J. Cheminform.*, vol. 9, no. 1, pp. 1–14, 2017.
[26] G. B. Goh, C. Siegel, A. Vishnu, N. O. Hodas, and N. Baker, "Chemception: a deep neural network with minimal chemistry knowledge matches the performance of expert-developed QSAR/QSPR models," *arXiv Prepr. arXiv1706.06689*, 2017.
[27] A. W. Senior *et al.*, "Improved protein structure prediction using potentials from deep learning," *Nature*, vol. 577, no. 7792, pp. 706–710, 2020.
[28] D. Merk, L. Friedrich, F. Grisoni, and G. Schneider, "De novo design of bioactive small molecules by artificial intelligence," *Mol. Inform.*, vol. 37, no. 1–2, p. 1700153, 2018.

[80] M. Wen *et al.*, "Deep-learning-based drug–target interaction prediction," *J. Proteome Res.*, vol. 16, no. 4, pp. 1401–1409, 2017.

[81] S. J. Capuzzi, R. Politi, O. Isayev, S. Farag, and A. Tropsha, "QSAR modeling of Tox21 challenge stress response and nuclear receptor signaling toxicity assays," *Front. Environ. Sci.*, vol. 4, p. 3, 2016.

[82] Y. Zhang, T. Ye, H. Xi, M. Juhas, and J. Li, "Deep learning driven drug discovery: tackling severe acute respiratory syndrome coronavirus 2," *Front. Microbiol.*, vol. 12, 2021.

[83] R. Das *et al.*, "Go for a walk and arrive at the answer: Reasoning over paths in knowledge bases using reinforcement learning," *arXiv Prepr. arXiv1711.05851*, 2017.

[84] H. Paulheim, "Knowledge graph refinement: A survey of approaches and evaluation methods," *Semant. Web*, vol. 8, no. 3, pp. 489–508, 2017.

[85] D. S. Himmelstein *et al.*, "Systematic integration of biomedical knowledge prioritizes drugs for repurposing," *Elife*, vol. 6, p. e26726, 2017.

[86] R. Zhang, D. Hristovski, D. Schutte, A. Kastrin, M. Fiszman, and H. Kilicoglu, "Drug repurposing for COVID-19 via knowledge graph completion," *J. Biomed. Inform.*, vol. 115, p. 103696, 2021.

[87] F. Van Veen and S. Leijnen, "The neural network zoo," *Asimov Inst.*, 2016.

[88] D. Castelvecchi, "Can we open the black box of AI?," *Nat. News*, vol. 538, no. 7623, p. 20, 2016.

[89] J. Gilmer, S. S. Schoenholz, P. F. Riley, O. Vinyals, and G. E. Dahl, "Neural message passing for quantum chemistry," in *International conference on machine learning*, 2017, pp. 1263–1272.

[90] K. Yang *et al.*, "Analyzing learned molecular representations for property prediction," *J. Chem. Inf. Model.*, vol. 59, no. 8, pp. 3370–3388, 2019.

[91] Z. Xiong *et al.*, "Pushing the boundaries of molecular representation for drug discovery with the graph attention mechanism," *J. Med. Chem.*, vol. 63, no. 16, pp. 8749–8760, 2019.

[92] Y. Song, S. Zheng, Z. Niu, Z.-H. Fu, Y. Lu, and Y. Yang, "Communicative Representation Learning on Attributed Molecular Graphs.," in *IJCAI*, 2020, vol. 2020, pp. 2831–2838.

[93] J. Jiménez-Luna, F. Grisoni, and G. Schneider, "Drug discovery with explainable artificial intelligence," *Nat. Mach. Intell.*, vol. 2, no. 10, pp. 573–584, 2020.

[94] A. Shrikumar, P. Greenside, and A. Kundaje, "Learning important features through propagating activation differences," in *International conference on machine learning*, 2017, pp. 3145–3153.

[95] A. Vaswani *et al.*, "Attention is all you need," *Adv. Neural Inf. Process. Syst.*, vol. 30, 2017.

[96] S. Lapuschkin, S. Wäldchen, A. Binder, G. Montavon, W. Samek, and K.-R. Müller, "Unmasking Clever Hans predictors and assessing what machines really learn," *Nat. Commun.*, vol. 10, no. 1, pp. 1–8, 2019.

[97] K. McCloskey, A. Taly, F. Monti, M. P. Brenner, and L. J. Colwell, "Using attribution to decode binding mechanism in neural network models for chemistry," *Proc. Natl. Acad. Sci.*, vol. 116, no. 24, pp. 11624–11629, 2019.

[98] J. Jiménez-Luna, F. Grisoni, N. Weskamp, and G. Schneider, "Artificial intelligence in drug discovery: Recent advances and future perspectives," *Expert Opin. Drug Discov.*, vol. 16, no. 9, pp. 949–959, 2021.

[99] W. Jin, R. Barzilay, and T. Jaakkola, "Junction tree variational autoencoder for molecular graph generation," *35th Int. Conf. Mach. Learn. ICML 2018*, vol. 5, pp. 3632–3648, 2018.

[100] J. Yu, J. Cao, and R. He, "Improving subgraph recognition with variational graph information bottleneck," in *Proceedings of the IEEE/CVF Conference on Computer Vision and Pattern Recognition*, 2022, pp. 19396–19405.

[101] B. Sanchez-Lengeling *et al.*, "Evaluating attribution for graph neural networks," *Adv. Neural Inf. Process. Syst.*, vol. 33, pp. 5898–5910, 2020.

[102] D. Stumpfe, Y. Hu, D. Dimova, and J. Bajorath, "Recent progress in understanding activity cliffs and their utility in medicinal chemistry: miniperspective," *J. Med. Chem.*, vol. 57, no. 1, pp. 18–28, 2014.

[103] J. Bajorath, S. Kearnes, W. P. Walters, N. A. Meanwell, G. I. Georg, and S. Wang, "Artificial intelligence in drug discovery: into the great wide open," *Journal of medicinal chemistry*, vol. 63, no. 16. ACS Publications, pp. 8651–8652, 2020.

[104] P. Linardatos, V. Papastefanopoulos, and S. Kotsiantis, "Explainable ai: A review of machine learning interpretability methods," *Entropy*, vol. 23, no. 1, p. 18, 2020.

[105] R. Rodríguez-Pérez and J. Bajorath, "Explainable Machine Learning for Property Predictions in Compound Optimization," *J. Med. Chem.*, vol. 64, no. 24, pp. 17744–17752, 2021, doi: 10.1021/acs.jmedchem.1c01789.

[106] P. E. Pope, S. Kolouri, M. Rostami, C. E. Martin, and H. Hoffmann, "Explainability methods for graph convolutional neural networks," in *Proceedings of the IEEE/CVF Conference on Computer Vision and Pattern Recognition*, 2019, pp. 10772–10781.

[107] R. R. Tice, C. P. Austin, R. J. Kavlock, and J. R. Bucher, "Improving the human hazard characterization of chemicals: a Tox21 update," *Environ. Health Perspect.*, vol. 121, no. 7, pp. 756–765, 2013.

[108] S. M. Lundberg and S.-I. Lee, "A unified approach to interpreting model predictions," *Adv. Neural Inf. Process. Syst.*, vol. 30, 2017.

[109] R. Rodríguez-Pérez and J. Bajorath, "Interpretation of compound activity predictions from complex machine learning models using local approximations and shapley values," *J. Med. Chem.*, vol. 63, no. 16, pp. 8761–8777, 2019.

[110] D. Weininger, "SMILES, a chemical language and information system. 1. Introduction to methodology and encoding rules," *J. Chem. Inf. Comput. Sci.*, vol. 28, no. 1, pp. 31–36, 1988.

[111] F. Grisoni and G. Schneider, "De novo molecular design with generative long short-term memory," *Chim. Int. J. Chem.*, vol. 73, no. 12, pp. 1006–1011, 2019.

[112] S. Hochreiter and J. Schmidhuber, "Long short-term memory," *Neural Comput.*, vol. 9, no. 8, pp. 1735–1780, 1997.

[113] S. Kearnes, K. McCloskey, M. Berndl, V. Pande, and P. Riley, "Molecular graph convolutions: moving beyond fingerprints," *J. Comput. Aided. Mol. Des.*, vol. 30, no. 8, pp. 595–608, 2016.

[114] P. Veličković, G. Cucurull, A. Casanova, A. Romero, P. Lio, and Y. Bengio, "Graph attention networks," *arXiv Prepr. arXiv1710.10903*, 2017.

[115] C. Shang *et al.*, "Edge attention-based multi-relational graph convolutional networks," *arXiv Prepr. arXiv 1802.04944*, 2018.

[116] S. Ryu, J. Lim, S. H. Hong, and W. Y. Kim, "Deeply learning molecular structure-property relationships using attention-and gate-augmented graph convolutional network," *arXiv Prepr. arXiv1805.10988*, 2018.

[117] C. W. Coley *et al.*, "A graph-convolutional neural network model for the prediction of chemical reactivity," *Chem. Sci.*, vol. 10, no. 2, pp. 370–377, 2019.

[118] T. Unterthiner, A. Mayr, G. Klambauer, and S. Hochreiter, "Toxicity prediction using deep learning," *arXiv Prepr. arXiv1503.01445*, 2015.

[119] Y. Xu, Z. Dai, F. Chen, S. Gao, J. Pei, and L. Lai, "Deep learning for drug-induced liver injury," *J. Chem. Inf. Model.*, vol. 55, no. 10, pp. 2085–2093, 2015.

[120] I. Kola and J. Landis, "Can the pharmaceutical industry reduce attrition rates?," *Nat. Rev. Drug Discov.*, vol. 3, no. 8, pp. 711–716, 2004.

[121] H. Van De Waterbeemd and E. Gifford, "ADMET in silico modelling: towards prediction paradise?," *Nat. Rev. Drug Discov.*, vol. 2, no. 3, pp. 192–204, 2003.

[122] F. Lombardo *et al.*, "In Silico absorption, distribution, metabolism, excretion, and pharmacokinetics (ADME-PK): utility and best practices. an industry perspective from the international consortium for innovation through quality in pharmaceutical development: miniperspective," *J. Med. Chem.*, vol. 60, no. 22, pp. 9097–9113, 2017.

[123] J. Ma, R. P. Sheridan, A. Liaw, G. E. Dahl, and V. Svetnik, "Deep neural nets as a method for quantitative structure–activity relationships," *J. Chem. Inf. Model.*, vol. 55, no. 2, pp. 263–274, 2015.

[124] B. Ramsundar *et al.*, "Is multitask deep learning practical for pharma?," *J. Chem. Inf. Model.*, vol. 57, no. 8, pp. 2068–2076, 2017.

[125] S. Sosnin, M. Vashurina, M. Withnall, P. Karpov, M. Fedorov, and I. V Tetko, "A survey of multi-task learning methods in chemoinformatics," *Mol. Inform.*, vol. 38, no. 4, p. 1800108, 2019.

[126] E. Griffen, A. G. Leach, G. R. Robb, and D. J. Warner, "Matched molecular pairs as a medicinal chemistry tool: miniperspective," *J. Med. Chem.*, vol. 54, no. 22, pp. 7739–7750, 2011.

[127] C. Kramer *et al.*, "Learning medicinal chemistry absorption, distribution, metabolism, excretion, and toxicity (ADMET) rules from cross-company matched molecular pairs analysis (MMPA) miniperspective," *J. Med. Chem.*, vol. 61, no. 8, pp. 3277–3292, 2017.

[128] E. J. Corey, A. K. Long, and S. D. Rubenstein, "Computer-assisted analysis in organic synthesis," *Science (80-. ).*, vol. 228, no. 4698, pp. 408–418, 1985.

[129] P. P. Plehiers *et al.*, "Artificial intelligence for computer-aided synthesis in flow: analysis and selection of reaction components," *Front. Chem. Eng.*, vol. 2, p. 5, 2020.

[130] Z. Wang, W. Zhao, G. Hao, and B. Song, "Mapping the resources and approaches facilitating computer-aided synthesis planning," *Org. Chem. Front.*, vol. 8, no. 4, pp. 812–824, 2021.

[131] A. Thakkar, S. Johansson, K. Jorner, D. Buttar, J.-L. Reymond, and O. Engkvist, "Artificial intelligence and automation in computer aided synthesis planning," *React. Chem. Eng.*, vol. 6, no. 1, pp. 27–51, 2021.

[132] T. J. Struble *et al.*, "Current and future roles of artificial intelligence in medicinal chemistry synthesis," *J. Med. Chem.*, vol. 63, no. 16, pp. 8667–8682, 2020.

[133] B. Liu *et al.*, "Retrosynthetic reaction prediction using neural sequence-to-sequence models," *ACS Cent. Sci.*, vol. 3, no. 10, pp. 1103–1113, 2017.

[134] C. W. Coley, L. Rogers, W. H. Green, and K. F. Jensen, "Computer-assisted retrosynthesis based on molecular similarity," *ACS Cent. Sci.*, vol. 3, no. 12, pp. 1237–1245, 2017.

[135] M. Sacha *et al.*, "Molecule edit graph attention network: modeling chemical reactions as sequences of graph edits," *J. Chem. Inf. Model.*, vol. 61, no. 7, pp. 3273–3284, 2021.

[136] T. Laugel, M.-J. Lesot, C. Marsala, X. Renard, and M. Detyniecki, "The dangers of post-hoc interpretability: Unjustified counterfactual explanations," *arXiv Prepr. arXiv1907.09294*, 2019.

[137] D. Alvarez Melis and T. Jaakkola, "Towards robust interpretability with self-explaining neural networks," *Adv. Neural Inf. Process. Syst.*, vol. 31, 2018.

[138] B. Hie, B. D. Bryson, and B. Berger, "Leveraging uncertainty in machine learning accelerates biological discovery and design," *Cell Syst.*, vol. 11, no. 5, pp. 461–477, 2020.

[139] S. E. Lazic and D. P. Williams, "Quantifying sources of uncertainty in drug discovery predictions with probabilistic models," *Artif. Intell. Life Sci.*, vol. 1, p. 100004, 2021.

[140] B. Lakshminarayanan, A. Pritzel, and C. Blundell, "Simple and scalable predictive uncertainty estimation using deep ensembles," *Adv. Neural Inf. Process. Syst.*, vol. 30, 2017.

[141] Z. C. Lipton, "The doctor just won't accept that!," *arXiv Prepr. arXiv1711.08037*, 2017.

[142] B. Goodman and S. Flaxman, "European Union regulations on algorithmic decision-making and a 'right to explanation,'" *AI Mag.*, vol. 38, no. 3, pp. 50–57, 2017.

# 12

# Automatic Segmentation of Spinal Cord Gray Matter from MR Images using a U-Net Architecture

**R. Polattimur[1] and E. Dandil[2]**

[1]Department of Electronics and Computer Engineering, Institute of Graduate, Bilecik Seyh Edebali University, Turkey
[2]Department of Computer Engineering, Faculty of Engineering, Bilecik Seyh Edebali University, Turkey
Email: rukiye.polattimur@ bilecik.edu.tr; emre.dandil@bilecik.edu.tr

## Abstract

The human spinal cord is a highly organized and complex part of the central nervous system. In particular, GM in the spinal cord is associated with many neurological diseases such as multiple sclerosis (MS), amyotrophic lateral sclerosis (ALS), etc. In addition, the accurate determination of GM in the spinal cord by volume is very important for the diagnosis of spinal cord lesions and other neurological diseases at an early stage. Clinical symptoms/signs, cerebrospinal fluid examinations, evoked potentials, and magnetic resonance imaging (MRI) findings are used in the diagnosis of neurological diseases in the spinal cord region. However, since the spinal cord area does not have a definite geometric shape and is not flat along the back, artifacts often occur in MR scans obtained from the region and it is more difficult to determine the boundaries of the spinal cord area and to detect the lesions in this region. In this chapter, automatic segmentation of spinal cord GM on MR images using U-Net deep learning architecture is proposed. Spinal cord gray matter segmentation challenge (SCGMC) publicly available dataset is used in the study for experimental studies. In this dataset, the spinal cord GM region is successfully segmented using the U-Net architecture. In experimental studies, score of 0.83 is achieved for the dice similarity coefficient (DSC) in

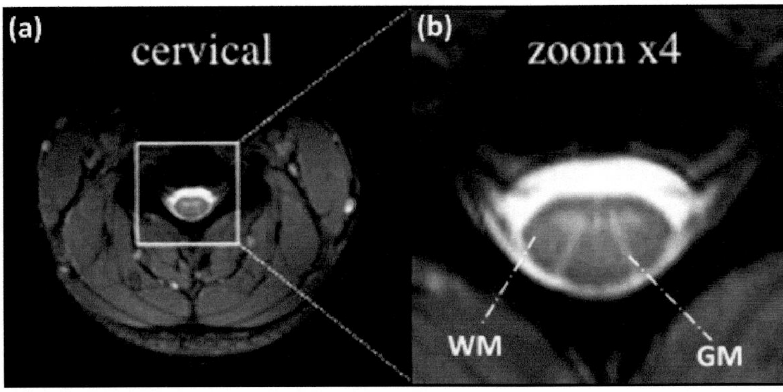


**Figure 12.1** (a) MR image obtained from the axial plane of the cervical region of the spinal cord. (b) GM and WM regions of the spinal cord with 4× zooming of the cross-sectional area [2].

segmentation of GM. As a result, it has been confirmed that the spinal cord GM can be segmented with high accuracy with the U-Net architecture proposed in the study.

## 12.1 Introduction

Neuroscientists generally divide the central nervous system (CNS) into two parts, the brain and spinal cord. Being responsible for connecting the brain and peripheral nervous system, the human spinal cord is about the thickness of an adult's pinky finger and consists of two basic nerve tissues, gray matter (GM) and white matter (WM) [1]. The human spinal cord is a highly organized and complex part of the CNS, and its function is to transmit neural signals from the brain (sensory information) to the peripheral nervous system (motor information) and from the peripheral nervous system to the brain. This information passes through myelinated motor and sensory axons in WM and is transmitted and controlled by spinal cord interneurons mostly found in GM [2]. The spinal cord GM resembles an H-shape in appearance, but also resembles a butterfly image [3]. Figure 12.1(a) shows an MR image obtained from the axial plane of the cervical region of the spinal cord, and in Figure 12.1(b), the GM and WM regions of the spinal cord can be clearly seen by 4× zooming of the cross-sectional area in this image.

As is known from histopathological studies, tissue changes in GM and WM appear to be related to many neurological-based diseases [4, 5]. While examining the prognosis of neurological diseases, structural defects in GM and WM can facilitate diagnosis and clinical follow-up by pointing out the

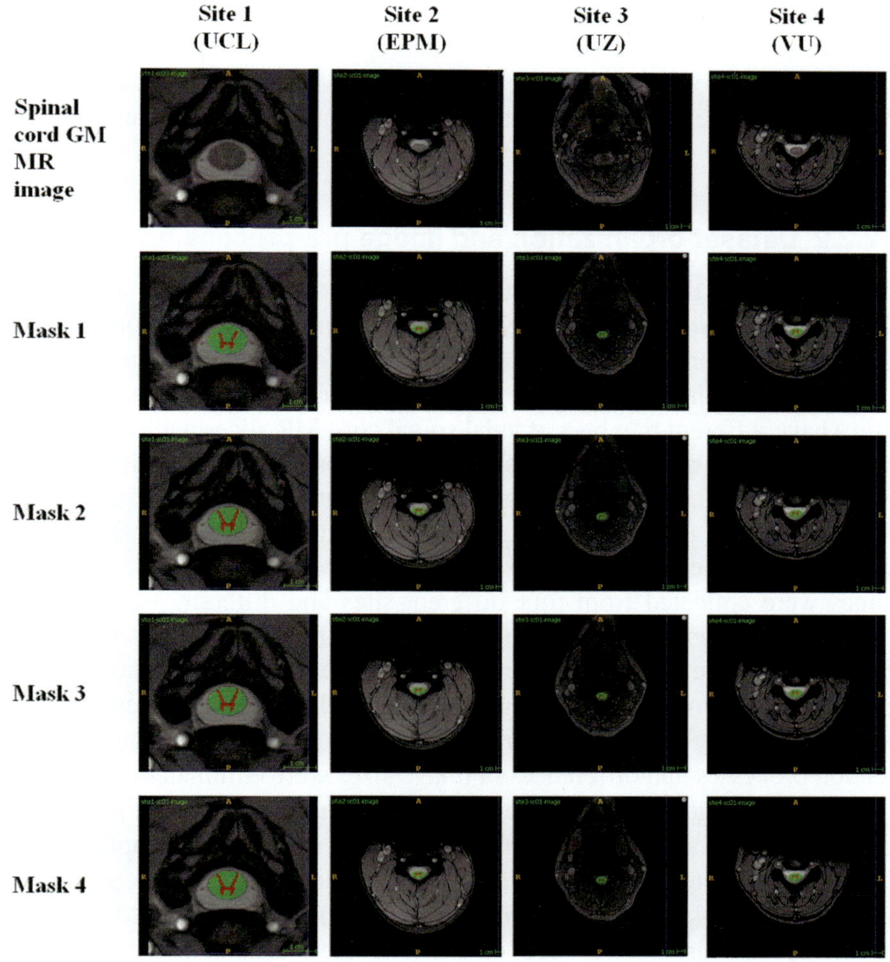


**Figure 12.3** Spinal cord GM MR images obtained from four different data centers (sites) in the SCGMC dataset and ground truth masks of four different raters.

The dataset was split into two sets such as training and test and includes MR images obtained from anatomical images of spinal cord regions of 20 healthy subjects for each site. Both training and test sets consist of 40 subject slices in total. In the dataset, each subject in each site contains 10 axial slices in total with spinal cord GM. The data in the challenge are shared from the CMIC [32] link. The MR images in the dataset were created separately from four different centers and 10 training and 10 test subject scans (images) from each. There are also spinal cord GM masks manually delineated by four different raters for each slice in the scans. In Figure 12.3, some sample slices obtained from four different sites in the SCGMC dataset and imported to the ITK-Snap [33] environment and the masks (ground truth) delineated by four different raters for these slices are shown. Here, Mask 1, Mask 2, Mask 3, and Mask 4 show the mask delineated by Rater 1, Rater 2, Rater 3, and Rater 4, respectively.

### 12.2.2 Dataset organization and image pre-processing

In the SCGMC dataset used in the study, axial MR images of spinal cord GM and masks are presented in NifTI format. Since the dataset contains four different MR scanners and slices of 10 scans by four different data providers, the sizes of the data are different from each other. Scans from data providers (site) have different numbers of axial spinal cord MR slices and masks of the spinal cord GM region of those slices. Since there is no GM region in some MR sections in the dataset, its mask was not created. For this study, a total of 424 MR images (382 for training and 42 for test) were selected from slices with masks in the dataset to be used in spinal cord segmentation. Since these slices were collected from four different sites and different MR scanners, they have different dimensions such as 100 × 100, 320 × 320, 774 × 654, and 560 × 560. While GM is clearer in 100 × 100 sized MR images, the region of interest (spinal cord GM region) gets smaller as the image size increases. For this, images were re-saved by performing image pre-processing and normalization processes and differences in image sizes were eliminated.

In all images used in the experimental studies, image pre-processing procedures such as cropping, normalization, and resizing were applied based on the mask center of region of interest. After the image pre-processing, the images were re-saved in .jpg format as 128 × 128 sized. GM MR images of the spinal cord in SCGMC dataset and their ground truth masks are shown in Figures 12.4(a) and 12.4(a1), and new images with crop and resizing after image pre-processing and their ground truth masks are shown in Figures 12.4(b) and 12.4(b1), respectively.

### 12.2.3 U-Net

Deep learning models are a very popular machine learning sub-field for researchers. Deep learning continues to develop rapidly in recent years, and this increases the motivation of researchers in many fields. In addition, deep network architectures provide a suitable basis for using in very large datasets, as they can perform feature extraction in artificial neural network studies within their own multi-layer structure. The most widely used and basic model

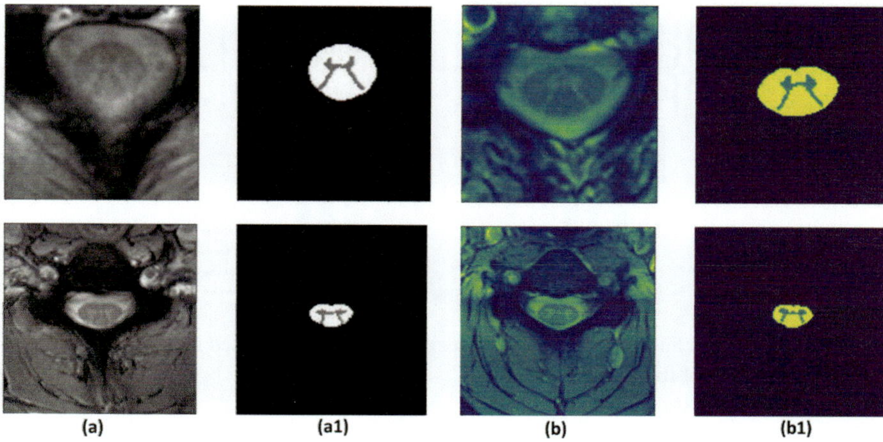


**Figure 12.4** (a) GM MR images of the spinal cord in SCGMC dataset and (a1) their ground truth masks, (b) GM MR images of the spinal cord with crop and resizing after image pre-processing and (b1) their ground truth masks.

in deep learning networks is CNN. In the CNN architecture, patterns with lower features such as horizontal–vertical edges are determined in the first layers and transferred to the network, and the learning processes begin with the transfer of the information obtained from these features to the network. In addition, deep learning also allows the use of pre-trained networks and models. Many models such as R-CNN [34], fast R-CNN [35], faster R-CNN [36], and mask R-CNN [37] have been developed in deep networks and are still being developed.

U-Net, a deep learning architecture, is another type of CNN approach and was first proposed in a biomedical image segmentation study [38]. The large datasets are needed for training in typical CNN architectures. The images in these datasets are labeled and presented to the network, and the network recognizes the images with this label information. Because biomedical images mostly require pixel-based approaches, the labeling process requires a lot of attention and this is quite difficult in some cases. In addition, the labeling process requires a lot of expert and hardware capacity. In addition, this process takes a lot of time and it is often impossible to reach this much data.

U-Net deep learning architecture offers pixel-based image segmentation with an architectural approach different from the traditional CNN structure in this regard [38]. U-Net is one of the most popular and successful deep learning models in biomedical image segmentation today. U-Net architecture consists of two symmetrical phases, encoder (contraction) in down-sampling

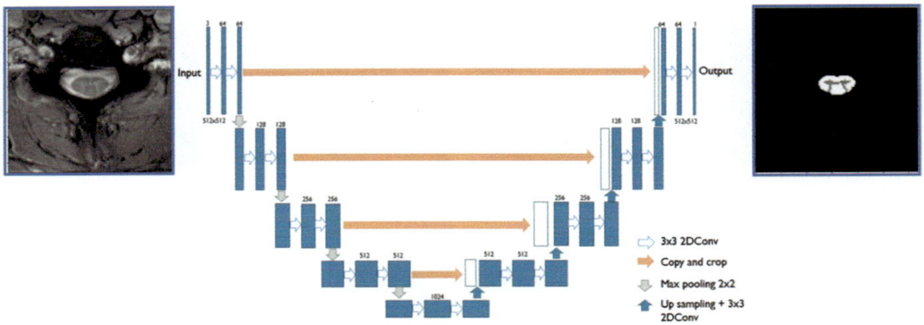


**Figure 12.5** The architecture of the U-Net deep learning network used in this study for automatic segmentation of the spinal cord GM.

and decoder (expansion) in up-sampling [39], and has a U-shaped layered structure. Besides, there is no fully connected layer in the U-Net model; only the convolution layer is used. The U-Net architecture used in this study is shown in Figure 12.5. In this model, each horizontal block contains three layers, and two unpadded 3 × 3 convolution layers and a rectified linear unit (ReLU) with a leakage factor of 0.1 of each layer are used. Also, the number of feature channels of the resulting image in each subsampling step is doubled. Moreover, a process called mirroring is applied to the inputs to estimate the pixels in the border region of the image so that the images can be segmented correctly.

## 12.3 Experimental Results

In this chapter, automatic segmentation of the spinal cord GM region using U-Net architecture was performed using MR images in the publicly available SCGMC dataset. In order to verify the performance of the proposed U-Net architecture, many experimental studies were carried out and the obtained results and findings were analyzed. All applications on the proposed model were carried out using the Python programming language. In experimental studies, for spinal cord GM segmentation, 382 (~90%) of a total of 424 MR slices selected from the SCGMC dataset were reserved for the training phase of the U-Net network and the remaining 42 (~10%) for the testing phase. In addition, for this study, delineated masks by Rater 4 were determined as ground truth reference masks in experimental studies. For the experimental studies, the computer whose hardware configurations are presented in Table 12.1 was used.

The compatibility of the hyperparameters with the model structure in the U-Net architecture positively affects the results of the experimental

**Table 12.1** Hardware specifications of the computer used for experimental studies in this study.

| **Hardware** | **Specifications** |
|---|---|
| CPU | Intel® Core™ i5-10600KF, 4.10 GHz, 6 Core/12 Thread |
| RAM (×2) | 16 GB (DDR4 3000 MHz) |
| Mainboard | ASUS B560 |
| GPU | NVIDIA RTX™ A4000 16 GB GDDR6 |
| Hard-disk driver | 1TB WD SATA 6G HDD + 500 GB PCIe NVMe M.2 SSD |

studies. The use of hyperparameters in the U-Net architecture differs from the parameters used in other CNN architectures. The U-Net architecture uses maximum pooling and ReLu activation function in its own layers, and differentiation in terms of use in hyperparameters is not possible in these stages. In addition, the fully connected layer in the last layer used in CNN is not included in the U-Net architecture. Therefore, the absence of this layer limits the parameter optimizations to be performed in the model.

In image segmentation, the success of the proposed method is calculated by measuring the similarity of the reference mask (ground truth) and the output image estimated (segmented) by the proposed method. Some numerical performance measures are used in the evaluations. These numerical measurements can be performed with pixel-based cluster similarity operations, or they can be calculated from the true positive (TP), false positive (FP), true negative (TN), and false negative (FN) values in the confusion matrix. In this study, the pixel-based similarity measures, Dice similarity coefficient (DSC) and Jaccard similarity index (JSI), were used to measure the performance of the proposed U-Net deep learning architecture for automatic spinal cord segmentation. The DSC metric is a similarity coefficient that specifies the rate of overlap between the reference area (ground truth mask) and the segmented area by the proposed method [40] and it is denoted in eqn (12.1). The intersection of the reference area and the segmented area divided by the total area is expressed by another similarity index [41], JSI, and it is presented in eqn (12.2). In the equations given for DSC and JSI criteria, the ground truth area is denoted by $A_{GT}$, and the area segmented by the proposed method is abbreviated as $A_{SEG}$.

$$\mathrm{DSC}\left(A_{\mathrm{SEG}}, A_{\mathrm{GT}}\right) = \frac{2\left|A_{\mathrm{SEG}} \cap A_{\mathrm{GT}}\right|}{\left|A_{\mathrm{SEG}}\right| \cup \left|A_{\mathrm{GT}}\right|} \tag{12.1}$$

$$\mathrm{JSI}\left(A_{\mathrm{SEG}}, A_{\mathrm{GT}}\right) = \frac{\left|A_{\mathrm{SEG}} \cap A_{\mathrm{GT}}\right|}{\left|A_{\mathrm{SEG}}\right| + \left|A_{\mathrm{GT}}\right| - \left|A_{\mathrm{SEG}} \cap A_{\mathrm{GT}}\right|}. \tag{12.2}$$

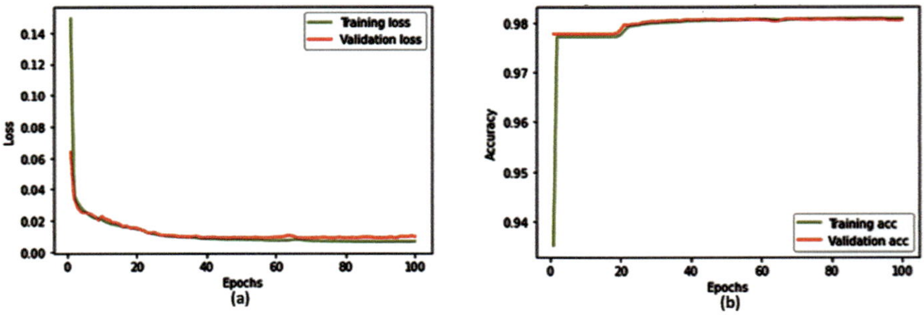


**Figure 12.6** Graph of change of training/validation accuracy and training/validation loss values of U-Net model for 100 epochs.

In this study, the performance of the proposed method for segmenting the spinal cord from MR images was also evaluated using the true positive rate (TPR), true negative rate (TNR), and positive predictive value (PPV) criteria calculated from the confusion matrix. Meanwhile, the TPR measure is also known as sensitivity, the TNR measure as specificity, and the PPV as precision. TPR, FNR, and PPV measures are denoted in eqn (12.3), (12.4), and (12.5), respectively.

$$\text{TPR}\left(A_{\text{SEG}}, A_{\text{GT}}\right) = \frac{\text{TP}}{\text{TP} + \text{FN}} \tag{12.3}$$

$$\text{TNR}\left(A_{\text{SEG}}, A_{\text{GT}}\right) = \frac{\text{TN}}{\text{FP} + \text{TN}} \tag{12.4}$$

$$\text{PPV}\left(A_{\text{SEG}}, A_{\text{GT}}\right) = \frac{\text{TP}}{\text{TP} + \text{FP}} \tag{12.5}$$

Figures 12.6(a) and 12.6(b) show the graphs of training loss/validation loss and training accuracy/validation accuracy values obtained after completing the 100 epoch training phase of the U-Net deep learning architecture proposed in experimental studies for automatic segmentation of the spinal cord. Here, it is seen that the training of the network was completed successfully and the loss value was decreased considerably as expected.

Figure 12.7 shows some successfully segmented MR slices in the dataset using the U-Net deep learning architecture in this study. Here, column (a) shows the original MR sections with the GM region of the spinal cord obtained from the axial plane after the image pre-processing. Column (b) shows the raters' reference masks (ground truth), while column (c) shows the GM masks segmented with the U-Net architecture proposed in this study. In

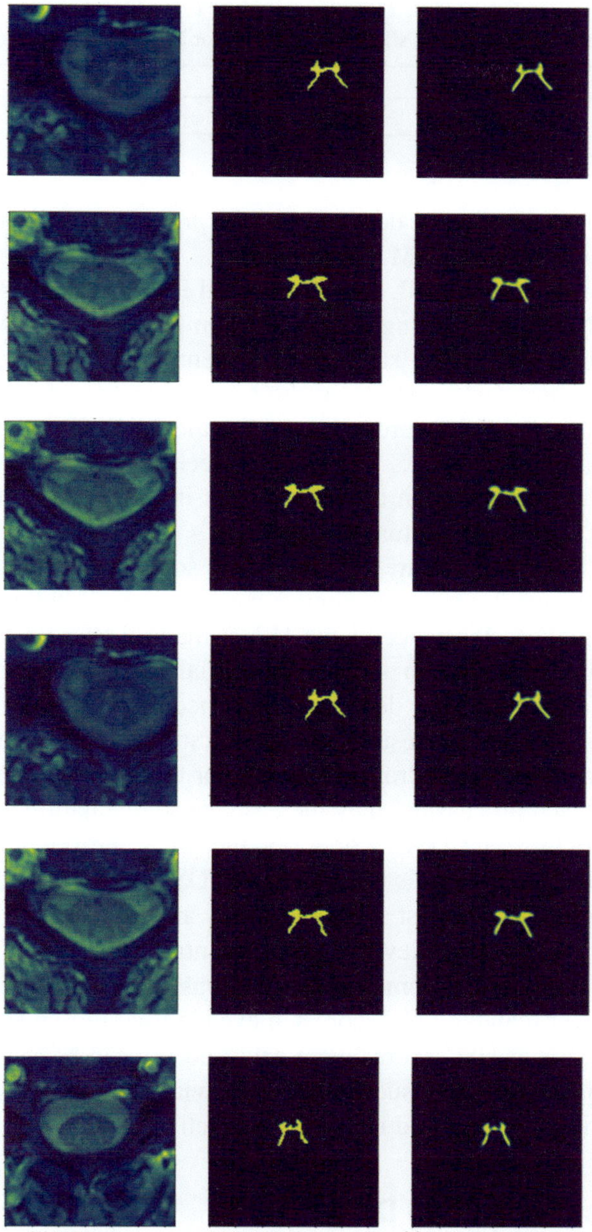


**Figure 12.7** Some successfully segmented MR slices in the dataset using the U-Net deep learning architecture in this study. (a) MR image. (b) Ground truth. (c) U-Net segmentation.

**Table 12.2** Results of DSC, JSI, TPR, TNR, and PPV metrics obtained for the proposed U-Net deep learning model on MR slices in the test set for 100 epochs in experimental studies.

| DSC | JSI | TPR | TNR | PPV |
|---|---|---|---|---|
| 0.83 | 0.71 | 0.98 | 0.98 | 0.72 |

Figure 12.7, it can be clearly deduced that the proposed U-Net architecture is successful for spinal cord GM segmentation.

The results of DSC, JSI, TPR, TNR, and PPV metrics obtained for the proposed U-Net deep learning architecture on MR slices in the test set for 100 epochs in experimental studies are presented in Table 12.2. Using the U-Net architecture for the slices in the test set, scores of 0.8267, 0.7078, 0.8267, 0.9801, and 0.72 were achieved for the DSC, JSI, TPR, TNR, and PPV metrics, respectively. As a result, it is seen that the spinal cord GM is successfully segmented from the MR images in the SCGMC dataset using the proposed U-Net architecture.

As can be seen in Figure 12.8, there are some slices of the spinal cord GM region that was not fully segmented in experimental studies. Particularly, the segmentation performance of the U-Net method decreases in the slices where the GM decreases in size in the spinal cord MR images obtained from the axial plane in the dataset. If it is necessary to evaluate the low-performance segmentation results obtained, first of all, it is evaluated that the large number of data in the training dataset for the U-Net model, which performs pixel-based processing, may increase the segmentation performance.

In Table 12.3, the DSC scores obtained in some previous studies on SCGMC dataset used in this study and the DSC score obtained using the U-Net architecture in the test set in this study are compared. In this study, a DSC score of 0.83 was achieved in experimental studies conducted with 42 test images. Although in some of the previously suggested studies, scores close to or lower than the DSC score achieved in this study were obtained, in some studies, lower DSC scores were achieved. As can be seen here, spinal cord GM can be segmented successfully and with a high DSC score on axial MR slices using the proposed U-Net-based architecture.

## 12.4 Conclusions and Discussions

Since the precise determination of the spinal cord boundary is relevant to many neurological disorders, automatic segmentation of the GM is very important. In this chapter, spinal cord GM was successfully segmented in the publicly available SCGMC dataset using U-Net deep learning architecture.

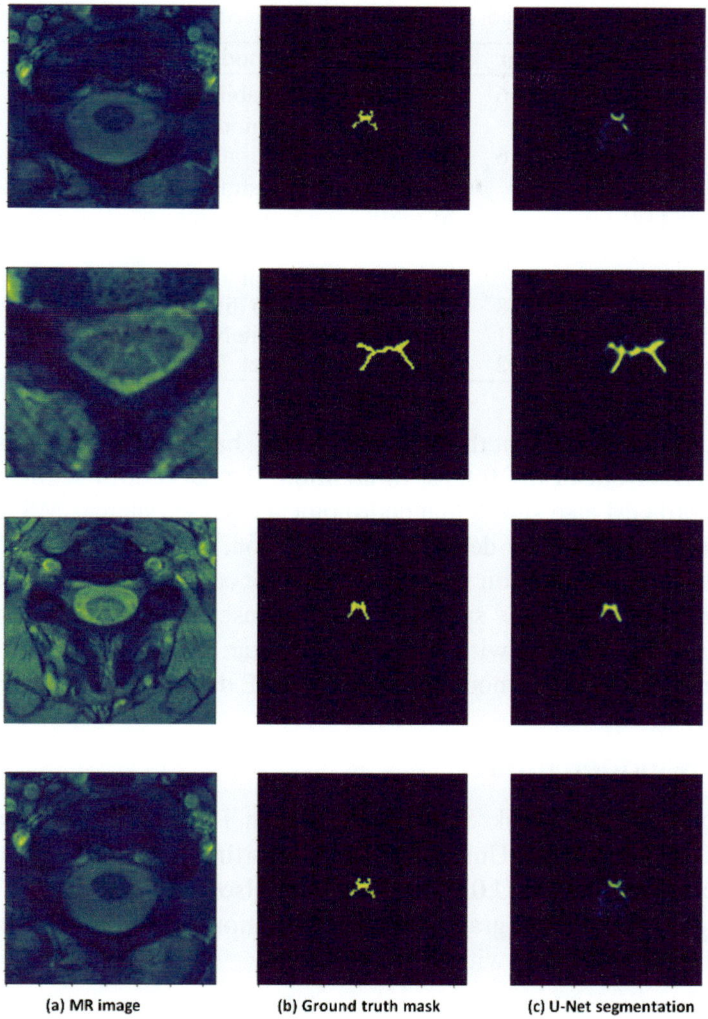


**Figure 12.8** Some slices of the spinal cord GM region that was not fully segmented in experimental studies.

In experimental studies conducted for automatic segmentation of the spinal cord GM, a DSC score of 0.83 was achieved, resulting in higher segmentation performance than some previously suggested studies. In conclusion, in this study, it has been seen that the spinal cord GM can be successfully segmented with computer-assisted automatic diagnosis approaches and a U-Net-based deep learning approach is presented, which physicians can use as a secondary support tool in decision-making processes.

**Table 12.3** Comparison of DSC scores obtained on the SCGMC dataset.

| Study | Year | Dataset | Method | DSC |
|---|---|---|---|---|
| Blaiotta et al. [42] | 2016 | SCGMC | Probabilistic clustering techniques | 0.61 |
| Dupont et al. [43] | 2016 | SCGMC | Multi-atlas-based template Registration framework | 0.69 |
| Datta et al. [12] | 2016 | SCGMC | Active contours | 0.75 |
| Prados et al.[5] | 2016 | SCGMC | Multi-atlas segmentation and fusion | 0.79 |
| Perone et al. [9] | 2018 | SCGMC | Deep dilated convolutions | 0.85 |
| Alsenan et al. [44] | 2021 | SCGMC | MobileNetV3 and U-Net | 0.78 |
| Proposed study | 2022 | SCGMC | U-Net | 0.83 |

It is considered that this study can give a basis for other works planned to be carried out in the future. In addition, the successful segmentation of spinal cord GM also shows that neurological diseases such as MS and tumor or tumor groups can be detected in this region. Moreover, it should not be overlooked that a decision support system that can assist clinical studies can be developed with a new spinal cord MR dataset. In addition, segmentation of the spinal cord GM with higher success can also be evaluated by using different deep learning models on the SCGMC dataset.

## Acknowledgements

We would like to thank Scientific Research Projects Coordinatorship of Bilecik Seyh Edebali University for supporting this study with Project Number: 2021-01.BŞEÜ.03-02. We would also like to thank the team for creating the spinal cord gray matter segmentation challenge (SCGMC) dataset and sharing the data with the researchers.

## References

[1] C.S. Perone, Deep Learning Methods for MRI Spinal Cord Gray Matter Segmentation, Ecole Polytechnique, Montreal (Canada), 2019.

[2] B. De Leener, M. Taso, J. Cohen-Adad, V. Callot, Segmentation of the human spinal cord, Magnetic Resonance Materials in Physics, Biology and Medicine, 29 (2016) 125–153.

[3] F. Prados, J. Ashburner, C. Blaiotta, T. Brosch, J. Carballido-Gamio, M.J. Cardoso, B.N. Conrad, E. Datta, G. Dávid, B. De Leener, Spinal cord grey matter segmentation challenge, Neuroimage, 152 (2017) 312–329.

[4] M. Calabrese, A. Favaretto, V. Martini, P. Gallo, Grey matter lesions in MS: from histology to clinical implications, Prion, 7 (2013) 20–27.

[5] F. Prados, M.J. Cardoso, M.C. Yiannakas, L.R. Hoy, E. Tebaldi, H. Kearney, M.D. Liechti, D.H. Miller, O. Ciccarelli, C.A. Wheeler-Kingshott, S. Ourselin, Fully automated grey and white matter spinal cord segmentation, Scientific reports, 6 (2016) 36151.

[6] C. Gros, B. De Leener, A. Badji, J. Maranzano, D. Eden, S.M. Dupont, J. Talbott, R. Zhuoquiong, Y. Liu, T. Granberg, Automatic segmentation of the spinal cord and intramedullary multiple sclerosis lesions with convolutional neural networks, Neuroimage, 184 (2019) 901–915.

[7] M.A. Horsfield, S. Sala, M. Neema, M. Absinta, A. Bakshi, M.P. Sormani, M.A. Rocca, R. Bakshi, M. Filippi, Rapid semi-automatic segmentation of the spinal cord from magnetic resonance images: application in multiple sclerosis, Neuroimage, 50 (2010) 446–455.

[8] M.C. Yiannakas, A.M. Mustafa, B. De Leener, H. Kearney, C. Tur, D.R. Altmann, F. De Angelis, D. Plantone, O. Ciccarelli, D.H. Miller, Fully automated segmentation of the cervical cord from T1-weighted MRI using PropSeg: application to multiple sclerosis, NeuroImage: Clinical, 10 (2016) 71-77.

[9] C.S. Perone, E. Calabrese, J. Cohen-Adad, Spinal cord gray matter segmentation using deep dilated convolutions, Scientific reports, 8 (2018) 1–13.

[10] B. De Leener, M. Taso, J. Cohen-Adad, V. Callot, Segmentation of the human spinal cord, Magma (New York, N.Y.), 29 (2016) 125–153.

[11] R.I. Grossman, F. Barkhof, M. Filippi, Assessment of spinal cord damage in MS using MRI, Journal of the neurological sciences, 172 (2000) S36–S39.

[12] E. Datta, N. Papinutto, R. Schlaeger, A. Zhu, J. Carballido-Gamio, R.G. Henry, Gray matter segmentation of the spinal cord with active contours in MR images, NeuroImage, 147 (2017) 788–799.

[13] S. Garg, S. Bhagyashree, Spinal Cord MRI Segmentation Techniques and Algorithms: A Survey, SN Computer Science, 2 (2021) 1–9.

[14] N. Losseff, S. Webb, J. O'riordan, R. Page, L. Wang, G. Barker, P.S. Tofts, W.I. McDonald, D.H. Miller, A.J. Thompson, Spinal cord atrophy and disability in multiple sclerosis: a new reproducible and sensitive MRI method with potential to monitor disease progression, Brain, 119 (1996) 701–708.

[15] M.-M. El Mendili, R. Chen, B. Tiret, N. Villard, S. Trunet, M. Pélégrini-Issac, S. Lehéricy, P.-F. Pradat, H. Benali, Fast and accurate semi-automated segmentation method of spinal cord MR images at 3T applied

to the construction of a cervical spinal cord template, PLoS One, 10 (2015) e0122224.
[16] T. Behrens, K. Rohr, H.S. Stiehl, Using an Extended Hough Transform Combined with a Kalman Filter to Segment Tubular Structures in 3D Medical Images, VMV, 2001, pp. 491–498.
[17] O. Coulon, S. Hickman, G. Parker, G. Barker, D. Miller, S. Arridge, Quantification of spinal cord atrophy from magnetic resonance images via a B-spline active surface model, Magnetic Resonance in Medicine: An Official Journal of the International Society for Magnetic Resonance in Medicine, 47 (2002) 1176–1185.
[18] B. De Leener, S. Kadoury, J. Cohen-Adad, Robust, accurate and fast automatic segmentation of the spinal cord, Neuroimage, 98 (2014) 528–536.
[19] J. Kawahara, C. McIntosh, R. Tam, G. Hamarneh, Globally optimal spinal cord segmentation using a minimal path in high dimensions, 2013 IEEE 10th International Symposium on Biomedical Imaging, IEEE, 2013, pp. 848–851.
[20] F.P. Bergo, M.C. França, C.F. Chevis, F. Cendes, SpineSeg: A segmentation and measurement tool for evaluation of spinal cord atrophy, 7th Iberian Conference on Information Systems and Technologies (CISTI 2012), IEEE, 2012, pp. 1–4.
[21] S. Pezold, K. Fundana, M. Amann, M. Andelova, A. Pfister, T. Sprenger, P.C. Cattin, Automatic segmentation of the spinal cord using continuous max flow with cross-sectional similarity prior and tubularity features, Recent Advances in Computational Methods and Clinical Applications for Spine Imaging, Springer2015, pp. 107–118.
[22] M. Chen, A. Carass, J. Oh, G. Nair, D.L. Pham, D.S. Reich, J.L. Prince, Automatic magnetic resonance spinal cord segmentation with topology constraints for variable fields of view, Neuroimage, 83 (2013) 1051–1062.
[23] S. Valverde, A. Oliver, E. Roura, S. González-Villà, D. Pareto, J.C. Vilanova, L. Ramió-Torrentà, À. Rovira, X. Lladó, Automated tissue segmentation of MR brain images in the presence of white matter lesions, Medical image analysis, 35 (2017) 446–457.
[24] S. Ma, Y. Huang, X. Che, R. Gu, Faster RCNN-based detection of cervical spinal cord injury and disc degeneration, Journal of Applied Clinical Medical Physics, 21 (2020) 235–243.
[25] D. McCoy, S. Dupont, C. Gros, J. Cohen-Adad, R. Huie, A. Ferguson, X. Duong-Fernandez, L. Thomas, V. Singh, J. Narvid, Convolutional neural network–based automated segmentation of the spinal cord and

contusion injury: Deep learning biomarker correlates of motor impairment in acute spinal cord injury, American Journal of Neuroradiology, 40 (2019) 737–744.

[26] J. Hong, B.-y. Park, M.J. Lee, C.-S. Chung, J. Cha, H. Park, Two-step deep neural network for segmentation of deep white matter hyperintensities in migraineurs, Computer methods programs in biomedicine, 183 (2020) 105065.

[27] Y. Zhang, W. Chen, Y. Chen, X. Tang, A post-processing method to improve the white matter hyperintensity segmentation accuracy for randomly-initialized U-net, 2018 IEEE 23rd International Conference on Digital Signal Processing (DSP), IEEE, 2018, pp. 1–5.

[28] J. Wu, Y. Zhang, K. Wang, X. Tang, Skip connection U-Net for white matter hyperintensities segmentation from MRI, IEEE Access, 7 (2019) 155194–155202.

[29] Y. Zhang, J. Wu, W. Chen, Y. Liu, J. Lyu, H. Shi, Y. Chen, E.X. Wu, X. Tang, Fully automatic white matter hyperintensity segmentation using U-Net and skip connection, 2019 41st Annual International Conference of the IEEE Engineering in Medicine and Biology Society (EMBC), IEEE, 2019, pp. 974–977.

[30] M. AskariHemmat, S. Honari, L. Rouhier, C.S. Perone, J. Cohen-Adad, Y. Savaria, J.-P. David, U-Net fixed-point quantization for medical image segmentation, Large-Scale Annotation of Biomedical Data and Expert Label Synthesis and Hardware Aware Learning for Medical Imaging and Computer Assisted Intervention, Springer2019, pp. 115–124.

[31] F. Paugam, J. Lefeuvre, C.S. Perone, C. Gros, D.S. Reich, P. Sati, J. Cohen-Adad, Open-source pipeline for multi-class segmentation of the spinal cord with deep learning, Magnetic resonance imaging, 64 (2019) 21–27.

[32] GM Spinal Cord Challenge Data Set 2016. Accessed 20.07.2021, http://cmictig.cs.ucl.ac.uk/niftyweb/challenge/.

[33] P.A. Yushkevich, J. Piven, H.C. Hazlett, R.G. Smith, S. Ho, J.C. Gee, G. Gerig, User-guided 3D active contour segmentation of anatomical structures: significantly improved efficiency and reliability, Neuroimage, 31 (2006) 1116–1128.

[34] R. Girshick, J. Donahue, T. Darrell, J. Malik, Rich feature hierarchies for accurate object detection and semantic segmentation, Proceedings of the IEEE conference on computer vision and pattern recognition, 2014, pp. 580–587.

[35] R. Girshick, Fast r-cnn, Proceedings of the IEEE international conference on computer vision, 2015, pp. 1440–1448.

[36] S. Ren, K. He, R. Girshick, J. Sun, Faster r-cnn: Towards real-time object detection with region proposal networks, Advances in neural information processing systems, 28 (2015).

[37] K. He, G. Gkioxari, P. Dollár, R. Girshick, Mask r-cnn, Proceedings of the IEEE international conference on computer vision, 2017, pp. 2961–2969.

[38] O. Ronneberger, P. Fischer, T. Brox, U-net: Convolutional networks for biomedical image segmentation, International Conference on Medical image computing and computer-assisted intervention, Springer, 2015, pp. 234–241.

[39] J. Zhang, C. Li, S. Kosov, M. Grzegorzek, K. Shirahama, T. Jiang, C. Sun, Z. Li, H. Li, LCU-Net: A novel low-cost U-Net for environmental microorganism image segmentation, Pattern Recognition, 115 (2021) 107885.

[40] L.R. Dice, Measures of the amount of ecologic association between species, Ecology, 26 (1945) 297–302.

[41] P. Jaccard, The distribution of the flora in the alpine zone. 1, New phytologist, 11 (1912) 37–50.

[42] C. Blaiotta, P. Freund, A. Curt, M. Cardoso, J. Ashburner, A probabilistic framework to learn average shaped tissue templates and its application to spinal cord image segmentation, Proceedings of the 24th Annual Meeting of ISMRM, Singapore, 2016.

[43] S.M. Dupont, B. De Leener, M. Taso, A. Le Troter, S. Nadeau, N. Stikov, V. Callot, J. Cohen-Adad, Fully-integrated framework for the segmentation and registration of the spinal cord white and gray matter, Neuroimage, 150 (2017) 358–372.

[44] A. Alsenan, B.B. Youssef, H. Alhichri, A Deep Learning Model based on MobileNetV3 and UNet for Spinal Cord Gray Matter Segmentation, 2021 44th International Conference on Telecommunications and Signal Processing (TSP), IEEE, 2021, pp. 244–248.

# 13

# XAI for Drug Discovery

**Ilhan Uysal[1] and Utku Kose[2]**

[1]Bucak Emin Gülmez Technical Sciences Vocational School, Burdur Mehmet Akif Ersoy University, Turkey
[2]Department of Computer Engineering, Faculty of Engineering, Suleyman Demirel University, Turkey
Email: iuysal@mehmetakif.edu.tr; utkukose@sdu.edu.tr

## Abstract

Since the improvement of a new drug is a complex, costly, and a quite over-long process, how to decrease prices and speed up new drug discovery has turned into a compelling and immediate problem in the industry. So, the importance of computer-aided drug discovery has been steadily increasing in recent times. Notwithstanding the increasing number of accomplished forward-looking practices, deep learning models need to be explainable as mathematical models are often difficult to interpret by the human mind. In this study, first, basic information about current explainable artificial intelligence (XAI) methods such as class activation mapping (CAM), local interpretable model-agnostic explanations (LIME), SHAP, Fairlearn, and Whitenoise is given. Afterward, XAI approaches used in the context of drug discovery such as feature attribution, instance-based, graph-convolution based, self-explaining, and uncertainty prediction are mentioned and predictions for future studies are made.

## 13.1 Introduction

Artificial intelligence techniques have become very popular today, as they take place in a wide variety of fields such as robotics, speech translation, and image analysis. Artificial intelligence is used in fields such as chemistry, biology, and pharmacy to design new organic synthetic schemes, understand complex biological systems, design new APIs, or develop new analytical, and diagnostic devices or methods. Artificial intelligence techniques can also be applied to nearly all aspects of drug discovery, drug development, drug repurposing, drug metabolism prediction, drug toxicity analysis, pharmaceutical productivity improvement, clinical trials, and pharmaceutical sciences. All of these techniques are collectively considered within the scope of artificial intelligence in drug discovery. These AI technologies are not yet routinely practical in computer-aided drug design but are used to solve complex drug discovery problems. Compared to ligand-based drug design and structure-based drug design, artificial intelligence in drug discovery is still under development [1–8].

The concepts of artificial intelligence, which has been frequently encountered in recent years, and machine learning and deep learning, which are its sub-branches, are becoming a part of life day by day. When it comes to the applicability of artificial intelligence, the concepts that shape today and the future in the technological context are known as machine learning and its sub-branch, deep learning. While machine learning makes predictions for the future by making use of existing data, deep learning works with artificial neural networks. The features that distinguish machine learning from deep learning are as follows [9]:

- Number of data: While machine learning uses small datasets, deep learning uses large datasets.
- Output: In machine learning, the outputs usually take numeric values, while in deep learning, the outputs can be in different formats such as text and audio apart from numeric values.
- Hardware dependency: While machine learning can run on low-spec machines, deep learning needs high-spec machines.
- Execution time: While machine learning systems take a short time to run, deep learning systems take longer to run because they contain many different layers.
- Contouring process: While the features must be defined and created correctly by the user in machine learning, deep learning can learn high-level features and create new features.

Models operating in an integrated system do not give any information about what they base their predictions on. For this reason, it is known as the black box. These concepts, which facilitate the usability and interpretability of big data with the development of technology, arouse curiosity with the algorithms they run in the background. Many questions such as what data reached

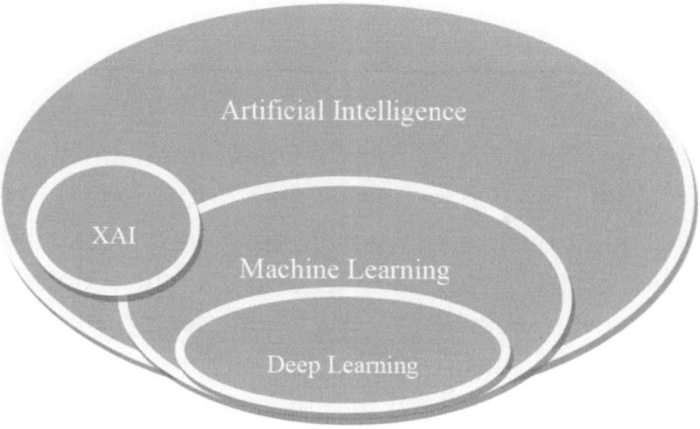


**Figure 13.1** The relationship between artificial intelligence, machine learning, deep learning, and explainable artificial intelligence [10].

the result, how reliable the result was, and how successful the established model was revealed the concept of XAI. The graph showing the relationship between artificial intelligence, machine learning, deep learning, and explainable artificial intelligence is given in Figure 13.1.

Drug discovery is a process that creates a therapeutically useful compound that is used to treat and cure diseases. Of late years, the popularity of computer-assisted drug discovery has been increasing, and, accordingly, drug discovery studies related to artificial intelligence have begun to emerge. De novo designs, structure- and ligand-based designs, a new compound design, prediction of the physicochemical and pharmacokinetic features of the drug, and machine learning algorithms for drug repurposing are used in computer-aided drug discovery. While deep learning approaches are employed to estimate output and features that depended on input data as well as to specify nonlinear input–output connections, machine learning algorithms emphasizing molecular explanatory raise drug discovery and cheminformatics synergies too. XAI has a great capacity to raise the understanding of the patterns that emerge from the input data and transform it into a human more explainable form. As the use of artificial intelligence in drug discovery and relevant areas becomes widespread, there will be an increasing requirement for the take advantage of XAI in the explanation of basic approaches. Besides mathematical approaches, XAI encourages the pattern of new drugs in the drug discovery process, subtraction of pharmacological actions from molecular structures, methods to generate fundamental decision-making clear, avoid false predictions, and increase interpretability, and the form of new bioactive composites with wanted features. It is thought that the rapidly developing use of XAI will also become widespread in drug discovery and pharmacological research soon [11–18].

## 13.2 Main Text

**Explainable artificial intelligence:**

Although technological structures made with artificial intelligence and used in most parts of life make life easier, they always create a question mark in mind. Is artificial intelligence having trouble distinguishing between a cake and a dog? The question has shaken the trust in artificial intelligence [9]. Artificial intelligence technologies used in areas where decisions that affect human life are made, especially in the health sector, must have a reliable structure. To increase the trust in artificial intelligence, it is important to present the decisions taken by artificial intelligence to the user together with the reasons. With XAI, this trust has begun to occur [19].

XAI can be expressed as presenting the way artificial intelligence technologies are used to make decisions for users, both textually and graphically. These systems tried to provide transparency and interpretability by producing answers to the questions created by artificial intelligence. With XAI, the question marks in the minds of users were resolved. XAI presents its results to users with an explanation interface, and this interface gives explanations about the reasons for the success or failure of the result produced by artificial intelligence.

The main purposes of XAI systems are as follows [20]:

- To produce explicable models while maintaining the accuracy of predictions with the high level of learning performance that artificial intelligence contains.
- It is to ensure that users can understand the result, interpret it, and make plans by relying on it.

XAI systems first aim to create models that can be explained at certain rates, and then models that can be fully explained. It improves the ability to understand future predictions by analyzing the strengths and weaknesses of the system. Figure 13.2 shows the solution process graph of XAI systems, which shows the processes that XAI systems go through until the accuracy is obtained after the training data is given to the system. The advantages of XAI can be listed as follows [9, 19, 20]:

- Increases confidence in artificial intelligence.
- It increases traceability by explaining the models.
- Explaining the decision with its justifications ensures that the effects of the changes on the decisions are revealed.

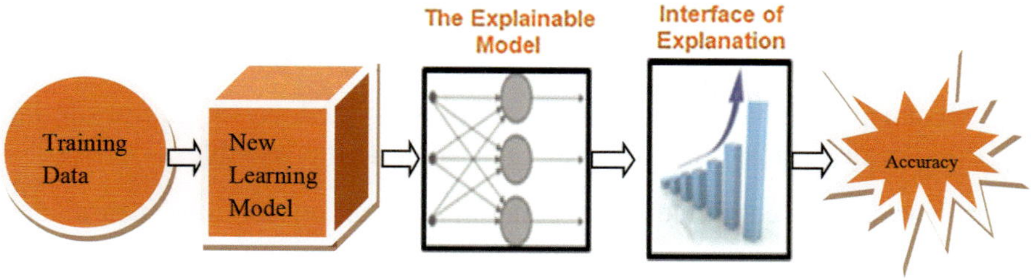


**Figure 13.2** Resolution process of XAI systems.

- It facilitates visual analysis by charting its outputs.
- It allows the differences between the endpoints to be seen more clearly.
- It allows for determining the success of the system.

There is an inverse relationship between the explainability of artificial intelligence and complexity (complex models). While complex artificial intelligence systems give more accurate results, it is difficult to explain, while less complex systems are easier to explain and give less accurate answers. For this reason, it is necessary to balance complexity and explainability in XAI systems.

### 13.2.1 The working principle of explainable artificial intelligence

Contrary to classical machine learning systems, solutions obtained with explainable artificial intelligence systems are met with a "glass box" approach that makes decision-making processes transparent. Accordingly, XAI aims to interfere with the typical learning process in machine learning or deep learning. When problem-solving is considered through image data such as medical diagnosis and object recognition, training data are created with many defined images, and the system learns to associate inputs with certain outputs by analyzing the data. When new data are entered into the system, the algorithm tries to reach the correct output by making use of the previous data. In this case, in the default solution, machine learning itself decides which points of the images to pay attention to and which points to ignore. It does not give any information about how it concluded. At this point, XAI makes it possible to provide the necessary order by integrating it into the existing solution model.

In XAI systems, the outputs provide evidence to the user with the explanation interface. Apart from these interfaces, texts and graphics:

- local explanations about how the model works in any field, and explanations based on an example from the training data the model uses;

- explanations through simplification, referring to a model that is simpler to interpret;
- it can also include explanations according to the level of feature similarity by measuring the effects of each input on the variables.

Deep-learning-based models are generally based on artificial neural networks. Artificial neural networks have a structure where neurons are connected. There are approaches to working in the network structure through hidden node layers. Therefore, the level of explainability is low.

### 13.2.2 Current methods in the scope of explainable artificial intelligence

The advancement of technology day by day and the frequent use of artificial intelligence have led to an increase in studies on XAI systems. There are many methods to explainable artificial intelligence. Some of the most notable methods developed in the field of XAI are as follows:

- **CAM:** Class activation mapping (CAM) is a method that is especially seen in deep learning models working on image data and is used to explain with heat maps which parts of the input images are focused. The CAM method brings together the weighted feature map components in the neural networks in which it is applied, in terms of the class options of the model, to create common activation maps and presents these maps with a heat map. The representation of the general structure of the CAM method on neural network architecture and its difference with the multi-class activation map (MultiCAM) are given in Figure 13.3.
- **LIME:** The LIME – local interpretable model-agnostic explanations – method describes the classifier for a single specific instance. It is more suitable for local assessments. It reveals the role of "explanatory" to be able to explain the predictions from each data sample. Although the model used according to LIME is very complex, it is easy to approach it from the environment of a feature [9]. Colored areas indicate decision regions for a complex binary classification model. The instance of interest is indicated by a black cross. Artificial data around the instance of interest are represented by dots. The dashed line represents a simple linear model describing the local behavior of the black box model around the instance of interest [22]. The output of a LIME model is shown in Figure 13.4.

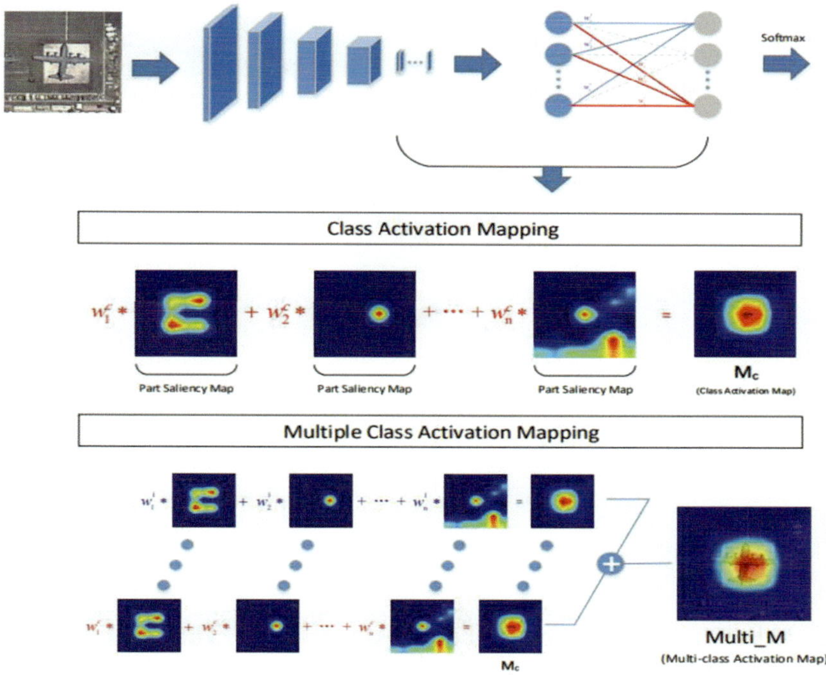


**Figure 13.3** Comparison between CAM and MultiCAM [21].

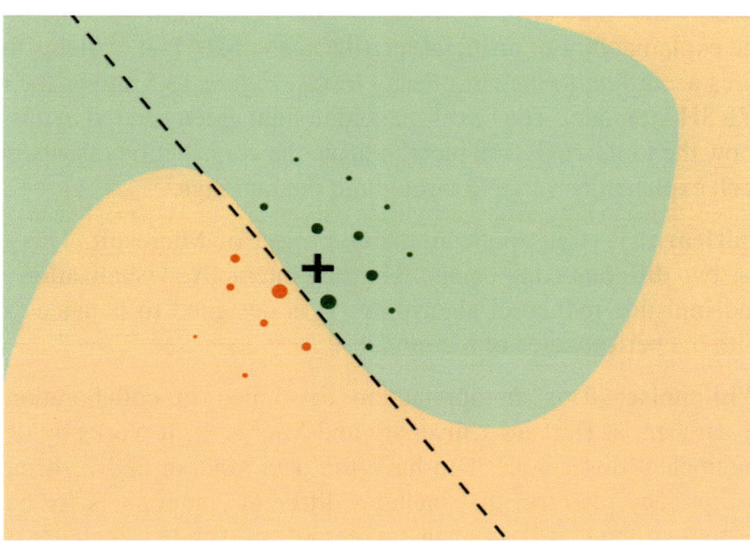

**Figure 13.4** The LIME method [22].

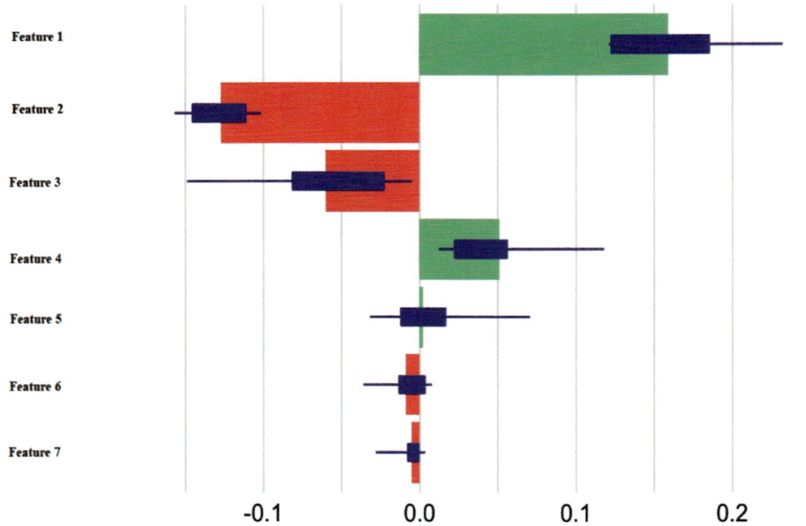


**Figure 13.5** The SHAP method [22].

- **SHAP:** This model combines the best inferences with local explanations based on the Shapley value in game theory and its extensions. The most important difference from locally interpretable models is the weighting of the instances in the regression model. LIME is used in simpler and less precise models, while SHAP is used in more complex models and more critical processes. One of the most used methods for the explainability of artificial intelligence is SHAP. It explains the features according to their similarity levels. Figure 13.5 shows the output of a SHAP model. The boxes marked in light green and red in this figure show the tools used. Box plots indicate the contribution distribution for each explanatory variable throughout the rankings.
- **Fairlearn:** It is an application-side project of Microsoft. This toolkit has two different components. They are interactive visualization boards and injustice reduction algorithms. It is designed to balance fairness with the performance of the model.
- **Whitenoise:** It is an application developed in collaboration with researchers at Harvard University and Microsoft. It works by defining parameters that enable it to have the data random and zero mean. It is a privacy platform that includes different components for building custom systems. It is an open-source project. While it includes privacy mechanisms with the Core library, it provides the necessary tools and

services for working with tables and relational data with the system library.

- **Eraser:** This model was developed by Salesforce. The model is aimed to evaluate rationalized natural language, and processing models. It focuses on snippets of text (justifications) extracted from source documents that provide sufficient evidence to predict the correct output. This model has class labels that include tasks such as sensitivity analysis, question answering, and natural language inference. Seven different language processing models consist of tasks that include human explanations of necessary explanations as supporting evidence for predictions from the dataset.

### 13.2.3 Approaches in XAI with drug discovery

There are five approaches in XAI to drug discovery such as feature attribution, instance-based, graph-convolution-based, self-explaining, and uncertainty estimation. These approaches and their sub-items are given in Figure 13.6.

#### 13.2.3.1 Feature attribution methods

The feature attribution approach produces an output showing the suitability of each input property for the final estimate computed by taking the inputs. It can be grouped into three categories as in Figure 13.7. The feature attribution method, which is widely used among deep learning applications, is to determine the derivative of the output of the neural network according to the input. Since the calculation of partial first-order derivatives in neural networks is done by backpropagation, the popularity of this model has increased [23–25].

Some noteworthy feature attribution techniques concern surrogate-model feature attribution, such as LIME, DeepLIFT (deep learning important features), SHAP, and layer-wise relevance propagation [26–30]. A subfamily of surrogate attribution methods and gradient-based methods offers local explanations. This explanation is not a common thought of the fundamental model but a review of each prediction separately. Initial endeavors were restricted to a family of tree-based ensemble techniques such as random forest; however, newer approaches can easily be applied to arbitrary deep learning models [31–33]. In perturbation-based approaches, it replaces or removes sections of the input by measuring the suitable alteration in the model output to assess the significance of the attribute. Perturbation-based approaches have the superiority of straight predicting the significance of attributes, but they are slow by calculation when the number of input attributes

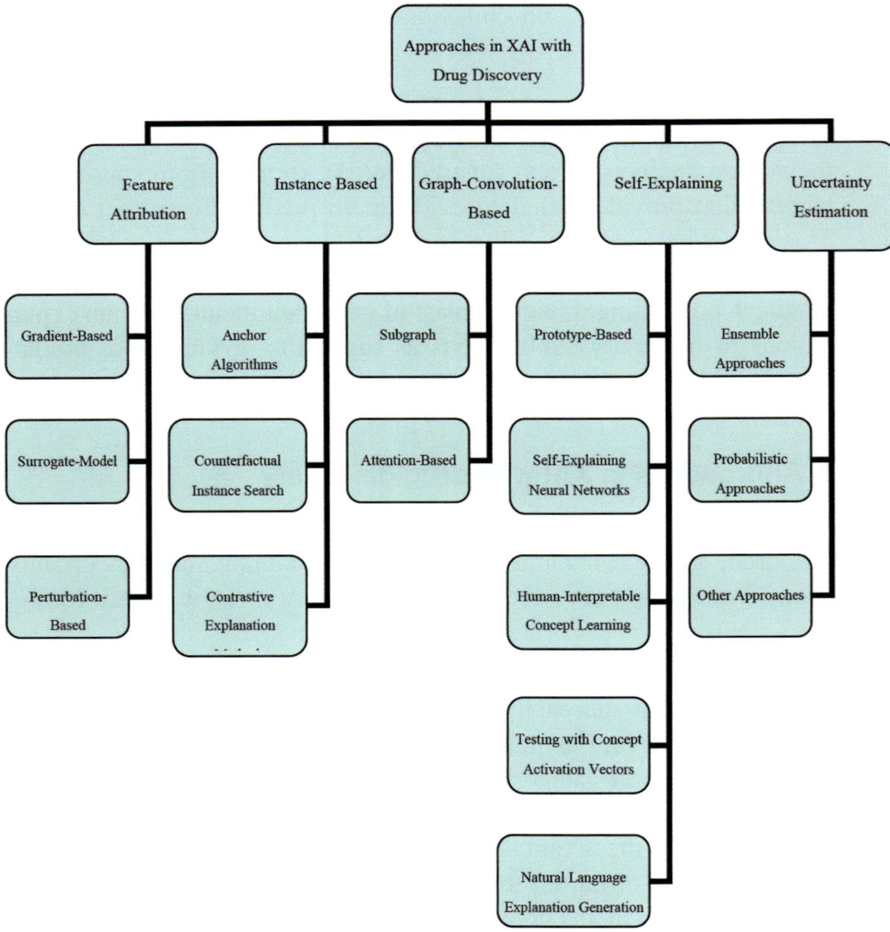


**Figure 13.6** Approaches in XAI with drug discovery.

raises and tend to be powerfully affected by the number of attributes that decay together [34, 35].

Feature attribution methods have recently become popular XAI techniques used in ligand- and structure-based drug discovery. For example, McCloskey et al. used a gradient-based feature to determine binding-related ligand pharmacophores [23, 36]. The study showed that models that were successful on the retained data were also able to learn fake correlations [36]. Pope et al. made suitable gradient-based feature attribution to identify functional groups of interest in the prediction of adverse effects [37–40]. Recently, SHAP has been used to interpret related properties for composite power and multi-target activity estimation [27, 41]. Hochuli et al., when comparing a

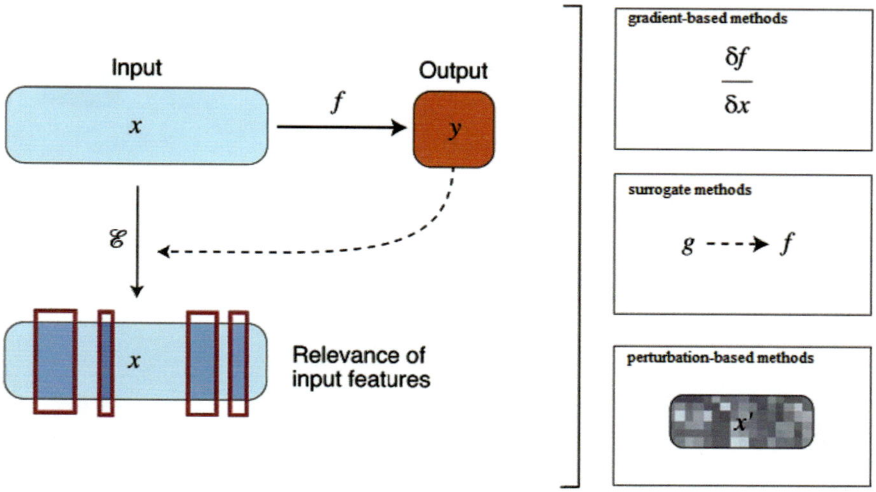


**Figure 13.7** The feature attribution methods [17].

few feature attribution methods, represented how to attribute visualization helps to differentiate and interpret three-dimensional convolutional neural networks and protein–ligand scoring [42–44].

### 13.2.3.2 Instance-based approaches

Instance-based methods calculate a subset of related samples that should or should not be present to alter the estimation of a certain design. An example may be real or constructed for the method [17]. The architecture of instance-based approaches in Figure 13.8 is given.

Anchor algorithms provide the interpretation regardless of the model in classifier models. They calculate a subset of the if–then rules according to one or more properties that specify the terms, to adequately secure the prediction of a given class. This is why anchors differ from many other local disclosure methods in that they clearly model the "scope" of the disclosure [45, 46].

Focusing on the realities we are in creates hypothetical images by presenting approaches with opposite facts. In XAI, counterfactual clarifications can be used to explain the estimations of individual samples. The inputs of a model can be seen as the reason for the estimation, even though the connection between the inputs and the outcome to be estimated is not causal. Counterfactuals are humane explanations because they are contrary to the present pattern and are selective; so, in general, they concentrate on a few feature changes [47].

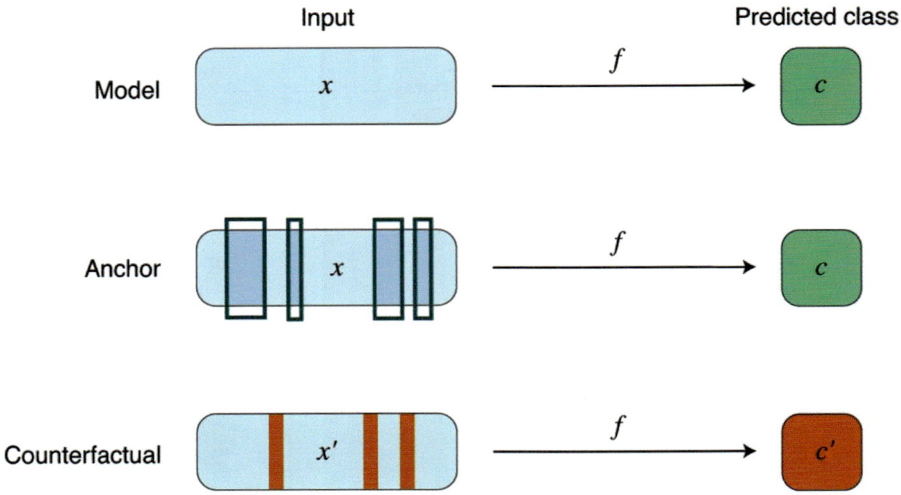


**Figure 13.8** The instance-based methods [17].

Contrasting annotation methods produce "related positive" and "related negative" sets, providing sample-based interpretability of classifiers. This technique is relevant to anchors as well as counterfactual research methods. Relevant positives are the smallest set of features in the sample so that the model can predict a "positive" outcome. Conversely, relevant negatives form the smallest set of properties that the model should not have to be adequately distinguished from other classes [17, 48].

Instance-based models can increase model transparency by specifying what molecular properties must be present to change or assure the model's prediction in drug discovery. Moreover, counterfactual thinking can support decision makers by providing new knowledge into base training data and the model [17].

#### 13.2.3.3 Graph-convolution-based methods

Molecular graphs are expressed as mathematical representations of atoms representing chemical bonds and nodes representing edges in molecular topology [50]. Their use in chemoinformatics and mathematical chemistry has been widespread since the late 1970s [51, 52]. For this reason, new graph convolutional neural networks, which join neural message forwarding algorithms, have increasing applications [53, 54]. The graph of the model is given in Figure 13.9. Convolution is a mathematical operation that combines two functions to produce a third function that expresses how one of the original functions affects the shape of the other. The resulting function is called the convolution of the

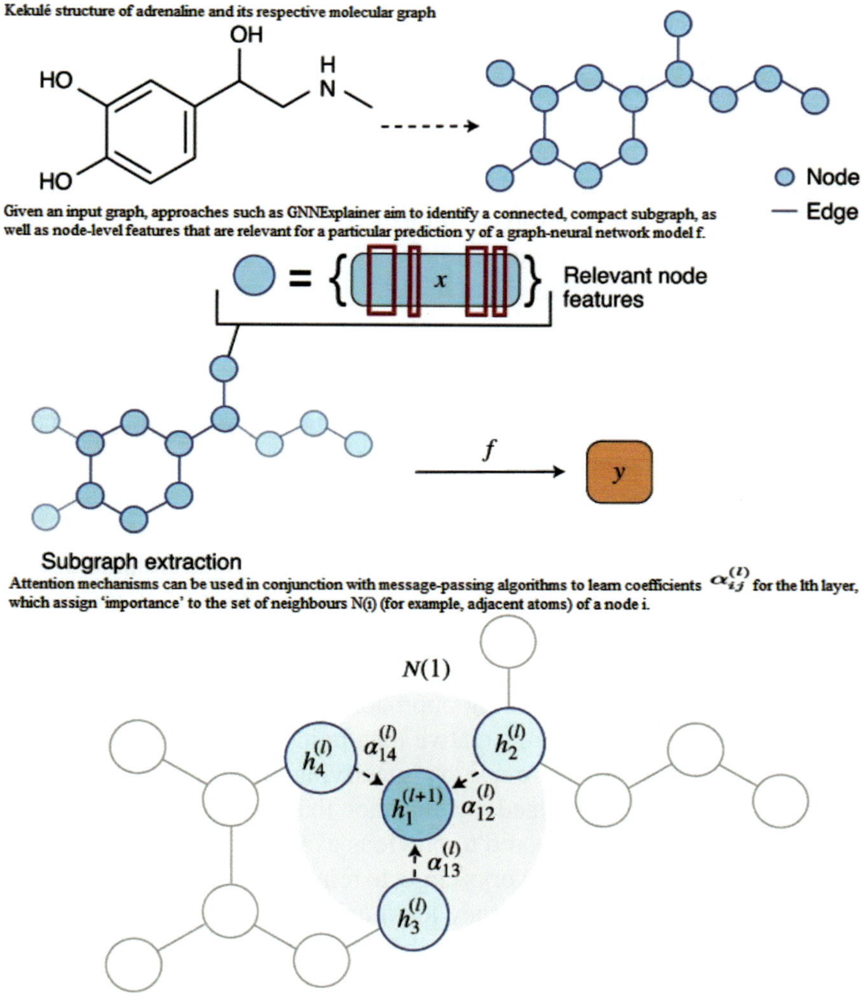


**Figure 13.9** The graph-convolution-based methods [17, 49].

two original functions and can be thought of as a measure of the amount of overlap between the two functions as one is shifted over the other. This notion is commonly used in convolutional neural networks for image analysis. Graph convolutions stretch the convolution process utilized in applications such as computer vision and natural language processing to randomly sized graphs [55, 56]. In drug discovery, molecular property estimation and graph curves are applied to manufacturer techniques for de novo drug discovery [57–59].

Approaches of subgraph identification focus on defining one or more components of a graph that are accountable for a certain estimation [17].

Attention-based methods are also the explication of graph-convolutional neural networks and take advantage of attentional mechanisms [60]. The main purpose here is to stack a few messages transmitting layers to acquire hidden node-level representations by first calculating the caution coefficients linked with a piece of the adjacent sides of a certain node appearing on the graph. Techniques of graphical convolutional are a potent device in drug discovery for chemists because of their direct and natural link to intuitive representations. Because of its intuitive connections with the two-size representation of molecules, graphical-convolution-based XAI can be applied to a few other prevalent modeling tasks in drug discovery [17].

#### 13.2.3.4 Self-explaining approaches

The self-explaining model is used to define techniques that prioritize explainability central piece of their project [17]. Self-explaining XAI methods can be classified as prototype-based reasoning, self-explaining neural networks, human-interpretable concepts, testing with concept activation vectors, and natural language explication generation. Explication formation methods can be applied to particular decision-making processes, like modifying animal testing and *in vitro* to *in vivo* extrapolation, where human-comprehensible annotations are a crucial element.

The prototype-based reasoning approach predicts forthcoming occurrences established especially informative data points. Prototypes adapted to make an estimate are usually made by specifying representative samples. These approaches are stimulated by the fact that estimations mimic the decision-making process compared to previous examples [61].

Self-explaining neural networks target to relate input or hidden attributes to semantic constructs. Together, they learn a class estimation and produce clarifications by taking advantage of attribute-to-construct mapping [62].

Human-interpretable concept learning defines the learning of high-level combinations of information items from data [63]. This approach is known to achieve human-like success on one-time learning [64, 65].

In concept activation vectors, the test calculates the directional derivatives of a concept concerning the input of the activations of a layer. Such derivatives measure the degree of the latter for a given classification [66].

The natural language annotation approach is used to generate descriptions for both the image and the class. However, to get expressive interpretations, this approach necessitates an important number of human-curated annotations for training, and, therefore, it can encounter restricted applicability in drug discovery [67].

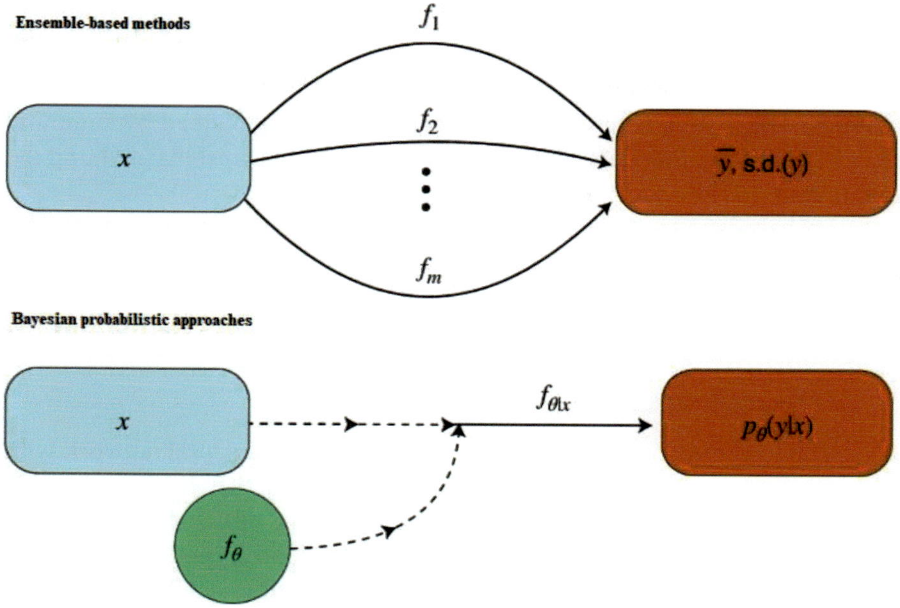


**Figure 13.10** The uncertainty estimation method [17].

#### 13.2.3.5 Uncertainty estimation

Uncertainty estimation is an approach to interpreting a model. It involves measuring the errors or inaccuracies in the model's predictions, which can provide insight into how reliable the model's output is. By estimating uncertainty, one can understand the range of potential outcomes for a given prediction and how confident the model is in its ability to make accurate predictions. Deep neural networks being insufficient at quantifying indefiniteness is one of the causes why struggles were dedicated to particularly quantifying indefiniteness in neural-network-based estimations [17]. Uncertainty prediction methods were successfully applied in drug discovery, frequently in conventional QSAR modeling, making use of either model that inherently deals with uncertainty or *post-hoc* methods [77–80]. Schwaller et al. suggested a transformer approach for the advanced chemical reaction estimation [81]. This method applies uncertainty prediction by calculating the result of the likelihoods of all estimated pointers in a SMILES array representing a molecule. Improving uncertainty prediction with transparency or justification is a key field of investigation for maximizing the dependability and efficacy of XAI in drug discovery [17]. The uncertainty estimation method graph is given in Figure 13.10.

One of the uncertainty estimation methods is the ensemble approach. Model ensembles can become standard for uncertainty estimations, improving whole prediction quality [68]. An uncertainty prediction can be derived from the relevant variance, while the final estimate is obtained by summing the estimates of all models. This model can then use "snapshots" to build the community [69].

Probabilistic techniques intend to predict the likelihood of a particular model output or execute *post-hoc* standardization. Gal *et al.* proposed the usage of the dropout arrangement to actualize estimated Bayesian inference, which was afterward enlarged to calculate epistemic and aleatoric uncertainty [70].

Other approaches are given below:

- The lower upper bound prediction method trains a neural network with two outputs matching the estimation top and nether borders. Instead of measuring the error of a single estimation, this approach utilizes simulated annealing and updates the model coefficients to accomplish maximal training computations inclusion and minimal estimation gap breadth [71].
- Ak et al. proposed measuring indefiniteness in neural network models by modeling interval-valued data [72].
- After union-based methods train a neural network model, they nourish its embeddings into a second model that accomplishes indefiniteness, like a Gaussian method or a random forest [73].
- Distance-based methods focus on predicting the predictive indefiniteness of a new "*x*" instance by computing the remoteness to the nearest instance in the training set, utilizing input attributes or a model-generated embedding [74–76].

## 13.3 Conclusion

In terms of drug discovery, it is difficult to achieve full intelligibility of deep learning models, although the predictions provided may still be beneficial to the applicator [82]. Endeavoring for clarifications that fit human instinct, it is critical to cautiously design a set of control tests to verify machine-driven assumptions and raise their trustworthiness and impartiality [83].

The current XAI confronts technical difficulties and ascertains the numerous possible clarifications and techniques practicable to a given task too. Most methods do not come as ready-to-use solutions but need to be adapted to every implementation [84]. Moreover, deep information on the issue is essential to determine which model decisions require further explanation, which types of replies are important to the user, and which are instead insignificant or anticipated. For people to decide, the clarifications formed with XAI need to be significant, non-artificial, and enlightening enough for the relevant scientific ensemble. Such resolutions necessitate the combined endeavors of deep learning experts, chemo informaticians and data scientists, chemists, biologists, and other field experts to provide that XAI techniques serve their aim and provide dependable replies [17].

It could be a step forward for chemists to construct explainable "low-level" molecular representations that have direct signification and are suitable for machine learning. Most researches lately base on well-founded molecular identifiers such as mixed binary fingerprints, and topochemical and geometric identifiers that capture structural attributes determined before [85–88]. The improvement of new explainable molecular representations for deep learning cannot be interpreted, but the development of sufficiently accurate predictions as well as self-explanatory methods to come through the barriers of explanations of information-rich descriptors will be an important field of research for years to come. In price and time susceptible scenarios such as drug discovery, deep learning experts have the liability to carefully examine and explain the estimations obtained from modeling selections. Considering the available possibilities and restrictions of XAI in drug discovery, the ongoing advancement of hybrid methods and different approaches that are easier to understand and in terms of calculating low-cost will not mislay their significance. In drug discovery, XAI should be an open community platform to share and develop software, explanation of techniques, and relevant training data through the energetic struggles of investigators from dissimilar scientific experiences. Enterprises such as the Machine Learning Ledger Orchestration for Drug Discovery (MELLODY) for non-central, combined model improving and safe data processing among drug firms are the initial move truly. Such collaborations are believed to support the improvement, verification, and admission of XAI and the related disclosures these devices supply [17].

## References

[1] McCarthy, J. Artificial intelligence, logic and formalizing common sense. In Philosophical logic and artificial intelligence; Springer: 1989, pp 161–190.

[2] McCarthy, J., From here to human-level AI. Artificial Intelligence2007, pp 1174–1182.

[3] https://www.ibm.com/in-en/cloud/learn/what-is-artificialintelligence
[4] Bharatam, P. V. Computer-aided drug design. In Drug Discovery and Development; Springer: 2021, pp 137–210.
[5] Zhang, Y.; Rajapakse, J. C., Machine learning in bioinformatics.John Wiley & Sons, Inc.; New Jersey, US: 2009; Vol. 4.
[6] Zupan, J.; Gasteiger, J., Neural networks in chemistry and drug design. John Wiley & Sons, Inc.; New Jersey, US: 1999.
[7] Gertrudes, J. C.; Maltarollo, V. G.; Silva, R.; Oliveira, P. R.; Honorio, K. M.; Da Silva, A., Machine learning techniques and drug design. Current Medicinal Chemistry 2012, 19, 4289–4297
[8] Sharma, V. K., & Bharatam, P. V. Artificial Intelligence in Drug Discovery (AIDD).
[9] Kaçar, T. (2021), "Explanaible Artificial Intelligence", ed. Kose, U., Ethics of Artificial Intelligence (1):99–115, Ankara, Nobel Publishing.
[10] Zhang, Y., Weng, Y., & Lund, J. (2022). Applications of Explainable Artificial Intelligence in Diagnosis and Surgery. Diagnostics, 12(2), 237.
[11] Deore A, Dhumane J, Wagh R, Sonawane R (2019) Asian J Pharm Res Dev 7:62
[12] Staszak M, Staszak K, Wieszczycka K, Bajek A, Roszkowski K, Tylkowski B (2021) Wiley Interdisciplinary Reviews:Computational Molecular Science Page 15/28
[13] Vamathevan J, Clark D, Czodrowski P, Dunham I, Ferran E, Lee G, Li B, Madabhushi A, Shah P, Spitzer M, Zhao S (2019) Nat Rev Drug Discov 18(6):463
[14] Lavecchia A (2015) Drug Discov Today 20(3):318
[15] Lo YC, Rensi SE, Torng W, Altman RB (2018) Drug Discov Today 23(8):1538
[16] Xue L, Bajorath J (2000) Comb Chem High Throughput Screen 3(5):363
[17] Jiménez-Luna, J., Grisoni, F., Schneider, G. (2020). Drug discovery with explainable artificial intelligence. Nature Machine Intelligence, 2(10), 573–584.
[18] Kırboğa, K. K., Küçüksille, E. U., Köse, U. (2022). Ignition of Small Molecule Inhibitors in Friedreich's Ataxia with Explainable Artificial Intelligence.
[19] Adadi, A., Berrada, M. (2018). Peeking inside the black-box: a survey on explainable artificial intelligence (XAI). IEEE Access, 6, 52138–52160.
[20] Arrieta, A. B., Díaz-Rodríguez, N., Del Ser, J., Bennetot, A., Tabik, S., Barbado, A., Herrera, F. (2020). Explainable Artificial Intelligence (XAI): Concepts, taxonomies, opportunities, and challenges toward responsible AI. Information fusion, 58, 82–115.

[21] Fu, K., Dai, W., Zhang, Y., Wang, Z., Yan, M., Sun, X. (2019). Multicam: Multiple class activation mapping for aircraft recognition in remote sensing images. Remote sensing, 11(5), 544.

[22] Biecek, P., Burzykowski, T. (2021). Explanatory model analysis: Explore, explain and examine predictive models. Chapman and Hall/CRC.

[23] Sundararajan, M., Taly, A., Yan, Q. (2017). Axiomatic attribution for deep networks. In Proc. 34th International Conference on Machine Learning Vol. 70, 3319–3328.

[24] Smilkov, D., Thorat, N., Kim, B., Viégas, F., Wattenberg, M. Smoothgrad. (2017). Removing noise by adding noise. Preprint at https://arxiv.org/abs/1706.03825.

[25] Rumelhart, D. E., Hinton, G. E. Williams, R. J. (1986). Learning representations by back-propagating errors. Nature 323, 533–536.

[26] Lipovetsky, S., Conklin, M. (2001). Analysis of regression in game theory approach. Appl. Stoch. Models Bus. Ind. 17, 319–330.

[27] Lundberg, S. M., Lee, S.-I. (2017). A unified approach to interpreting model predictions. Adv. Neural Inf. Process. Syst. 30, 4765–4774.

[28] Ribeiro, M. T., Singh, S., Guestrin, C. (2016). "Why should I trust you?" Explaining the predictions of any classifier. In Proc. 22nd ACM SIGKDD International Conference on Knowledge Discovery and Data Mining 1135–1144.

[29] Shrikumar, A., Greenside, P., Kundaje, (2017). A. Learning important features through propagating activation differences. In Proc. 34th International Conference on Machine Learning Vol. 70, 3145–3153.

[30] Bach, S., Binder, A., Montavon, G., Klauschen, F., Müller, K. R., Samek, W. (2015). On pixel-wise explanations for non-linear classifier decisions by layer-wise relevance propagation. PloS one, 10(7), e0130140.

[31] Lakkaraju, H., Kamar, E., Caruana, R., Leskovec, J. (2017). Interpretable & explorable approximations of black box models. arXiv preprint arXiv:1707.01154.

[32] Deng, H. (2019). Interpreting tree ensembles with intrees. International Journal of Data Science and Analytics, 7(4), 277–287.

[33] Bastani, O., Kim, C., Bastani, H. (2017). Interpreting black box models via model extraction. arXiv preprint arXiv:1705.08504.

[34] Zintgraf, L. M., Cohen, T. S., Adel, T., Welling, M. (2017). Visualizing deep neural network decisions: Prediction difference analysis. arXiv preprint arXiv:1702.04595.

[35] Ancona, M., Ceolini, E., Öztireli, C., Gross, M. (2017). Towards better understanding of gradient-based attribution methods for deep neural networks. arXiv preprint arXiv:1711.06104.

[36] McCloskey, K., Taly, A., Monti, F., Brenner, M. P., Colwell, L. J. (2019). Using attribution to decode binding mechanism in neural network models for chemistry. Proceedings of the National Academy of Sciences, 116(24), 11624–11629.

[37] Pope, P. E., Kolouri, S., Rostami, M., Martin, C. E., Hoffmann, H. (2019). Explainability methods for graph convolutional neural networks. In Proceedings of the IEEE/CVF Conference on Computer Vision and Pattern Recognition (pp. 10772–10781).

[38] Selvaraju, R. R., Cogswell, M., Das, A., Vedantam, R., Parikh, D., Batra, D. (2017). Grad-cam: Visual explanations from deep networks via gradient-based localization. In Proceedings of the IEEE international conference on computer vision (pp. 618–626).

[39] Zhang, J., Bargal, S. A., Lin, Z., Brandt, J., Shen, X., Sclaroff, S. (2018). Top-down neural attention by excitation backprop. International Journal of Computer Vision, 126(10), 1084–1102.

[40] Tice, R. R., Austin, C. P., Kavlock, R. J., & Bucher, J. R. (2013). Improving the human hazard characterization of chemicals: a Tox21 update. Environmental health perspectives, 121(7), 756–765.

[41] Rodríguez-Pérez, R., Bajorath, J. (2019). Interpretation of compound activity predictions from complex machine learning models using local approximations and Shapley values. Journal of medicinal chemistry, 63(16), 8761–8777.

[42] Hochuli, J., Helbling, A., Skaist, T., Ragoza, M., Koes, D. R. (2018). Visualizing convolutional neural network protein-ligand scoring. Journal of Molecular Graphics and Modelling, 84, 96–108.

[43] Jiménez-Luna, J., Skalic, M., Martinez-Rosell, G. De Fabritiis, G. KDEEP: protein-ligand absolute binding affinity prediction via 3D-convolutional neural networks. J. Chem. Inf. Model. 58, 287–296 (2018).

[44] Jiménez-Luna, J., Pérez-Benito, L., Martinez-Rosell, G., Sciabola, S., Torella, R., Tresadern, G., De Fabritiis, G. (2019). DeltaDelta neural networks for lead optimization of small molecule potency. Chemical science, 10(47), 10911–10918.

[45] Ribeiro, M. T., Singh, S., Guestrin, C. (2016). " Why should i trust you?" Explaining the predictions of any classifier. In Proceedings of the 22nd ACM SIGKDD international conference on knowledge discovery and data mining (pp. 1135–1144).

[46] Ribeiro, M. T., Singh, S., Guestrin, C. (2018). Anchors: High-precision model-agnostic explanations. In Proceedings of the AAAI conference on artificial intelligence (Vol. 32, No. 1).

[47] Dandl, S., Molnar, C., Binder, M., & Bischl, B. (2020, September). Multi-objective counterfactual explanations. In International Conference on Parallel Problem Solving from Nature (pp. 448–469). Springer, Cham.

[48] Dhurandhar, A., Chen, P. Y., Luss, R., Tu, C. C., Ting, P., Shanmugam, K., Das, P. (2018). Explanations based on the missing: Towards contrastive explanations with pertinent negatives. Advances in neural information processing systems, 31.

[49] Ying, Z., Bourgeois, D., You, J., Zitnik, M., Leskovec, J. (2019). Gnnexplainer: Generating explanations for graph neural networks. Advances in neural information processing systems, 32.

[50] Consonni, V., Todeschini, R. (2009). Molecular Descriptors for Chemoinformatics: Volume I: Alphabetical Listing/Volume II: Appendices, References. John Wiley & Sons.

[51] Randić, M., Brissey, G. M., Spencer, R. B., Wilkins, C. L. (1979). Search for all self-avoiding paths for molecular graphs. Computers & Chemistry, 3(1), 5–13.

[52] Bonchev, D., Trinajstić, N. (1977). Information theory, distance matrix, and molecular branching. The Journal of Chemical Physics, 67(10), 4517–4533.

[53] Duvenaud, D. K., Maclaurin, D., Iparraguirre, J., Bombarell, R., Hirzel, T., Aspuru-Guzik, A., Adams, R. P. (2015). Convolutional networks on graphs for learning molecular fingerprints. Advances in neural information processing systems, 28.

[54] Gilmer, J., Schoenholz, S. S., Riley, P. F., Vinyals, O., Dahl, G. E. (2017, July). Neural message passing for quantum chemistry. In International conference on machine learning (pp. 1263–1272). PMLR.

[55] Krizhevsky, A., Sutskever, I., Hinton, G. E. (2012). Imagenet classification with deep convolutional neural networks. Advances in neural information processing systems, 25.

[56] Zhang, Y., Wallace, B. (2015). A sensitivity analysis of (and practitioners' guide to) convolutional neural networks for sentence classification. arXiv preprint arXiv:1510.03820.

[57] Kearnes, S., McCloskey, K., Berndl, M., Pande, V., Riley, P. (2016). Molecular graph convolutions: moving beyond fingerprints. Journal of computer-aided molecular design, 30(8), 595–608.

[58] Wu, Z., Ramsundar, B., Feinberg, E. N., Gomes, J., Geniesse, C., Pappu, A. S., Pande, V. (2018). MoleculeNet: a benchmark for molecular machine learning. Chemical science, 9(2), 513–530.

[59] Jin, W., Barzilay, R., Jaakkola, T. (2018). Junction tree variational autoencoder for molecular graph generation. In International conference on machine learning (pp. 2323–2332). PMLR.

[60] Veličković, P., Cucurull, G., Casanova, A., Romero, A., Lio, P., Bengio, Y. (2017). Graph attention networks. arXiv preprint arXiv:1710.10903.
[61] Leake, D. B. (1996). Case-based reasoning: experiences, lessons, and future directions.
[62] Alvarez Melis, D., Jaakkola, T. (2018). Towards robust interpretability with self-explaining neural networks. Advances in neural information processing systems, 31.
[63] Goodman, N. D., Tenenbaum, J. B., Gerstenberg, T. (2014). Concepts in a probabilistic language of thought. Center for Brains, Minds, and Machines (CBMM).
[64] Vinyals, O., Blundell, C., Lillicrap, T., Wierstra, D. (2016). Matching networks for one shot learning. Advances in neural information processing systems, 29.
[65] Altae-Tran, H., Ramsundar, B., Pappu, A. S., Pande, V. (2017). Low data drug discovery with one-shot learning. ACS central science, 3(4), 283–293.
[66] Kim, B., Wattenberg, M., Gilmer, J., Cai, C., Wexler, J., Viegas, F. (2018). Interpretability beyond feature attribution: Quantitative testing with concept activation vectors (tcav). In International conference on machine learning (pp. 2668–2677). PMLR.
[67] Hendricks, L. A., Akata, Z., Rohrbach, M., Donahue, J., Schiele, B., Darrell, T. (2016). Generating visual explanations. In European conference on computer vision (pp. 3–19). Springer, Cham.
[68] Hansen, L. K., Salamon, P. (1990). Neural network ensembles. IEEE transactions on pattern analysis and machine intelligence, 12(10), 993–1001.
[69] Huang, G., Li, Y., Pleiss, G., Liu, Z., Hopcroft, J. E., Weinberger, K. Q. (2017). Snapshot ensembles: Train 1, get m for free. arXiv preprint arXiv:1704.00109.
[70] Gal, Y., Ghahramani, Z. (2016). Dropout as a bayesian approximation: Representing model uncertainty in deep learning. In international conference on machine learning (pp. 1050–1059). PMLR.
[71] Khosravi, A., Nahavandi, S., Creighton, D., Atiya, A. F. (2010). Lower upper bound estimation method for construction of neural network-based prediction intervals. IEEE transactions on neural networks, 22(3), 337–346.
[72] Ak, R., Vitelli, V., Zio, E. (2015). An interval-valued neural network approach for uncertainty quantification in short-term wind speed prediction. IEEE transactions on neural networks and learning systems, 26(11), 2787–2800.

[73] Huang, W., Zhao, D., Sun, F., Liu, H., Chang, E. (2015, June). Scalable Gaussian process regression using deep neural networks. In: Twenty-fourth international joint conference on artificial intelligence.

[74] Sheridan, R. P., Feuston, B. P., Maiorov, V. N., Kearsley, S. K. (2004). Similarity to molecules in the training set is a good discriminator for prediction accuracy in QSAR. Journal of chemical information and computer sciences, 44(6), 1912–1928.

[75] Liu, R., Wallqvist, A. (2018). Molecular similarity-based domain applicability metric efficiently identifies out-of-domain compounds. Journal of Chemical Information and Modeling, 59(1), 181-189.

[76] Janet, J. P., Duan, C., Yang, T., Nandy, A., Kulik, H. J. (2019). A quantitative uncertainty metric controls error in neural network-driven chemical discovery. Chemical science, 10(34), 7913–7922.

[77] Scalia, G., Grambow, C. A., Pernici, B., Li, Y. P., Green, W. H. (2020). Evaluating scalable uncertainty estimation methods for deep learning-based molecular property prediction. Journal of chemical information and modeling, 60(6), 2697–2717.

[78] Obrezanova, O., Csányi, G., Gola, J. M., Segall, M. D. (2007). Gaussian processes: a method for automatic QSAR modeling of ADME properties. Journal of chemical information and modeling, 47(5), 1847–1857.

[79] Schroeter, T. S., Schwaighofer, A., Mika, S., Ter Laak, A., Suelzle, D., Ganzer, U., Müller, K. R. (2007). Estimating the domain of applicability for machine learning QSAR models: a study on aqueous solubility of drug discovery molecules. Journal of Computer-aided molecular design, 21(9), 485–498.

[80] Bosc, N., Atkinson, F., Felix, E., Gaulton, A., Hersey, A., Leach, A. R. (2019). Large scale comparison of QSAR and conformal prediction methods and their applications in drug discovery. Journal of cheminformatics, 11(1), 1–16.

[81] Schwaller, P., Laino, T., Gaudin, T., Bolgar, P., Hunter, C. A., Bekas, C., Lee, A. A. (2019). Molecular transformer: a model for uncertainty-calibrated chemical reaction prediction. ACS central science, 5(9), 1572–1583.

[82] Schneider, P., Schneider, G. (2016). De novo design at the edge of chaos: Miniperspective. Journal of medicinal chemistry, 59(9), 4077–4086.

[83] Sheridan, R. P. (2019). Interpretation of QSAR models by coloring atoms according to changes in predicted activity: how robust is it?. Journal of chemical information and modeling, 59(4), 1324–1337.

[84] Lipton, Z. C. (2017). The doctor just won't accept that! arXiv preprint arXiv:1711.08037.

[85] Rogers, D., Hahn, M. (2010). Extended-connectivity fingerprints. Journal of chemical information and modeling, 50(5), 742–754.

[86] Awale, M., Reymond, J. L. (2014). Atom pair 2D-fingerprints perceive 3D-molecular shape and pharmacophores for very fast virtual screening of ZINC and GDB-17. Journal of chemical information and modeling, 54(7), 1892–1907.

[87] Todeschini, R., Consonni, V. (2010). New local vertex invariants and molecular descriptors based on functions of the vertex degrees. MATCH Commun. Math. Comput. Chem, 64(2), 359–372.

[88] Katritzky, A. R., Gordeeva, E. V. (1993). Traditional topological indexes vs electronic, geometrical, and combined molecular descriptors in QSAR/QSPR research. Journal of chemical information and computer sciences, 33(6), 835–857.

# 14

# Explainable Intelligence Enabled Smart Healthcare for Rural Communities

**Soumyadeep Chanda, Rohan Kumar, Aditya Kumar Singh, and Sushruta Mishra**

Kalinga Institute of Industrial Technology, Deemed to be University, India
Email: 20051368@kiit.ac.in; 20051374@kiit.ac.in; 2006305@kiit.ac.in; sushruta.mishrafcs@kiit.ac.in

## Abstract

The Internet of Things (IoT) is based on intelligent health monitoring systems that could be a new idea for India. Doctors and adequate and bare minimum medical facilities are out of reach in rural India. Almost 56% of the total population lives in rural areas. Residents of rural India are suffering greatly because they do not receive proper medical services. Therefore, IoT-based intelligent medical services are critical in our country, especially in rural areas.

With the wide use of advanced technologies, it can establish a more vital and more innovative health supply system as the Internet of Things (IoT) is revolutionizing the healthcare industry by adding up new and advanced technologies to form healthcare efficiency, improve access to worry, increase quality, and reduce care cost. This research paper's main objective is to suggest some models using IoT to confirm better healthcare facilities for poor people. Furthermore, it will take a vital role in delivering healthcare to people present in remote areas by observing the healthcare systems through Internet connectivity, providing emergency notifications, and supplying accurate data in real time for making better or more accurate health decisions.

## 14.1 Introduction

IoT (Internet of Things) makes things easier. Information and communication technologies (ICTs) have great potential to address some of the challenges developed and developing countries face in furnishing accessible, cost-effective, and high-quality healthcare services.

ICTs are analogous to computers, the Internet, and cell phones, revolutionizing the self-identity of people who communicate with each other to seek information that helps enrich their lives. These technologies have great potential to solve today's worldwide health problems [1]. One such benefit is telemedicine, which plays a specific role in providing emergency medical services. Telemedicine offers healthcare using information and communication technology.

Tracking people in real time was impossible, especially in rural areas. Simultaneous treatment of multiple patients in a short period of time and frequent and repeated doctor visits are problematic and expensive at this time and space. Health monitoring is the key to enriching the living standards in rural areas. It displays data such as body temperature and heart rate graphically on the page at the request of authorized persons [2]. Wired Ethernet connected to heart rate sensor and Arduino helps to maintain mobility in monitoring patients at nursing homes. Citations include performance, implementation, and analysis of information and healthcare [3].

The IoT is entering the healthcare industry by adding pioneering technologies to optimize healthcare, improve access to healthcare, improve healthcare quality, and reduce healthcare costs – it will start a revolution. It plays an essential role in providing healthcare to people in remote areas by monitoring health systems via Internet connections, providing emergency alerts and accurate real-time data, and making better healthcare decisions. Reducing mortality rates in rural areas could lead to better healthcare [4].

In India, mainly in rural areas, people are not aware of technologies like IoT. So, proper guidance is a prerequisite. For example, IoTs can tell them in which season they have to cultivate crops and suggest the same according to the condition of the soil. With the help of such technologies, now they can predict the weather too.

IoTs not only help in the agricultural sector but also in the medical field. Some of them are explained below, expanding on how it will help them in upcoming years and how it is best from the existing models [5].

The main aim of the paper is to provide a better healthcare facility in rural areas of India. The main objectives of our models are as follows:

- To provide a reliable ambulance service at the time of emergency using XAI.
- To provide adequate health insurance to farmers.

- To provide a bridge between NGOs and hospitals to provide healthcare facilities collectively using an app and a toll-free number.
- To discuss the impact of explainable AI on smart healthcare in rural regions.

## 14.2 Relevant Models for Smart Rural Healthcare

In recent times, some modern smart healthcare models have been developed, but most of them are designed to operate in urban zones. Rural regions are still neglected. People in rural areas need effective healthcare facilities with a substantial explanation. In such scenarios, explainable AI can be of great help [6]. This section discusses three advanced models using XAI in rural healthcare.

### 14.2.1 An interpretable emergency ambulance response model

In the present technical era, where almost every work is done on smartphones, efficient and quick services are essential, especially when it comes to medical services [7]. Efficient and effective medical services are critical in today's society. However, these services are not always available in cases of severe illness and emergency. Due to a lack of knowledge, rural people suffer greatly. The lack of such attention and information leads to severe casualties [8]. The challenges range from unstructured addresses to poor road connectivity to non-arrival of ambulances leading to loss of lives. The main aim of this model is to reduce the waiting time for the patient and the ambulance to search for each other and provide the best medical service in a brief time interval by using a GPS signal. This model designs and implements a system prototype using mobile application technologies to offer cost-effective and fast ambulances during emergencies [9].

The benefits of the model include the following:

- Reduces operator calls and reports every detail accurately.
- When someone is stuck in a new location and calls an ambulance, it provides reliable information about the site.
- To reduce the number of fraudulent calls.
- It takes a long time to reach the hospital because the current system needs to dispatch an ambulance correctly, and it is difficult for the driver to arrive at the accident scene urgently due to traffic jams.

**Table 14.1** Comparison of the current and the proposed model.

| Current model | Proposed XAI model |
|---|---|
| • Computer phone system is expensive | • Android app is cheaper than the current model |
| • Dispatching emergency service to the location takes a long time | • Computer assistance – emergency call with GPS system faster |
| • Local information system | • Double tap to request ambulance ambulance or hospital |
| • One emergency line (101) | • Sends notification request to nearest ambulance or hospital |
| • The ambulance gets all details of the exact location and the estimated time of the user or patient's ambulance who cannot find the location and estimated time | • The user and driver receives all the details of each other along with the address with the help of Google maps |

Constraints of the model include:

- A user may accidentally provide incorrect information, or an operator may fill up some false information.
- The user must call and provide their exact location so that the ambulance can track and contact the patient timely.
- The user must check the availability of an ambulance and wait for the ambulance to be vacant.
- Many inquiries about fraud lead to the abuse of resources.

Table 14.1 describes the difference between the challenges of the current model and possible freedom in the proposed XAI-based model.

The android application allows the user to book an ambulance and send the location of the accident to the administrator. Administrators can use the links on the user page to get the received GPS address. This area is assigned to the driver. The driver then sends a notification to the administrator. If possible, the administrator informs the driver of the location of the nearest hospital.

Figure 14.1 shows the medical needs of rural areas. It focuses on providing the fastest and most effective medical facilities. This app allows ambulance drivers to register their availability and location. Alternatively, the user is asked to log in by providing their phone number and signing in from their

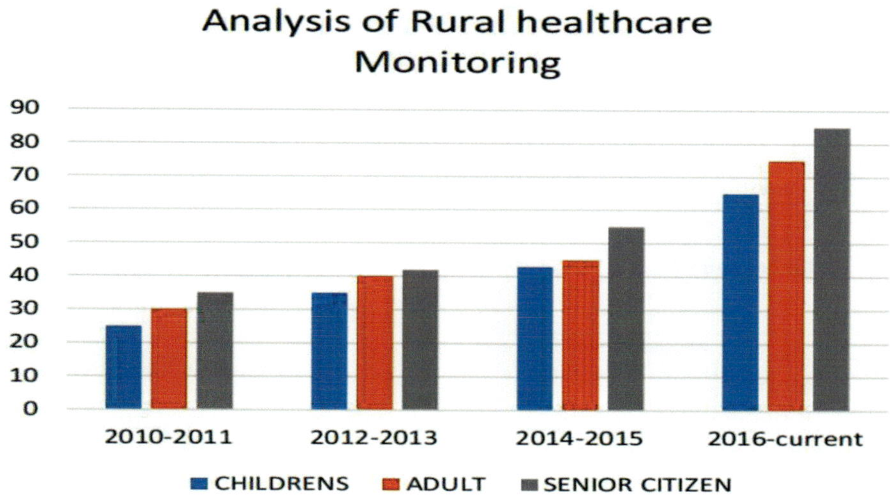


**Figure 14.1** Analysis of rural healthcare monitoring.

Google account. First, the user's location is recorded on Google Maps. Next, the user identifies the nearest ambulance on the map. When the patient enters the identified ambulance station and sends it to the administrator, the location is assigned to the ambulance driver, and the list of hospitals allows the administrator to select the nearest hospital and bring the patient to the hospital on time. Now the user sends the danger zone to the manager.

Figure 14.2 explains the working of the application. First, the area is displayed on the website, and the driver gives the administrator a location after the officer informs the driver of the site of the accident. Then, upon arriving at the accident scene, the driver sends a notice to the supervisor, after which the patient can reach the hospital grounds. Finally, the driver can control the traffic lights on the route of the oncoming ambulance.

#### 14.2.1.1 Software used in this model

Google's official integrated development platform (IDE) for the Android operating system – Android Studio – was created upon IntelliJ, IDEA, and JetBrains' software and manufactured specifically for Android development [10].

It is downloadable for Windows, Mac-OS, and Linux operating systems. It replaces Eclipse Android Development Tools (ADT) as the default native IDE for Android application development.

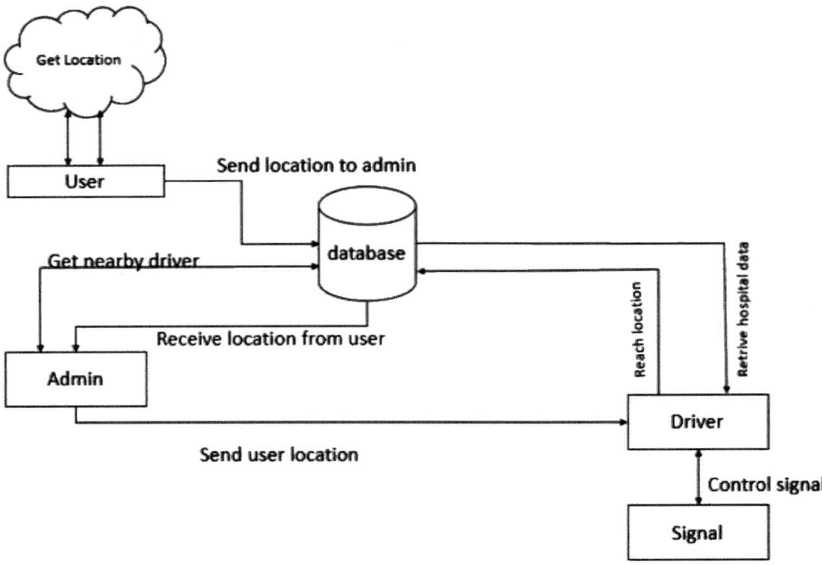


**Figure 14.2** Flow diagram of emergency ambulance response model.

#### 14.2.1.2 Detailed process for managing the execution of applications by users, ambulances, and administrators

The system works as follows:

When the user clicks on the find ambulance icon in the app, a notification is sent to the rescue guidance system.

- Users do not need to call to check the ambulance availability; it is shown via Google maps.
- Notifications sent by users include the user's GPS location as well as the user's pre-registered address.
- Ambulances will track their location via GPS.

The detailed execution flow is discussed here:

Step 1. Users must register.

This is the first function that opens when the user installs the application. First, the user must enter the correct contact number and password [11]. If the information provided to the user matches the data in the site table and the user tries to log in again to the application, a login error will be displayed, and the user must re-enter the correct information. Next, the link to the registration feature is for registering new users.

Step 2. Administrator.

The administrator finds the location of the user's accident, which is shared with the ambulance driver.

The administrator checks the driver's availability and counts the latitude and longitude values. When the driver arrives at the location, the driver sends a notification to the supervisor. The supervisor assigns hospitals according to latitude and the maximum longitude the driver must reach.

Step 3. Driver.

The driver delivers a notification to the system mainframe.

After sending the notification himself, he finds the location of the hospital to reach. The driver may change the signal of the ambulance's approach route by changing the red alert to green depending on the emergency [12].

#### 14.2.1.3 Future applications with conclusion of the model

The rescue service system has multiple features and offers the users additional benefits. For example, advanced features such as ambulance tracking help managers track ambulance drivers. This makes users and drivers feel more comfortable [13].

For future improvements in the mobile application platform, we can add Google voice commands to the app. Additional voice commands will be implemented using the voice implementation system. Hence, the user is directly in contact with the person on the other end of the system chain. Furthermore, this voice command could be integrated and linked to the Android watch. These improvements will allow the user to enable notifications and send a request to the administrator with a tap on his watch.

### 14.2.2 An explainable farmer health insurance model

The cost of treatment for lower income groups has become prohibitive with the exorbitant hospital bills that they need to pay for any significant surgeries [14].

Hence, the Farmer Health Insurance Model is structured to provide financial security to low-income groups, which does not consider the beneficiaries' premiums or user fees, simultaneously allowing these people to access state-of-the-art facilities of private healthcare.

#### 14.2.2.1 Comparing existing models relevant to our proposed model

Here, we compare how this model is better than the existing model:

- General policies provide critical insurance but take a long time to process. But this policy provides critical care insurance for a limited time.
- In general, health insurance is costly, and the cost of premiums depends on which coverage we choose, but in this model, we only provide insurance to people who are very poor and have no money for surgery and any major treatments.
- In the existing model, there is no option to go cashless. However, the proposed model provides a patient party to make cashless transactions.
- In the existing model, if they have any query regarding insurance, they have to contact a specific person, and if he is not available, they have to wait.

But in the aforementioned model, if a patient party needs any help, they can reach out through the app or call on the toll-free number.

#### 14.2.2.2 Benefits of the model over existing models

The benefits of the model are listed below:

- The model provides insurance to cardholders who subscribe to BPL (below the poverty line). They need to upload their details in the government portal for the insurance verification required for the model. This model provides an easy way for insurance and is a fast process.
- A health insurance plan is essential for people below the poverty line.
- Access to tertiary healthcare.
- All medical expenses are covered.
- Cashless treatment.
- Critical illness covered.

Figure 14.3 graph (panel 1) shows that every type of illness in male patients is more than that in female patients. The number of male cancer patients is more than that of female cancer patients. In total, the healthcare expenditure is approximately 120,000 rupees.

Figure 14.3 graph (panel 2) depicts average healthcare expenditure and duration of hospital stay. One notices that there is a surge in hospital bills per day. Even in this graph, the male indicator is high.

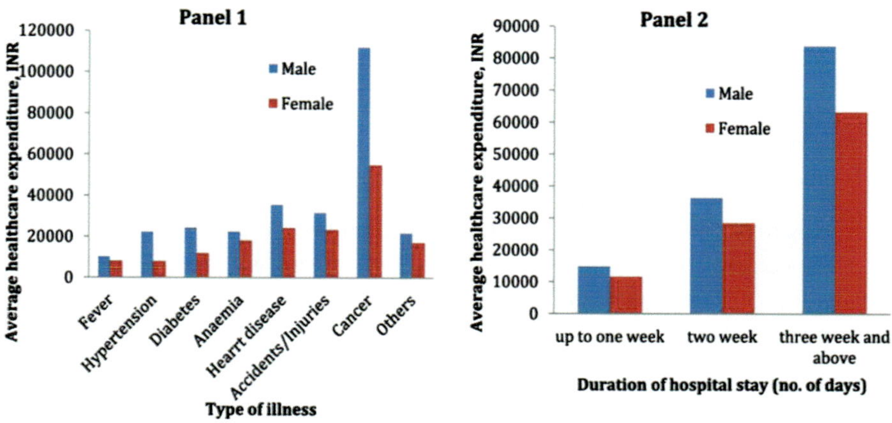


**Figure 14.3** Comparison between the types of illness and days spent in hospital.

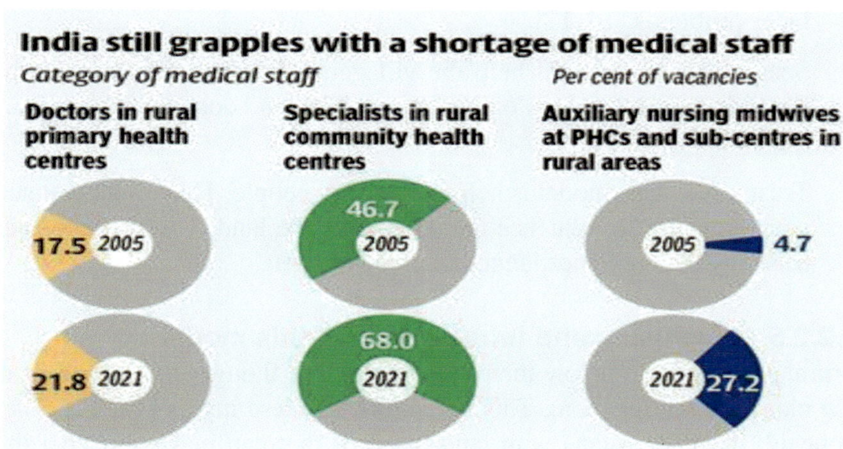


**Figure 14.4** Shortage of medical staff in rural areas.

Hence, this indicates that panel 2 depends on panel 1, i.e., hospital bills rely on the type and intensity of an illness.

Figure 14.4 indicates several health facilities in the country functioning without doctors and healthcare [15]. In 2005, 17.5% of the primary health centers and sub-centers functioned without doctors. This is one of the major reasons people avoid going to government hospitals and private hospitals have their game level upped. However, the majority of the public cannot afford its service.

#### 14.2.2.3 Some BPL health insurance policies created by government

1. Ayushman Bharat: Pradhan Mantri Jan Arogya Yojana (PMJAY) aims to serve the poor and deprived society. Each family pays an annual insurance premium of 500,000 and it represents 30% of their yearly income.
2. Rashtriya Svastya Bima Yojana (RSBY): This is also for the BPL group, especially for the informal sector. This system is extended to a maximum of 1 million won for workers and their families – 30,000 per year per family.

#### 14.2.2.4 Challenges of the model

A) Flood area: Flooding is the primary challenge for this model because it affects their land, and if they claim the insurance earlier, the company suffers. Currently, they cannot take land for treatment, and this model faces problems [16, 17].

B) Scam: This model will help the villagers. However, every model has flaws that scammers exploit by forging fake land documents and claiming insurance.

C) Trust issue: This model is helpful for rural people. They think that such companies try to influence them and take the land. They do not easily trust any new schemes launched in the market.

#### 14.2.2.5 Conclusion and future scope of this model

In rural areas, people below the poverty line have thought that health insurance plans are not for them. This model breaks these myths [18, 19]. There are health insurance plans with land or crops that can make sure that they receive proper medical care irrespective of their economic status.

### 14.2.3 A bridge between NGO and hospitals model

India is said to be a country of villages. According to a survey conducted in 2011, it is estimated that about three-fourth of our people live in villages. In many parts of the country, rural communities face a lack of digital connectivity compared to urban areas regarding broadband quality. In this scenario, it is not easy to introduce telemedicine practices in rural areas. Most people are used to using their cell phones as calling devices. The toll-free model intermediates between a simple villager and an NGO/hospital [20].

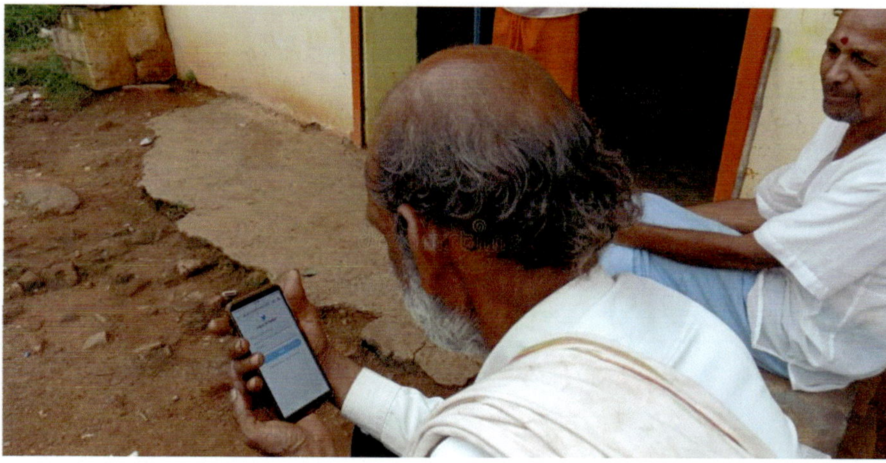

**Figure 14.5** Digitization in rural India.

The concept supports whoever in need to call on the toll-free number, and then the receivers at the other end will contact NGOs/hospitals, villagers, and helpers and try to coordinate through the website (Figure 14.5).

The main aim of this model is to guide villagers during any medical conditions in their families. For example, if they have any medical condition, they send messages in their local language, or they can call us at our toll-free number. If they need small help, then we guide them on the phone. If it is an emergency, we contact the nearest NGOs to provide them with proper medical service. As it is already known, many villagers do not know what to do in such an emergency. In such conditions, our model works.

The purpose of this study is also to find out the villagers' main problems. So here are the solutions that we need to work out.

- The time it takes an NGO to reach a place.
- There is no fee.
- The NGO was not contacted at a time when the individual was responsible for everything that happened to the patient.
- Someone is unable to pay for treatment.
- Drugs are free.

In the current model, it is impossible to say how long it will take for NGOs to provide healthcare, as villagers have difficulty obtaining adequate first aid kits unless villagers accurately describe a patient's condition. In addition, we

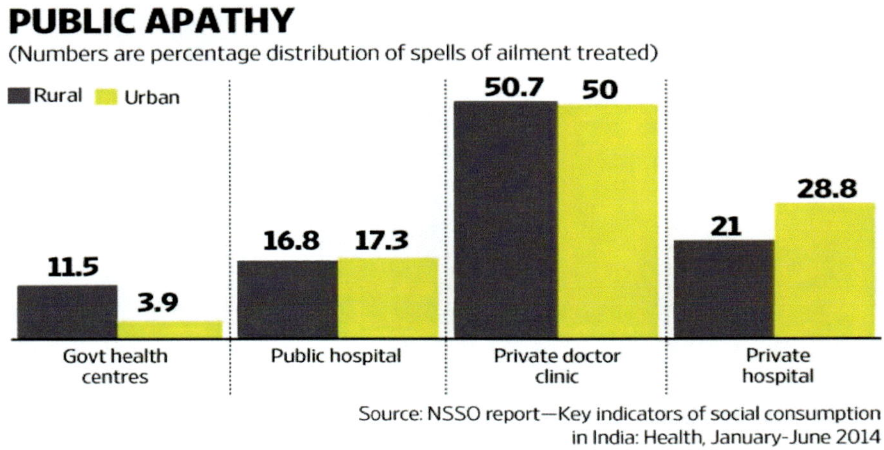


**Figure 14.6** Graph comparing the treatment of urban and rural residents.

know that some village routes have no recognition on Google Maps; so it may take some time to reach the destination [21]. All these things are to give farmers a healthy life. Farmers are the backbone of our country.

Figure 14.6 shows that public institutions do not meet the criteria for rural residents. Public and private hospitals are in better condition than government hospitals, but rural residents cannot afford the cost. Therefore, this model will help rural residents and provide better conditions.

#### 14.2.3.1 Comparison of existing work-related models to the proposed model

- As we know, free ambulances 102 and 108 are successful models in Korea.

The 108 free GPS models installed by major ambulances in different locations guarantee an average response time of 35 minutes.

- A vehicle's average response time (site visit) must be at most 35 minutes in any month.

The average response time in our model should be at most 25 minutes. Another important thing that improves our model is using volunteers (or helpers). A volunteer is a person who seeks help if the caller needs a medical emergency. And another advantage of this model is the NGO/hospital response [22].

The person in need will get a reply from NGOs/hospitals in their regional language, which we will share with the help of the website. So this

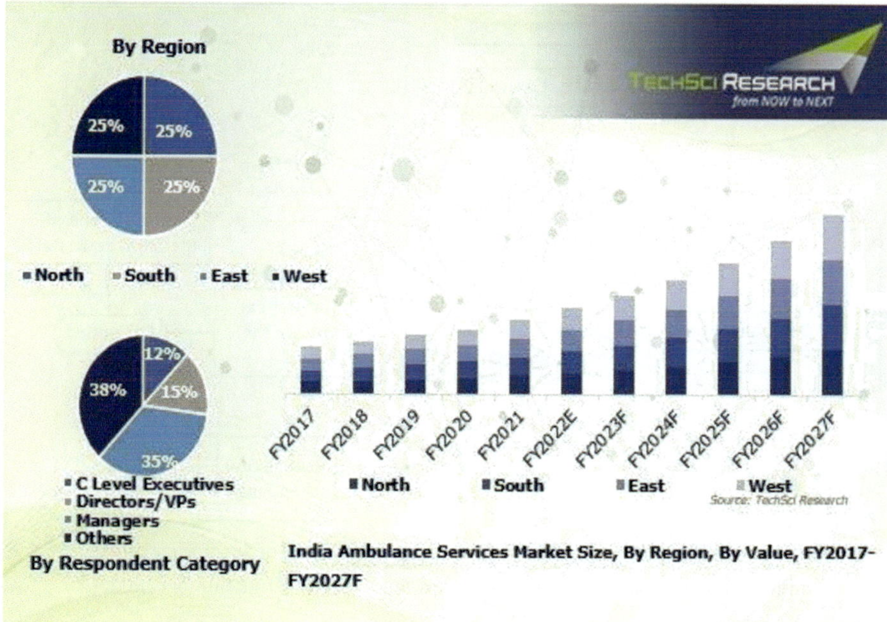


**Figure 14.7** Graph showing Indian ambulance service market size, by region, and by value.

facility will help those people who find it challenging to communicate in Hindi or English.

Figure 14.7 shows us that in the last five years, the market size of the Indian ambulance service has increased rapidly, and in the coming five years, it is expected to double as compared to the current financial year [23].

This model will also work for those types of people (Figure 14.8). This will be a straightforward process to get the proper medical help. Many people do not consult a doctor not because they do not have money for their visiting fees or because they do not consider some diseases a disease; instead, they view them as a lifestyle. In addition, they do not want to visit the doctors because they are unwilling to wait for a very long time in the medical registration system. This model will also work for those types of people.

Many NGOs work for villagers' welfare; so a team of volunteers will contact them and connect them with our website. Then it will generate a toll-free number and advertise pertinent things like what they (the villagers) should do with that number. As we know, many villagers do not know how to use a smartphone. But everyone knows how to control the phone with the keypad. So they need to call our toll-free number and report a problem. They can speak their local language, and our people contact NGOs to report their

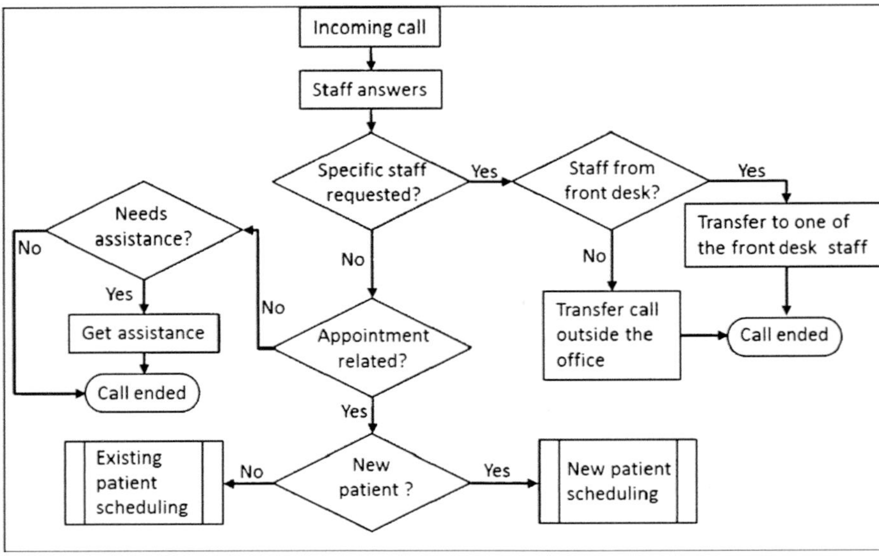


**Figure 14.8** Flow diagram for the working of the toll-free number model.

status. Now it is up to them to decide whether they can help them or not. Our job is to connect them [24].

This is the way we go if NGOs help.

Residents → our toll-free number → NGO → residents

This is the way we go when the first NGO cannot help:

Residents → Our toll-free number → 1

NGO (cannot help) → 2. NGO → villager

In the first route, we will see that the villagers can call or message the toll-free number. It then uploads information about health urgency to the website, along with state and town names. In doing so, NGOs will help those in need.

On the second route, we saw an NGO come forward to help, but after a few minutes, the meeting was canceled. In this case, they contact other NGOs to share information about needy villagers.

Our model does not require the Internet, and language will not be a barrier in this model. So if they (villagers) have a smartphone, it is good, and if they know how to operate it, it is also good. And if someone (a villager) does not have a smartphone and uses a keypad phone, they can also avail themselves of our service at no cost.

#### 14.2.3.2 Challenge of the model

As we know, a coin has two sides. Similarly, this model has some challenges, or we can say that these are the disadvantages of the model, which we need to identify and rectify. However, before proceeding, we should know what those challenges are so that the solutions can be provided:

(i) The major challenge is that customers are left on hold. Whenever we called a business, we found ourselves on hold for excessive time. Reducing the number of times customers answer calls speeds up processing and increase caller satisfaction.

(ii) Another problem is that there needs to be a concept of voicemail. In many developed countries, this concept is widely used. If a caller places a call on a ringing line without voicemail, the number of minutes waiting for a representative to make a call will affect the overall rate.

## 14.3 An Explainable AI Approach to Smart Rural Healthcare

Smart healthcare refers to using technologies such as cloud computing, the Internet of Things (IoT), and AI to enable an efficient, convenient, and personalized healthcare system. Such technologies facilitate real-time health monitoring using healthcare applications on smartphones or wearable devices, encouraging individuals to be in control of their well-being. Health information collected at a user level can also be shared with clinicians for further diagnosis and, together with AI, can be used in health screening, early diagnosis of diseases, and treatment plan selection. In the healthcare domain, the ethical issue of transparency associated with AI and the lack of trust in the black-box operation of AI systems create the need for AI models that can be explained. These Interpretable techniques used for explaining AI models along with their predictions are known as explainable AI (XAI) methods

The benefits of XAI models in rural smart healthcare are as follows:

- Increased transparency: As XAI methods explain why an AI system arrived at a specific decision, it increases transparency in how AI systems operate and can lead to increased levels of trust.
- Outcome tracking: You can use XAI-generated descriptions to track factors influencing AI systems to predict outcomes.
- Model enhancement: AI systems learn from data to make predictions. Sometimes the learned rules need to be corrected and can lead to erroneous predictions.

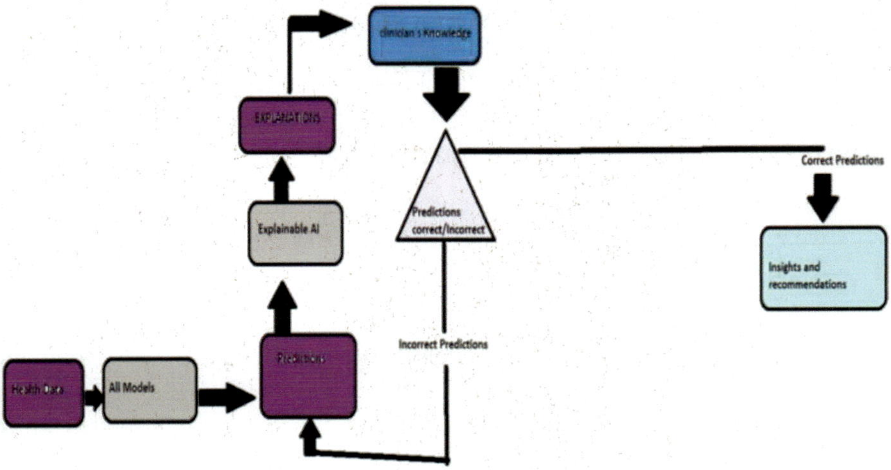


**Figure 14.9** Generating insights using XAI and clinical expertise.

- The explanations obtained by the XAI method help to understand the learned rules so that errors in the rules can be identified and the model can be improved.

This article proposes combining existing XAI models with clinical knowledge to utilize AI-based systems' benefits further. As in the Figure 14.9, the approach presented using XAI is described as follows. The intelligent healthcare application collects information about people's health and uses a trained artificial intelligence model to predict the likelihood of a specific anomaly or disease. XAI methods can be used to generate descriptions with the help of health data predictions.

## 14.4 Conclusion

Fast Internet and seamless communication networks have made it possible to deliver e-health even in remote areas lacking modern healthcare facilities. Digital health is a new concept, and many people in India live in villages. It is essential to let these people know about their health. Therefore, the private sector also needs state support. Healthcare is a big area for people and is very important.

In the first model, the passerby must book the ambulance for that location wherever the accident happens. This is as simple as booking Ola and Uber, and the main benefit of the model is that it changes the red traffic signal to green when the patient is inside the ambulance. The primary purpose of the second model is that no one is being treated well because they have no money. This method is designed and implemented in rural areas as rural residents do not pay for private hospitals. We provide fast service through the application, a toll-free number created by our team, and it is secure.

The scheme empowers eligible participants to receive free treatment for various targets, primarily cancer, surgery, and neurology. In the last model, when anyone has an emergency, they can dial the toll-free number and get an immediate response from the tech team. This model is for those villagers who panic during an emergency and need help deciding what step to take. Because of this, they lose their close ones. By this model, they just need to dial the toll-free number and then the tech team will contact them. Despite the first organizations in the industry facing many challenges in providing healthcare-based IoT services in India, we must explore the right solution for this issue. Our main goal is to decide whether this approach will bring about a reasonable reduction in death, disability, and disaster healthcare costs (e.g., healthcare costs that put money at risk safety of patients and their families) in different settings and cultures. They believe that such evidence would provide a solid basis for raising all disadvantaged people in regional communities and many other places in the world, impacting for health and well-being of billions of people. Although health research has had its drawbacks affecting the accessibility, usability, and feasibility of healthcare delivery models in rural areas, it should be encouraged to provide an improved understanding of what works and what does not work in rural areas. Opportunities are provided with information and communication technologies (including telemedicine) that are closing gaps in rural and remote areas.

## References

[1] Al-Fuqaha, A., Guizani, M., Mohammadi, M., Aledhari, M., & Ayyash, M. (2015). Internet of things: A survey on enabling technologies, protocols, and applications. IEEE Communications Surveys & Tutorials, 17(4), 2347–2376.

[2] Zarkogianni, K., Litsa, E., Mitsis, K., Wu, P. Y., Kaddi, C. D., Cheng, C. W., ... & Nikita, K. S. (2015). A review of emerging technologies for the management of diabetes mellitus. IEEE Transactions on Biomedical Engineering, 62(12), 2735–2749.

[3] Mishra, S., Raj, A., Kayal, A., Choudhary, V., Verma, P., & Biswal, L. (2012). Study of cluster based routing protocols in wireless sensor networks. International journal of scientific and engineering research, 3(7). 2

[4] Mishra, S., Jena, L., & Pradhan, A. (2012). Fault tolerance in wireless sensor networks. International Journal, 2(10), 146–153.

[5] Fernandes, D., Cabral, J., & Rocha, A. M. (2016, March). A smart wearable system for sudden infant death syndrome monitoring. In 2016 IEEE International Conference on Industrial Technology (ICIT) (pp. 1920–1925). IEEE.

[6] Ullah, K., Shah, M. A., & Zhang, S. (2016). Effective ways to use the Internet of Things in the field of medical and smart health care. In 2016 International Conference on Intelligent Systems Engineering (ICISE) (pp. 372–379). IEEE.

[7] Ukil, A., Bandyopadhyay, S., Puri, C., & Pal, A. (2016, March). IoT Healthcare Analytics: The Importance of Anomaly Detection. In 2016 IEEE 30thInternational Conference on Advanced Information Networking and Applications (AINA) (pp. 994–997). IEEE

[8] Mishra, S., Mahanty, C., Dash, S., & Mishra, B. K. (2019). Implementation of BFS-NB hybrid model in intrusion detection system. In Recent developments in machine learning and data analytics (pp. 167-175). Springer, Singapore.

[9] S.Yoon and L. A. Albert, "A dynamic ambulance routing model with multiple response," Transp. Res. Part E Logist. Transp. Rev., vol. 133, no. November, pp. 1–18, 2020, DOI: 10.1016/j.tre.2019.11.001.

[10] Mishra, S., Mallick, P. K., Tripathy, H. K., Jena, L., & Chae, G. S. (2021). Stacked KNN with hard voting predictive approach to assist hiring process in IT organizations. The International Journal of Electrical Engineering & Education, 0020720921989015.

[11] A.Yogaraj, M.R Ezilarasan, Dr.Anuroop. RV and C.S.Sivanthiram, "IOT Based Smart Healthcare Monitoring System for Rural/Isolated Areas" in International Journal of Pure and Applied Mathematics Volume 114 No. 12 2017.

[12] Sahoo, S., Das, M., Mishra, S., & Suman, S. (2021). A hybrid DTNB model for heart disorders prediction. In Advances in electronics, communication and computing (pp. 155-163). Springer, Singapore.

[13] Zarkeshev and C. Csiszár, "Patients' Willingness to Ride on a Driverless Ambulance: A Case Study in Hungary," Transp. Res. Procedia, vol. 44, no. 2019, pp. 8–14, 2020, DOI: 10.1016/j.trpro.2020.02.002.

[14] Wajid, N. Nezamuddin, and A. Unnikrishnan, "Optimizing Ambulance Locations for Coverage Enhancement of Accident Sites in South Delhi," Transp. Res. Procedia, vol. 48, pp. 280–289, 2020, doi: 10.1016/j.trpro.2020.08.022.

[15] 1R. R. Al-Hakim, E. Rusdi, and M. A. Setiawan, "Android Based Expert System Application for Diagnose COVID-19 Disease : Cases Study of Banyumas Regency," J. Intell. Comput. Heal. Informatics, vol. 1, no. 2, pp. 1–13, 2020, DOI: 10.26714/jichi.v1i2.5958.

[16] Dutta, A., Misra, C., Barik, R. K., & Mishra, S. (2021). Enhancing mist assisted cloud computing toward secure and scalable architecture for smart healthcare. In Advances in Communication and Computational Technology (pp. 1515-1526). Springer, Singapore.

[17] M.Ranjith Kumar, Prabu S, "Smart Healthcare Monitoring System for Rural Area using IOT " International Journal of Pharmacy & Technology Vol. 8 Issue No.4 Dec-2016.

[18] Sahoo, S., Das, M., Mishra, S., & Suman, S. (2021). A hybrid DTNB model for heart ` disorders prediction. In Advances in electronics, communication and computing (pp. 155–163). Springer, Singapore.

[19] Abhishek, Tripathy, H.K., Mishra, S. (2022). A Succinct Analytical Study of the Usability of Encryption Methods in Healthcare Data Security. In: Tripathy, B.K., Lingras, P., Kar, A.K., Chowdhary, CL (eds) Next Generation Healthcare Informatics. Studies in Computational Intelligence, vol 1039. Springer, Singapore. https://doi.org/10.1007/978-981-19-2416-3_7

[20] Mohapatra, S. K., Mishra, S., Tripathy, H. K., Bhoi, A. K., & Barsocchi, P. (2021). A Pragmatic Investigation of Energy Consumption and Utilization Models in the Urban Sector Using Predictive Intelligence Approaches. Energies, 14(13), 3900.

[21] Mohanty, A., & Mishra, S. (2022). A Comprehensive Study of Explainable Artificial Intelligence in Healthcare. In Augmented Intelligence in Healthcare: A Pragmatic and Integrated Analysis (pp. 475-502). Springer, Singapore.

[22] Patnaik, M., & Mishra, S. (2022). Indoor Positioning System Assisted Big Data Analytics in Smart Healthcare. In Connected e-Health (pp. 393–415). Springer, Cham.

[23] De, A., & Mishra, S. (2022). Augmented Intelligence in Mental Health Care: Sentiment Analysis and Emotion Detection with Health Care Perspective. Augmented Intelligence in Healthcare: A Pragmatic and Integrated Analysis, 205–235.

[24] Chattopadhyay, A., Mishra, S., & González-Briones, A. (2021). Integration of machine learning and IoT in healthcare domain. In Hybrid artificial intelligence and IoT in healthcare (pp. 223–244). Springer, Singapore.

# 15

# Explainable Artificial Intelligence in Drug Discovery for Biomedical Applications

**Godwin M. Ubi[1,4], Edu N. Eyogor[1], Hannah E. Etta[2], Nkese D. Okon[1], Effiom B. Ekeng[3], and Imabong S. Essien[3]**

[1]Department of Genetics and Biotechnology, Faculty of Biological Science, University of Calabar, Nigeria
[2]Department of Pharmacy, Faculty of Pharmaceutical Science, University of Calabar, Nigeria
[3]Department of Guidance and Counselling, Faculty of Education, University of Calabar, Nigeria
[4]Biggmade Scientific Research Academy, Esierebom, Calabar, Nigeria

## Abstract

This chapter reveals the ease with which artificial intelligence (computer-based simulations and algorithms) can be applied in the discovery, identification, and explanation of carfentanil, rispiridine, naltrexone, buprenorphine, naloxone, and morphine as having the same biomedical applications and effects on CYP206 and OPRM2 major genes and CHRNA7, SLC5A4, and OPED7 minor genes as alternative drugs for Tramadol in biomedical applications. It also revealed that artificial intelligence can be used to discover and explain that omega-3-fatty acid, 1,1-dimethetyl, rimonabant, 1-naphthalenyl, HU-210, 2-arachidonyl and anandamide are alternative drugs with same biomedical applications and effects as Cannabinol drug on CD5 major and minor CNR1and CNR2 genes. It was also discovered that Verdanafil and Tadalafil have same and similar biological applications and effect on CYP25 OPRD1, and HTR7 major genes and PRKG2 and CAVI minor genes and are discovered as alternative drugs to Sildenafil drug. The study revealed that GDP-mannose, uridine phosphate, and guanosine diphosphate possess same and similar biological applications and effect on DNAI2 major gene and EPGN and ALGI1 minor genes and are discovered as alternative drugs to the Praziquantel drug used as anthelminthic drug in biomedical applications. Such discovered drugs can be properly harnessed, reconstituted, redesigned, refocused, and utilized as potential prophylactic or therapeutic drug (single or in combinations) for the prevention and treatment of diseases, which is a cardinal focus and target for the pharmaceutical industries. Hence, a computational-based algorithm that utilizes bioinformatics tools will therefore provide the much needed validation approach for the discovery and provides better explanations for the applications of small molecules as potential drugs for the prevention and cure of most health-related ailments and biomedical applications.

## 15.1 Introduction

A drug is any substance that is inhaled, injected, smoked, consumed, or absorbed through a patch on the skin or dissolved under the tongue causing a philosophical change in the body. A drug is also any substance (exception of food and water) that, when taken into the body, alters the body functions either physically or psychologically [1]. Drugs may be legal, e.g., alcohol caffeine, or tobacco or illegal, e.g., cannabis, cocaine, heroin, etc. All medicines are drugs, but not all drugs are medicines. A medicine is a chemical substance used to treat, cure, prevent, and diagnose a disease so as to promote an individual wellbeing [2].

Plants contain chemicals with potential economic values that are not only used for mere satisfaction or sustenance of hunger but also for the maintenance of good health. Phytochemicals have remained the best sources of natural products where they form the major parts of recipe for all human endeavors of drug discovery [3].

The action of chemical substances (drugs) in the genes of biological recipients (humans, animals, or plants) triggers and elicits the corresponding immune responses required to subdue pains and uncomfortable situations in the biological systems [4].

This action is achieved through the interactions of the chemical substances (drugs) and major genes and minor (polygenes) genes, which tend to cause the actions and inactions leading to pains and cures in biological systems [5].

The use of computer-based algorithms and simulations in simply identifying drug and protein (genes) interactions makes it easy to know drugs with similar actions on the same major and minor genes in different biological systems. This also provides the basis for the easy identification of chemical drugs with similar prophylactic and therapeutic potentials [6].

Hence, the use of computer-based intelligence in this regard provides an explainable easy means of discovery drugs with similar prophylactic and therapeutic potentials (similar actions on same major and minor genes), through this simple approach [7].

In contemporary drug discovery processes, secondary metabolites (chemical derivatives of artificial or natural origin) with previously unknown biomedical activities are widely evaluated in a series of approaches including *in silico*, *in vitro*, and *in vivo* processes and taking several years to achieve approval as drugs for biomedical applications [8]. This has often resulted in huge capital and financial losses, which impact a cumulative hike in the prices of drugs due to unavoidable trials and errors associated with the processes [9].

The opportunity offered by the applications of artificial intelligence in discovering drugs for biomedical applications eliminated the trials and errors in drug development process and invariably and significantly reduced the cost of drug production [10].

So using computer-based simulations to simply identify drugs with similar effects on different biological systems easily explains the simple mechanisms with which drugs used in biomedical applications can be discovered [11]. This has ushered in a major renewal of interest and boasted the utilization of artificial intelligence or computer-based approach in the discovery of drugs for biomedical applications.

Drug usage in biomedical applications remains significantly important in both developing and developed nations of the world as a recipe and solutions for the treatment of various diseases and health challenges confronting mankind in the 21st century and has continued to play a critical role in protecting lives and maintaining good human health. This chapter has become ultimately indispensable especially with the advent of the global pandemic that has sent more than 50 million people to their early graves [12–14].

The importance of this chapter emphasizes the relative ease with which the pharmacist can apply this artificial intelligence approach to explain and suggest alternative drugs with same functions to patients for biomedical applications while physicians can also utilize this simple and easy explainable approach in the prescription of drugs with similar gene actions to patients for biomedical applications.

## 15.2 Methodology

***In silico* identification of alternative drugs in biomedical applications:** The Click2drug option of Swiss drug design online interactive program of expasy.org was adopted in order to determine the *in silico* drug–protein gene interactions for selected drugs like Tramadol, Cannabinol, Paracetamol, Postinor, Oxytocin, Ascorbate, Sildenafil (Viagra), and Praziquantel with the several protein receptor genes of the human biological systems. The approach

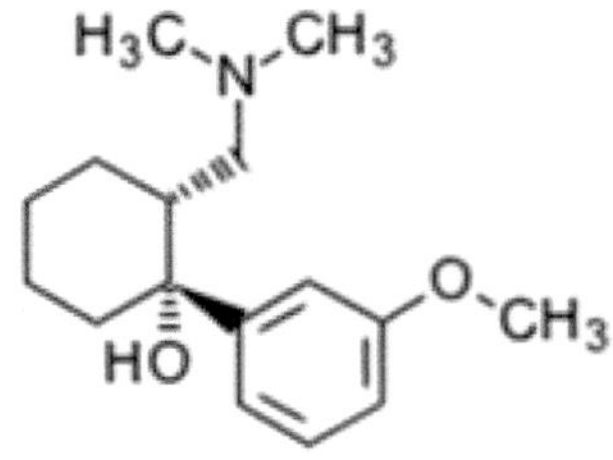


**Figure 15.1** Showing chemical structure of Tramadol drug.

can be used as explainable artificial intelligence for any drug of interest in biomedical applications.

The pathway database of stitch in expasy.org of the Swiss institute of Bioinformatics (SIB) was used to achieve the drugs (chemicals) and protein (genes) interactions and the associated networks using related computer-based algorithms and bioinformatics tools.

Big circles with thick and bold lines indicate the major genes affected and the direct interaction of drugs with the proteins, while the small circles with thin and normal lines indicate minor genes affected and indirect interactions between the drugs and the protein targets.

The red rectangular shape represents the main drug of interest while other gray colored rectangular shapes represent alternative drugs with same and similar actions on the major and minor genes like the main drug upon which this study was based.

**Results:**

## 15.2.1 Tramadol drug

### 15.2.1.1 Tramadol

Tramadol (Figure 15.1) has a brand name known as Ultram. Tramadol is an opioid pain medication used to treat moderate to moderately severe pain. It has the molecular formula of $C_{16}H_{25}NO_2$ and a molecular weight of 263.38 g/mol. Tramadol acts on CYP206, OPRK1, and OPRM2 major genes and CHRNA7, SLC5A4, SLC6A4, HTR7, HTR2A, and OPED7 minor genes in its mode of action in suppressing pains in biomedical applications.

### 15.2.1.2 Biological processes of major genes affected by Tramadol and other alternative drugs

*15.2.1.2.1 CYP206*

CYP206 is a major gene called cytochrome p450 (Figure 15.2 and Table 15.1). It is D – polypeptide 6 gene that functions in the utilization (build up and breaking down) of many drugs including Tramadol and other

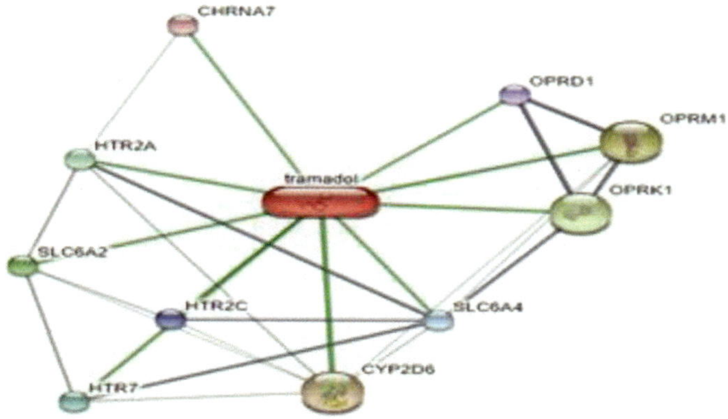


**Figure 15.2** Showing interactions of major and minor genes with tramadol drug via XAI.

**Table 15.1** Major and minor genes affected by Tramadol and alternative drugs.

| Drug name | Major genes affected | False discovery rate (score) | Minor genes affected | False discovery rate (score) | Alternative drugs with same effects on major and minor genes as revealed by XAI |
|---|---|---|---|---|---|
| Tramadol | OPRM1 | 0.968 | CHRNA7 | 0.800 | Morphine |
| | OPRK1 | 0.926 | HTR2A | 0.899 | Naltrexone |
| | CYP206 | 0.991 | SLC6A2 | 0.914 | Buprenorphine |
| | | | HTR2C | 0.835 | Naloxone |
| | | | HTR7 | 0.897 | Carfentanil |
| | | | OPRD1 | 0.820 | Nor-BNI |
| | | | SLC6A4 | 0.842 | DAMGO |
| | | | | | Endormorphine-2 |
| | | | | | Paroxetine |
| | | | | | Rispiridine |

chemical compounds that it oxidizes [16]. Tramadol is known to be involved in the metabolism of drugs, such as antiarrhythmic, adrenocetor, antagonists, and tricyclic antidepressants. The CYP206 gene is affected by ingestion of Tramadol and the other alternative drugs (Figures 15.3 and 15.4).

### *15.2.1.2.2 OPRKI*

OPRKI is an opioid receptor kappa 1 gene (Figure 15.5 and Table 15.1) that inhibits neurotransmitter release by reducing calcium ion currents and increasing potassium ion conductance. It functions as a dynorphin receptor and plays a major role in the erection and regulation of neuroendocrine

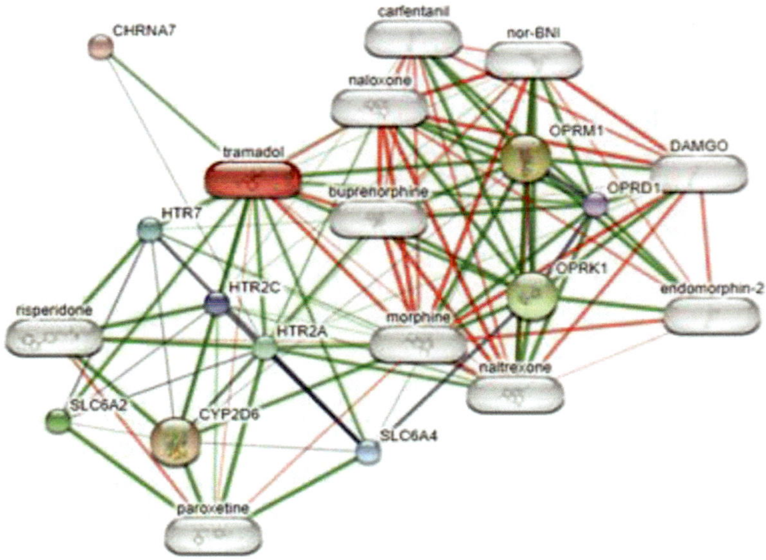


**Figure 15.3** Showing alternatives drugs interactions with same major and minor genes as tramadol via XAI.

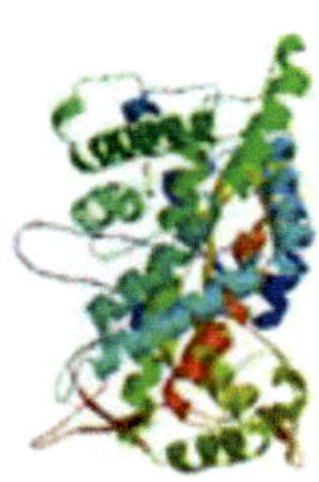

**Figure 15.4** Protein structure of CYP206 major gene.

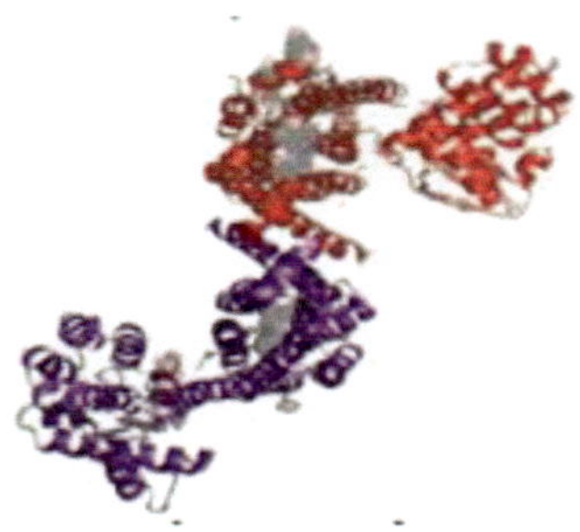

**Figure 15.5** Protein structure of OPKR1 major gene.

and automatic functions [17]. The OPRK1 gene is affected by ingestion of Tramadol and the other alternative drugs (Figures 15.6 and 15.7).

### *15.2.1.2.3 OPRM1*

OPRM1 is an opioid receptor 1 gene Figure 15.8 and Table 15.1), which also increases potassium ion conductance. It further plays a role in dynorphin receptor protein and plays a critical function in the erection and regulation of neuroendocrine and automatic functions [18]. The OPRM1 gene is affected

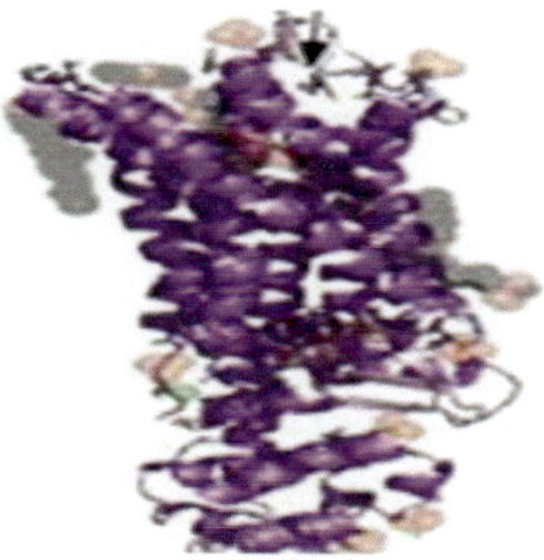

**Figure 15.6** Protein structure of OPRM1 major gene.

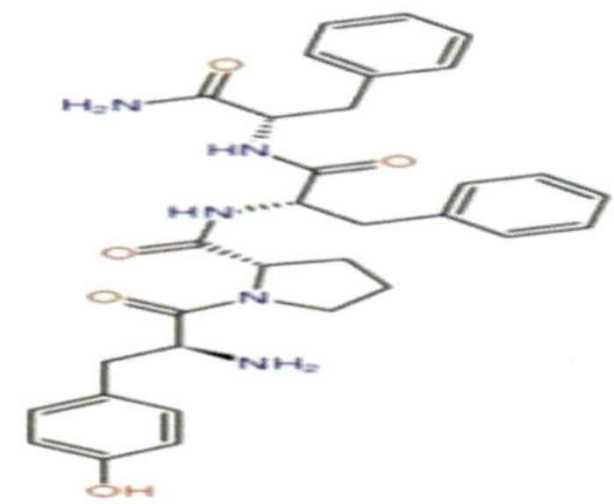

**Figure 15.7** Chemical structure of Endomorphin – 2 drug as alternative to tramadol drug

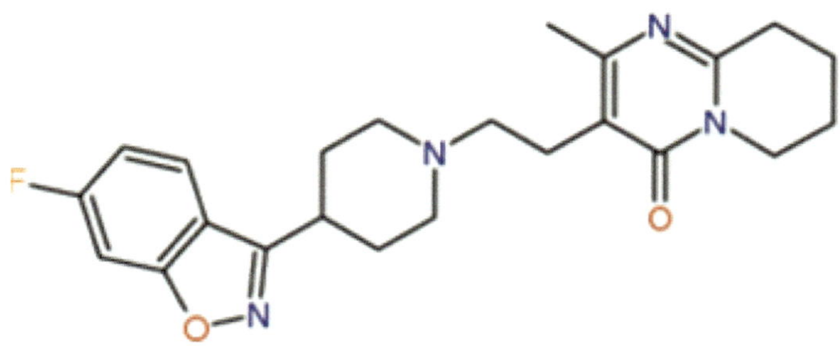

**Figure 15.8** Chemical structure of Risperidine drug as alternative to tramadol drug.

by ingestion of Tramadol and the other alternative drugs (Figures 15.9 and 15.10).

#### 15.2.1.3 Discovery of alternative drugs affecting major and minor genes as Tramadol based on XAI for biomedical applications

*15.2.1.3.1 Endomorphin-2*

Endomorphin-2 (Figures 15.11 and Table 15.1) is an endogenous opioid peptide like Tramadol and also one of the Endomorphins. The drug has high affinity for opioid reception and, if combined with Endomorphin-1, acts as an endogenous ligand to the opioid receptor [19]. This drug produces analgesic in human biological systems where its action usually occurs in the spinal cord, thus producing a measure of drug aversion, an effect which is dynorphins-A-dependent. Endomorphin-2 acts on CYP206, OPRK1, and OPRM2 major genes and CHRNA7, SLC5A4, SLC6A4, HTR7, HTR2A,

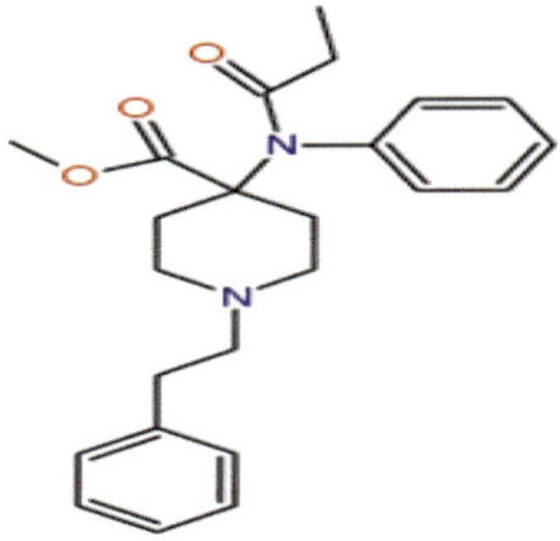

**Figure 15.9** Chemical structure of Carfentanil drug as alternative to tramadol drug.

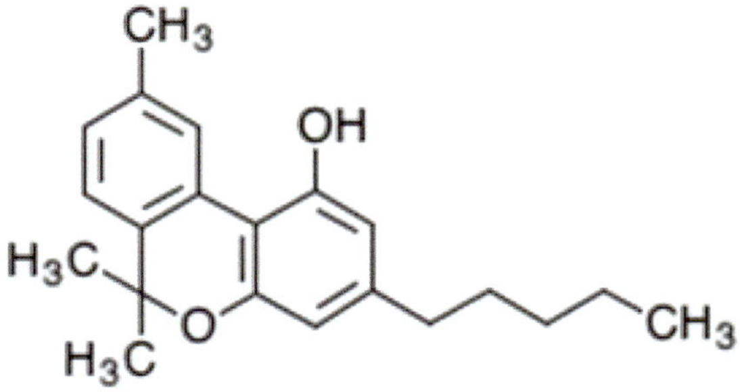

**Figure 15.10** Chemical structure of cannabinol drug.

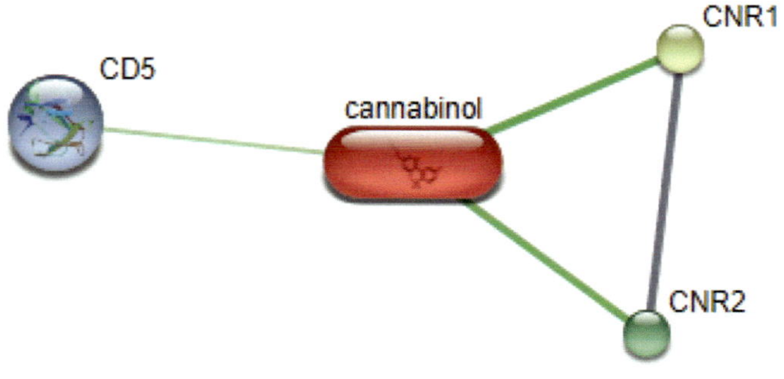


**Figure 15.11** Showing interactions of major and minor genes with cannabinol drug via XAI.

and OPED7 minor genes as alternative drugs for Tramadol in its mode of action in suppressing pains in biomedical applications.

*15.2.1.3.2 Rispiridine*

Rispiridine (Figures 15.12 and Table 15.1), formally called Risperdal or generics, is an antipsychotic drug mainly used to treat schizophrenia and

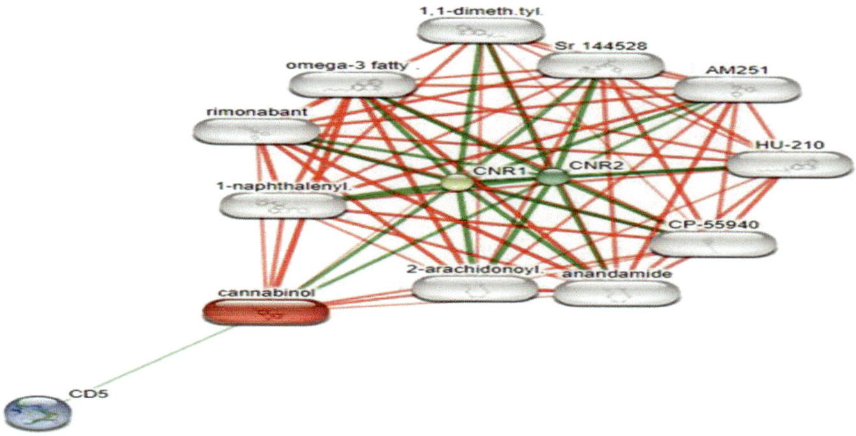


**Figure 15.12** Showing alternatives drugs interactions with same major and minor genes as cannabinol via XAI.

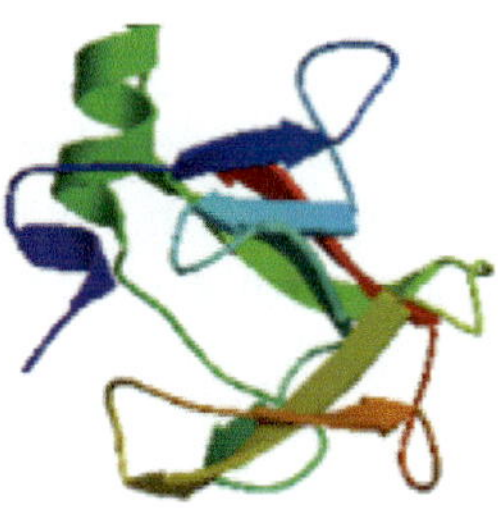

**Figure 15.13** Protein structure of CD5 major gene.

schizoaffective disorder, bipolar disorders, and irritability in people with autism [20]. Rispiridine acts on CYP206, OPRK1, and OPRM2 major genes and CHRNA7, SLC5A4, SLC6A4, HTR7, HTR2A, and OPED7 minor genes as alternative drugs for Tramadol in its mode of action in suppressing pains in biomedical applications.

### *15.2.1.3.3 Carfentanil*

Carfentanil (Figure 15.13 and Table 15.1) is a synthetic opioid analgesic fentanyl, which is one of the most potent opioids used commercially. Its potency is 10,000-fold greater than morphine and 100-fold greater than fentanyl. Its activity in humans is about 1 microgram from start [21]. It is used as a general anesthetic agent in large animals whose use is intended only and not good for humans. Carfentanil acts on CYP206, OPRK1, and OPRM2 major genes and CHRNA7, SLC5A4, SLC6A4, HTR7, HTR2A, and OPED7 minor

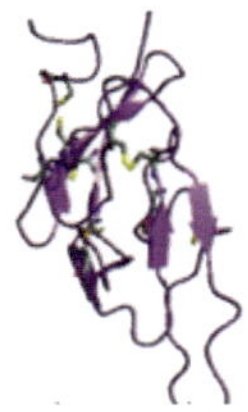

**Figure 15.14** Protein structure of CNR1 minor gene.

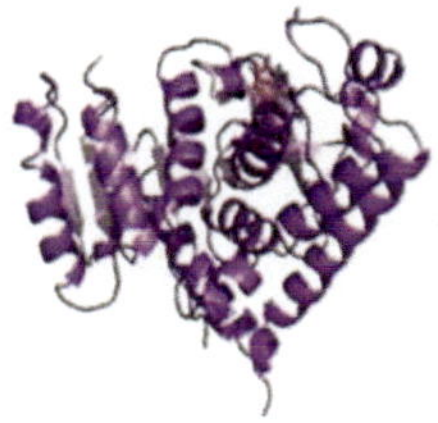

**Figure 15.15** Protein structure of CNR2 minor gene.

genes as alternative drugs for Tramadol in its mode of action in suppressing pains in biomedical applications.

### 15.2.2 Cannabinol drug

#### 15.2.2.1 Cannabinol

Cannabinol (CBN) (Figure 15.14 and Table 15.1) is considered as a weak psychoactive cannabinoid obtained in trace amounts only in *Cannabis indica* and *Cannabis saliva* and is mostly a metabolite of tetrahydrocannabinol (THC) [22]. Cannabinol acts as a weak agonist of CB1 receptors, with lower affinities in comparison to THC. The Cannabinol drug acts on major CD5 and minor CNR1and CNR2 genes in its mode of action in exerting its effects in biomedical applications.

#### 15.2.2.2 Biological activities of major genes affected by Cannabinol and other alternative drugs

*15.2.2.2.1 CD5*

CD5 (Figure 15.5 and Table 15.1) is a biological macro-molecule that usually acts as a binding receptor gene that functions in regulating the proliferation of T-cells [24]. The CD5 major gene is affected by ingestion of Cannabinol and the other alternative drugs.

*15.2.2.2.2 CNR1*

CNR1 (Figure 15.16 and Table 15.2) is a cannabinoid receptor 1 gene that functions predominantly as brain receptor gene in humans [25]. The CNR1 gene is affected by ingestion of Cannabinol and the other alternative drugs.

*15.2.2.2.3 CNR2*

CNR2 (Figure 15.17 and Table 15.2) is a cannabinoid receptor 2 gene (macrophage). It is a heterotrimetric G protein-couple receptor for endocannabinoid

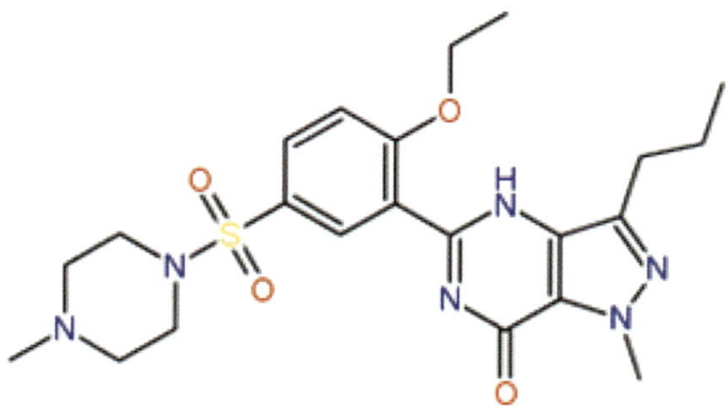

**Figure 15.16** Chemical structure of Sildenafil drug.

**Table 15.2** Major and minor genes affected by Cannabinol and alternative drugs.

| Drug name | Major genes affected | False discovery rate (score) | Minor genes affected | False discovery rate (score) | Alternative drugs with same effects on major and minor genes as revealed by XAI |
|---|---|---|---|---|---|
| Cannabinol | CD5 | 0.533 | CNR1<br>CNR2 | 0.904<br>0.855 | Omega-3-fatty acid<br>1, 1-dimethyl<br>Rimonabant<br>1-naphthalenyl<br>AM251<br>Hu-210<br>CP-55940<br>2-arachidonnyl<br>Anandamide<br>Sr 144528 |

2-arachidonyl glycerol that acts as a mediator that inhibits adenylate cyclase [26]. It also plays a major role in the inflammatory responses, nociceptive transmission, and bone homeostasis. The CNR2 gene is affected by ingestion of Cannabinol and the other alternative drugs.

### 15.2.3 Sildenafil (Viagra) drug

#### 15.2.3.1 Sildenafil

Sildenafil (Figure 15.18 and Table 15.3) is also regarded as a vasoactive ingredient utilized in the correction of erectile dysfunction and reduces the pains suffered by patients having pulmonary arterial hypertension (PAH). Sildenafil has been reported to increase the level of the second messenger known as cGMP by stopping its catabolism using phosphodiesterol type 5

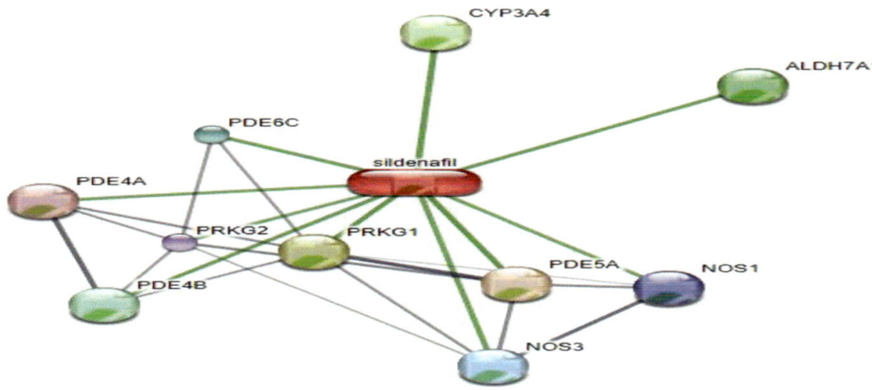


**Figure 15.17** Showing interactions of major and minor genes with Sildenafil drug via XAI.

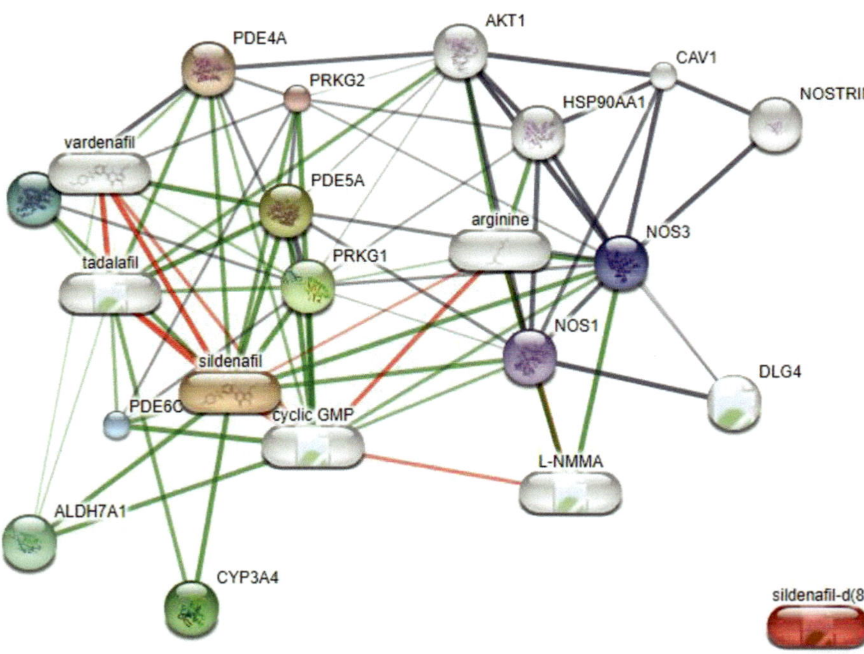


**Figure 15.18** Showing alternatives drugs interactions with same major and minor genes as Sildenafil drug via XAI.

(PDE5) [27]. PDE5 is found in particularly high concentrations in the corpus cavernosum, which is the erectile tissue of the male reproductive organ. It is also found in the retina and vascular endothelium increasing cGMP, resulting in vasodilation that facilitates generation and maintenance of erection [28]. The vasodilation effects of Sildenafil also help reduce symptoms

**Table 15.3** Major and minor genes affected by Sildenafil and alternative drugs.

| Drug name | Major genes affected | False discovery rate (score) | Minor genes affected | False discovery rate (score) | Alternative drugs with same effects on major and minor genes as revealed by XAI |
|---|---|---|---|---|---|
| Sildenafil | NOS1 | 0.996 | PRKG2 | 0.865 | Verdanafil |
| | NOS3 | 0.953 | PDE6C | 0.687 | Tadalafil |
| | CYP3A | 0.998 | CAVI | 0.553 | Cyclic GMP |
| | PRKG1 | 0.865 | | | Arginine |
| | PDE4A | 0.896 | | | L-NMMA |
| | PDE4B | 0.886 | | | Carfentanil |
| | ALDH7A1 | 0.903 | | | |
| | PRKG2 | 0.871 | | | |

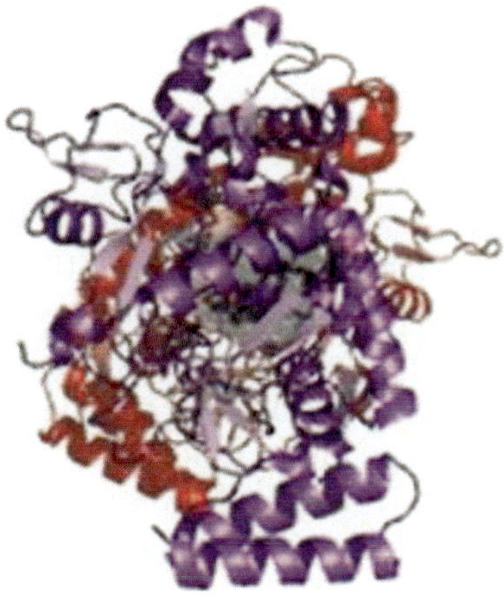

**Figure 15.19** Protein structure of NOS1 major gene.

of PAH. Sildenafil acts on CYP256, OPRM1, OPRK1, OPRD1, and HTR7 major genes and PRKG2, PDE6C, and CAVI minor genes in its mode of action in delaying production of phosphodiesterol in males in biomedical applications.

#### 15.2.3.2 Biological activities of major genes affected by Sildenafil and other alternative drugs

*15.2.3.2.1 NOS1*

NOS1 (Figure 15.19 and Table 15.3) is nitric oxide synthase 1 (neuronal) gene that releases nitric oxide (NO) as messenger molecule with different functions throughout the human body [29]. Nitrous oxide displays many properties of a neurotransmission in the brain and peripheral nervous system and probably

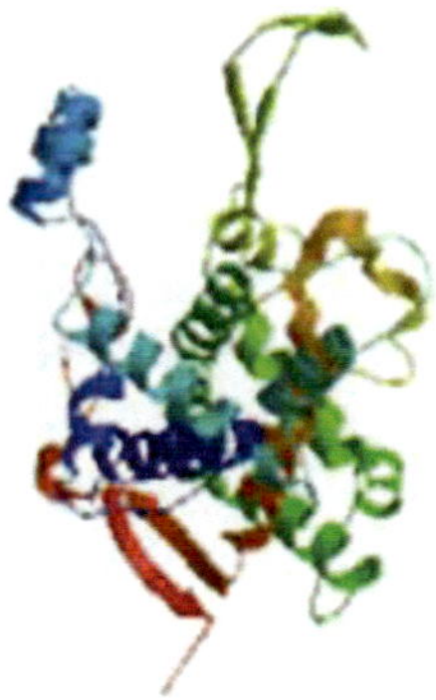

**Figure 15.20** Protein structure of CYP34A major gene.

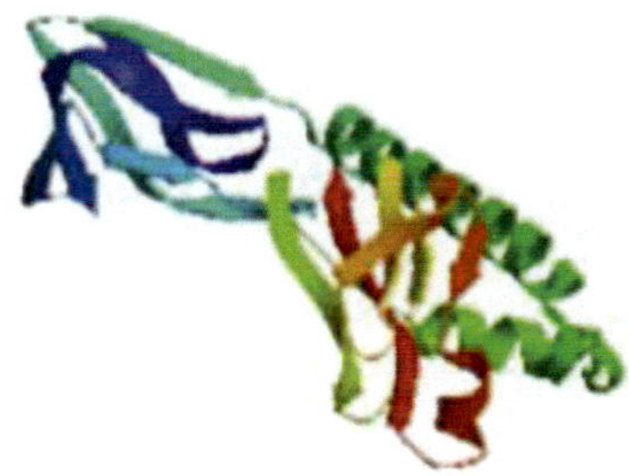

**Figure 15.21** Protein structure of PRKG1 major gene.

shows nitrosylase activity, which also mediates cysteine S-nitrosylation of cytoplasmic target proteins such as SSR [30]. The NOS1 gene is affected by ingestion of Sildenafil and the other alternative drugs.

*15.2.3.2.2 CYP3AA*

CYP3AA is also known as cytochrome P450 family 3 subfamily A polypeptide 4 gene (Figure 15.20 and Table 15.3). Thus, cytochromes P450 are a group of heme-thiolate monooxygenases. In liver microsomes, this protein enzyme is involved in an NADPH-dependent electron transport pathway [31]. It performs a variety of oxidation reactions of structurally unrelated compounds including steroids, fatty acids, and xenobiotic. It also acts as a 1, 8-cineole 2-exo-monooxygenases and also hydroxylates etoposide in human [32]. The CYP3AA gene is affected by ingestion of Sildenafil and the other alternative drugs.

*15.2.3.2.3 PRKG1*

PRKG1 is protein kinase cGMP-dependent type 1 gene (Figure 15.21 and Table 15.3) or serine/threonine protein kinase that functions as a key mediator of the nitric oxide (NO)/cGMP signaling pathway. The GMP binding protein activates the PRKG1 gene which phosphorylates Serine and Threonine amino acids in most of the calcium-based cells, but however, the contribution of each of these targets [33]. Proteins that are phosphorylated by PRKG1 regulate platelets activation and adhesion, smooth muscle contraction, cardiac function, and gene expression. The PRKG1 gene is affected by ingestion of Sildenafil and the other alternative drugs.

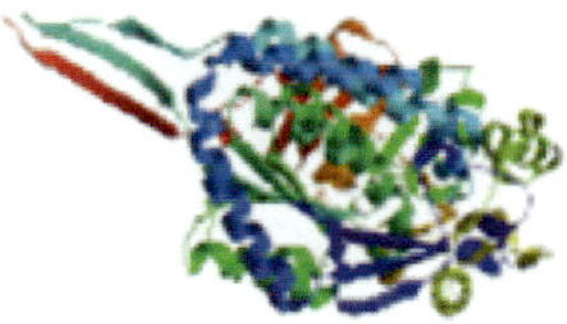

**Figure 15.22** Protein structure of ALDH7A1 major gene.

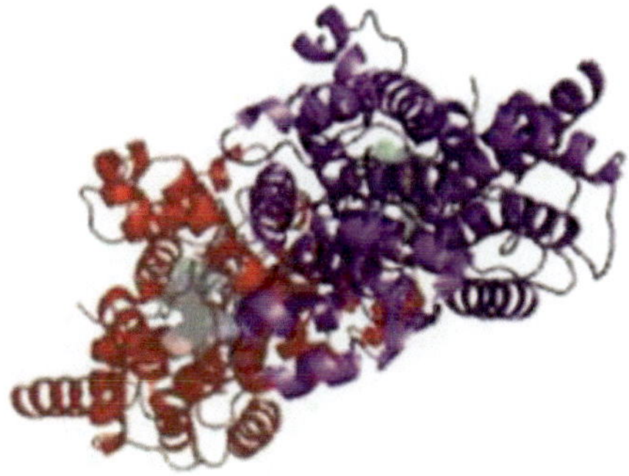

**Figure 15.23** Protein structure of PDE4B major gene.

### *15.2.3.2.4 ALDH7A1*

ALDH7A1 is aldehyde dehydrogenase 7 family member A1 gene (Figure 15.22 and Table 15.3). A functional enzyme with multipurpose activity, some of which includes mediating important protective effects [34]. It metabolizes betaine aldehyde to betaine, which is an important cellular osmolyte and a methyl donor. It also protects cells from oxidative stress by metabolizing a number of lipid peroxidation-derived aldehydes. It is also involved in lysine catabolism in humans [35]. The ALDH7A1 gene is affected by ingestion of Sildenafil and the other alternative drugs.

### *15.2.3.2.5 PDE4B*

PDE4B is phosphodiesterase 4B, cGMP gene (Figure 15.23 and Table 15.3); specifically, it hydrolyzes the messenger cAMP in quick succession as second-phase activity. This is the key regulator of many important physiological processes [36]. PDE4B takes part in mediating central nervous system effects of therapeutic agents ranging from antidepressants to antiasthmatic and anti-inflammatory agents. The PDE4B gene is affected by ingestion of Sildenafil and the other alternative drugs.

### *15.2.3.2.6 NOS3*

NOS3 (Figure 15.24 and Table 15.3) is nitric oxide synthase 3 (endothelial cell) gene, which produces nitric oxide. Nitric oxide exhibits many properties of a neurotransmitter and probably mediates cysteine S-nitrosylation and nitrosylase activity of cytoplasmic target proteins [37, 38]. The NOS3 gene is affected by ingestion of Sildenafil and the other alternative drugs.

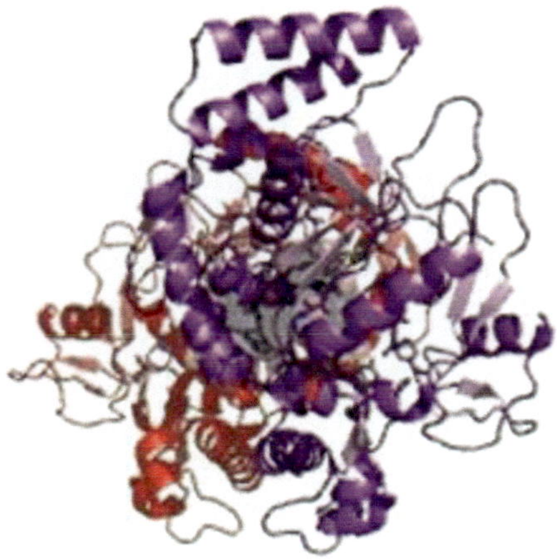

Figure 15.24 Protein structure of NOS3 major gene.

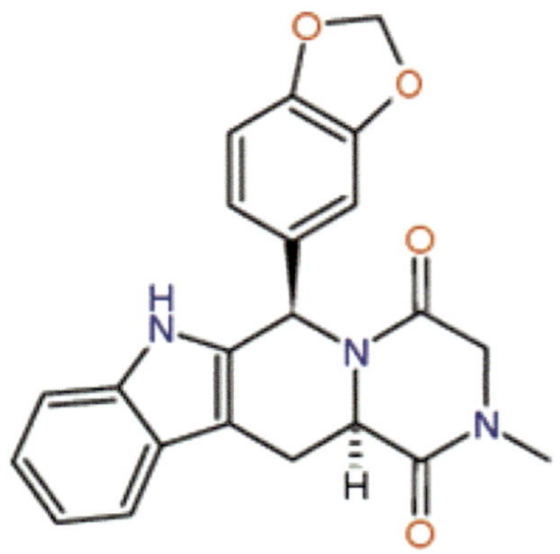


Figure 15.25 Chemical structure of Tadalafil drug.

### 15.2.3.3 Discovery of alternative drugs affecting major and minor genes as Sildenafil based on XAI for biomedical applications

*15.2.3.3.1 Tadalafil*

Tadalafil (Figure 15.25 and Table 15.3) is a phosphodiesterol-5 inhibitor usually traded as tablets and used for treating erectile dysfunction (ED). Tadalafil is also traded as Cialis with the name ad circa, which is used for the treatment of pulmonary arterial hypertension [39]. It is also used for treating the signs and symptoms of benign prostatic hyperplasia (BPH) as well as a combination of BPH and erectile dysfunction [40]. Tadalafil has same and similar biological applications and effects on CYP256, OPRM1, OPRK1, OPRD1, and HTR7 major genes and PRKG2, PDE6C, and CAVI minor genes in its mode of action in prolonging ejaculation in males in biomedical applications.

*15.2.3.3.2 Verdanafil*

Verdanafil (Figure 15.26 and Table 15.3) is another phosphodiesterol-5, inhibitor utilized for the treatment of erectile dysfunction. It is marketed as Levitra drug [41]. Verdanafil has same and similar biological applications and effects on CYP256, OPRM1, OPRK1, OPRD1, and HTR7 major genes and PRKG2, PDE6C, and CAVI minor genes in its mode of action in prolonging ejaculation in males in biomedical applications.

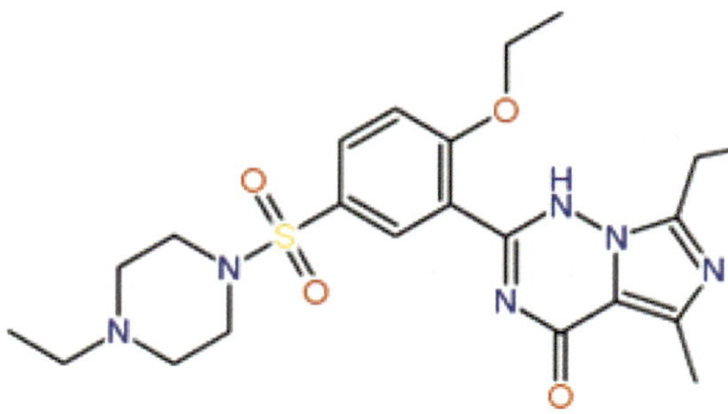


**Figure 15.26** Chemical structure of Verdanafil drug.

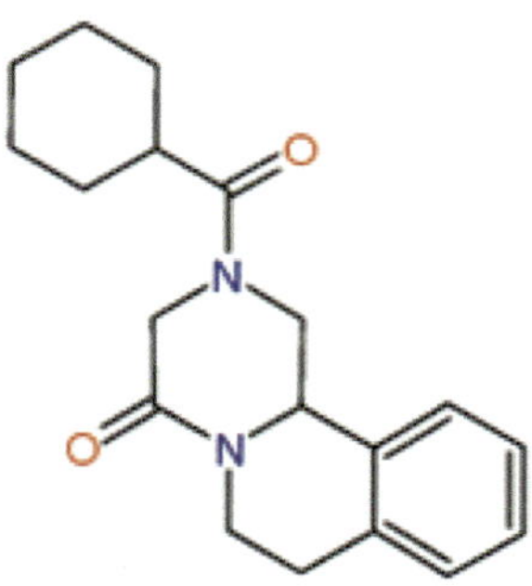


**Figure 15.27** Chemical structure of Praziquantel drug.

## 15.2.4 Praziquantel drug

### 15.2.4.1 Praziquantel

Praziquantel (Bitricide) is an anthelminthic drug (Figure 15.27 and Table 15.4) used in humans and animals for the treatment of tapeworm and flukes infections [42]. Specifically, it is effective against schistosoma, *Clonorchis sinensis*, and for the fish tapeworm *Diphyllotrium latum.* Praziquantel acts on DNAI2 major gene and EPGN, FBRS, and ALGI1 minor genes in its mode of action in truncating the development of human urinary schistosomiasis in biomedical applications.

### 15.2.4.2 Biological activities of major genes affected by Praziquantel and other alternative drugs

*15.3.4.2.1 DNA12*

DNA12 is Dyneal Axonemal intermediate chain 2 gene (Figure 15.28 and Table 15.4). This is a protein coding gene in humans for diseases associated with DNAI2, some of which includes ciliary dyskinesia of the respiratory tract [43]. It is part of the dynein complex of respiratory cilia and sperm

**Table 15.4** Major and minor genes affected by Praziquantel and alternative drugs.

| Drug name | Major genes affected | False discovery rate (score) | Minor genes affected | False discovery rate (score) | Alternative drugs with same effects on major and minor genes as revealed by XAI |
|---|---|---|---|---|---|
| Praziquantel | DNAI2 | 0.996 | EPGN | 0.865 | GDP-mannose |
| | | | FBRS | 0.687 | Uridine diphosphate |
| | | | ALGI1 | 0.553 | Guanosine diphosphate |
| | | | Smp 150200 | 0.882 | Phosphate |
| | | | Smp 052330 | 0.968 | mgATP |
| | | | Smp 131100 | 0.884 | R-Praziquantel |
| | | | Smp 177080 | 0.990 | S-Praziquantel |

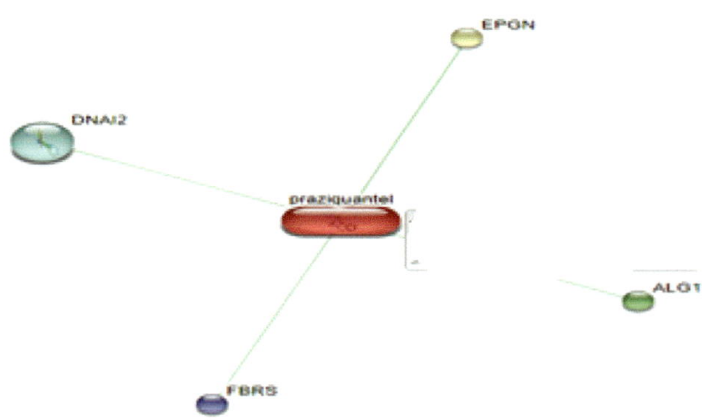


**Figure 15.28** Showing interactions of major and minor genes with Praziquantel drug via XAI.

flagella [44]. The DNAI2 gene is affected by ingestion of Praziquantel and the other alternative drugs (Figures 15.28 and 15.29).

Figure 15.30 shows the protein structure of DNAI2 major gene.

### *15.2.4.2.2 EPGN*

EPGN is also called an epithelial mitogen gene (Figure 15.31 and Table 15.4). It is a protein coding gene in humans directly associated with epithelial growth factor family of proteins [45]. Its primary function is in cell survival preventing apoptosis. It works to help repair and fix cells, thus ensuring that they survive longer, proliferate, and in cell migration [46]. The EPGN gene is affected by ingestion of Praziquantel and the other alternative drugs.

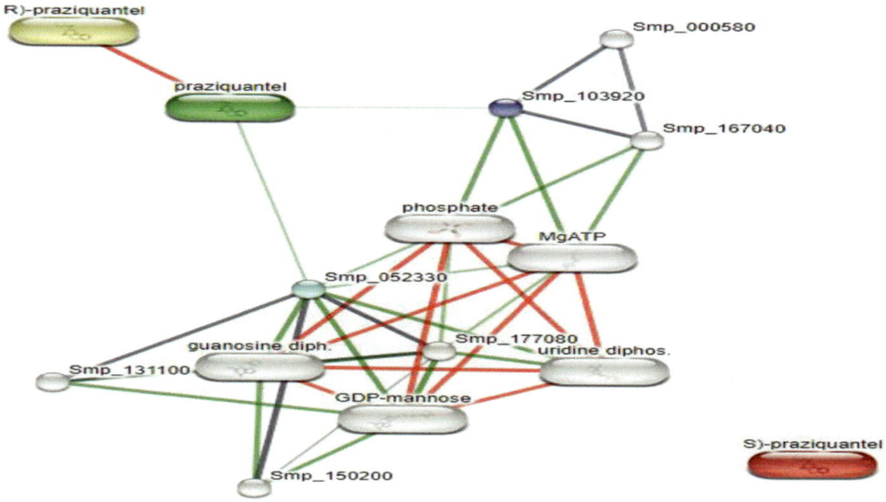


**Figure 15.29** Showing alternatives drugs interactions with same major and minor genes as Praziquantel drug via XAI.

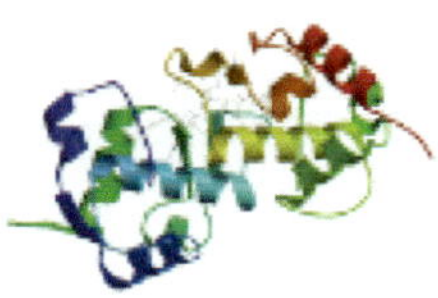

**Figure 15.30** Protein structure of DNAI2 major gene.

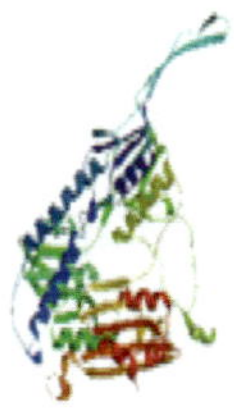

**Figure 15.31** Protein structure of EPGN major gene.

### *15.2.4.2.3 FBRS*

FBRS, also known as fibrosin (Figure 15.32 and Table 15.4), is a protein coding gene. It functions in the treatment of diseases associated with FBRS, which include labyrinthitis and WB syndrome. It is a long transcript protein called fibrosin-1. Fibrosin is a lymphokine secreted by activated lymphocytes that induces fibroblast proliferation [47]. The FBRS gene is affected by ingestion of Praziquantel and the other alternative drugs.

### *15.2.4.2.4 ALGII*

ALGII, also known as acetylase gene (Figure 15.33 and Table 15.4), is a pseudomonas protegens found in both pathogenic and non-pathogenic organisms [48]. The ALGI1 gene is affected by ingestion of Praziquantel and the other alternative drugs.

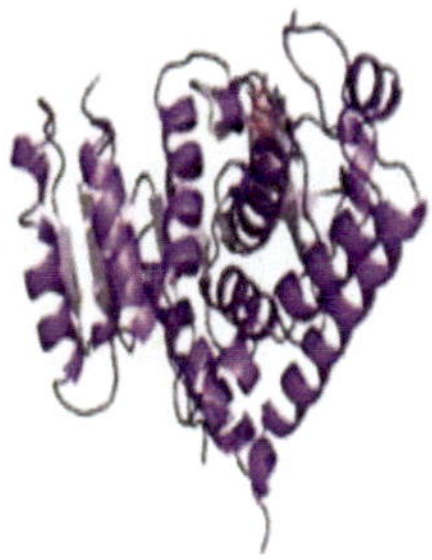

**Figure 15.32** Protein structure of FBRS major gene.

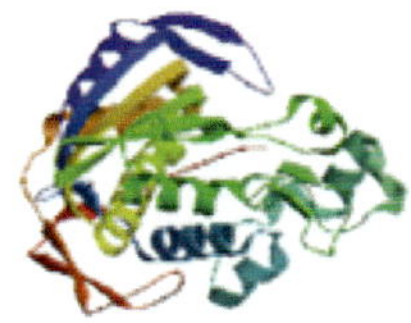

**Figure 15.33** Protein structure of ALGI1 major gene.

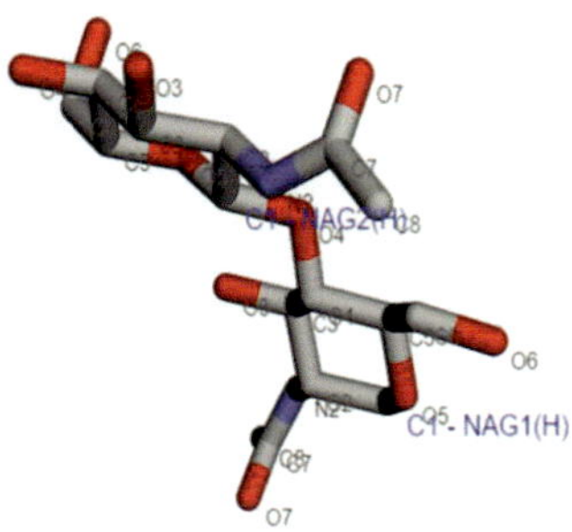


**Figure 15.34** Chemical structure of GDP - mannose drug.

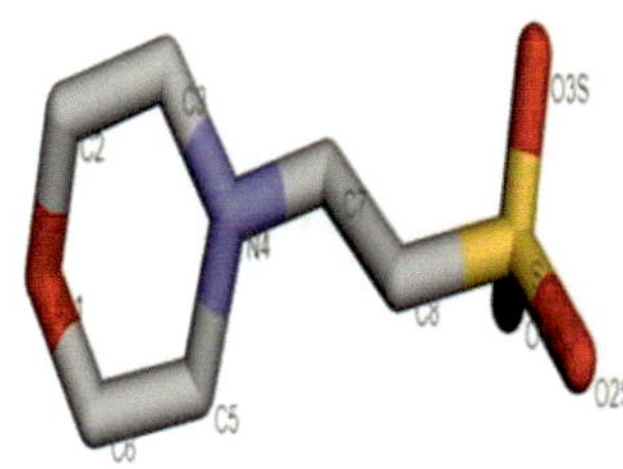


**Figure 15.35** Chemical structure of MgATP drug.

### 15.2.4.3 Discovery of alternative drugs affecting same major and minor genes as Praziquantel based on XAI for biomedical applications

*15.2.4.3.1 GDP mannose or Guanosine diphosphate mannose*

GDP mannose or guanosine diphosphate mannose (Figure 15.34 and Table 15.4) is a nucleotide sugar that is a substrate for glycosyltransferase reactions in metabolism [49]. This drug is a substrate for enzymes known as mannosyltransferases. It is a conjugate acid of GDP alpha D mannose. It is a druggable protein involved in host cell interactions [50]. It has a molar mass of 605.341 g/mol. GDP mannose drug exhibits same and similar biological applications and effect on DNAI2 major gene and EPGN, FBRS, and ALGI1 minor genes and are discovered as alternative drugs to Praziquantel drug used as anthelminthic drug in biomedical applications.

*15.2.4.3.2 MgATP*

MgATP is an adenine nucleotide (Figure 15.35 and Table 15.4) containing three phosphate groups esterified to the sugar moiety [51]. It plays a

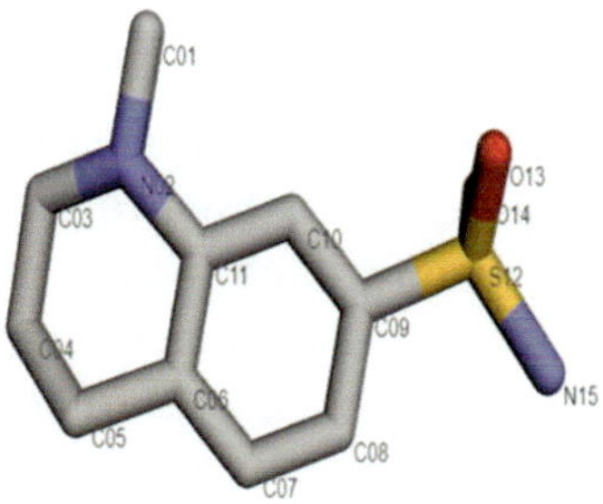


**Figure 15.36** Chemical structure of uridine diphosphate drug.

crucial role in metabolism of adenosine triphosphate. It is L-ascorbic acid 2-phosphate magnesium salt, which is a vitamin C derivative. Its molecular weight is 529.47 g/mol. MgATP drug induces same and similar biological applications and effect on DNAI2 major gene and EPGN, FBRS, and ALGI1 minor genes and are discovered as alternative drugs to Praziquantel drug used as anthelminthic drug in biomedical applications.

*15.2.4.3.3 Uridine diphosphate*

Uridine diphosphate (Figure 15.36 and Table 15.4) is designated as UDP and is a nucleotide diphosphate, which is an ester of pyrophosphate acid with the nucleoside uridine [52]. It consists of a pyrophosphate group, pentose sugar ribose, and the uracil nucleobase. It plays a role in *Escherichia coli* and mouse metabolites [53]. Its molecular weight is 404.16 g/mol. Uridine diphosphate has similar biological applications and effect on DNAI2 major gene and EPGN, FBRS, and ALGI1 minor genes and is discovered as an alternative drug to Praziquantel drug used as anthelminthic drug in biomedical applications.

## 15.3 Discussion

The selected medicines, drugs, or small molecules, as revealed from the chapter study, function effectively in the biosynthesis of secondary metabolite, small and large molecules metabolism, protein metabolism, as well as in coordination of biological processes in the human body, medicinal and small molecular transmembrane transporter activity, target–ligand binding, and ion binding. The structural models of the major and minor gene interactions with different drug structures are shown in the respective figures. This result reveals the protein target sites that interact with the different medicines or drugs target compounds for prevention, treatment, normalization, optimization, and complex formation, which guarantees healing [54, 55].

## 15.4 Conclusion

Explainable artificial intelligence for biomedical applications was achieved using bioinformatics tools of expasy.org. The technique was used to easily discover alternative drugs with same and similar effects on major and minor genes as main drugs in biological systems of humans and other living things. The study showed the relative ease with which the use of artificial intelligence (computer-based simulations and algorithms) can be adopted in the discovery and identification of carfentanil, rispiridine, endomorphine-2, naltrexone, buprenorphine, DAMGO, paroxetine, Nor-BNI, naloxone, and morphine with same biomedical applications and effects on CYP206, OPRK1, and OPRM2 major genes and CHRNA7, SLC5A4, SLC6A4, HTR7, HTR2A, and OPED7 as alternative drugs for Tramadol in biomedical applications.

Also artificial intelligence was used to discover and explain that omega-3-fatty acid, 1,1-dimethetyl, rimonabant, 1-naphthalenyl, AM 251, HU-210, CP-55940, 2-arachidonyl, and anandamide are alternative drugs with same biomedical applications and effects as Cannabinol drug on selected major CD5 and minor CNR1 and CNR2 genes. It was also discovered that Verdanafil, Carfentanil, and Tadalafil have same and similar biological applications and effect on CYP256, OPRM1, OPRK1, OPRD1, and HTR7 major genes and PRKG2, PDE6C, and CAVI minor genes and are discovered as alternative drugs to Sildenafil drug.

The study revealed that GDP-mannose, uridine diphosphate, phosphate, MgATP, and guanosine diphosphate possess same and similar biological applications and effect on DNAI2 major gene and EPGN, FBRS, and ALGI1 minor genes and are discovered as alternative drugs to Praziquantel drug used as anthelminthic drug in biomedical applications.

It is therefore easy to discover and explain drugs for biomedical applications using artificial intelligence. Such discovered drugs can be properly harnessed, reconstituted, redesigned, refocused, and utilized as potential prophylactic or therapeutic drug (single or in combinations) for the prevention and treatment of diseases, which remains a focal point and target of pharmaceutical industries. Thus, a computational-based algorithm that utilizes bioinformatics tools will therefore provide the much needed validation approach for the discovery and further provides better explanations for the applications of small molecules as potential drugs for the prevention and cure of most health-related ailments and biomedical applications.

## Acknowledgements

The authors wish to acknowledge the CEO of Biggmade Scientific Research Academy for the useful advice and criticism as well as the provision of great assistance in laboratory bench and bioinformatics tools/software, which helped in the accomplishment of this chapter.

## References

[1] Whittaker M (2004). The role of bioinformatics in target validation. Drug Discovery To-Clinical trial registration: a statement from the International Committee of Medical Journal Editors. Medical Journal of Australia; 181: 293–4.

[2] Lengauer M (2002). Bioinformatics.From Genomes to Drugs.Wiley-VCH, Weinheim, Germany.

[3] Lipinski D (2004). Lead and drug-like compounds: the rule-of-five revolution. Drug Discovery Today: Technologies; 1(4): 337–341.

[4] Leeson P D, Davis A M, Steele J (2004). Drug-like properties: Guiding principles for design – or chemical prejudice? Drug Discovery Today: Technologies; 1(3): 189–195.

[5] Hou T. Xu X (2004). Recent development and Application of Virtual Screening in Drug Discovery: An Overview. Current Pharmaceutical Design; 10: 1011–1033.

[6] Klebbe G (2004). Lead Identification in Post-Genomics: Computers as a Complementary Alternative. Drug Discovery Today: Technologies; 1(3): 225–215.

[7] GisbertSchneider, Uli Fechner (2005). Computer-based de novo design of drug-like molecules.Nature. Reviews. Drug Discovery; 4(8): 649–663.

[8] Ubi, GM, Ebigwai, KJ, Udensi, OU and Essien, IS (2021) Drug Discovery with Computational Intelligenc Against COVID – 19: In Computational Intelligence for COVID -19 and future pandemics – Emerging applications and strategies: Springer publishers 2021.

[9] Ubi, GM, Ikpeme, E.V, and Essien, IS (2021) Essentials of COVID 19 Coronavirus. Data Science for COVID 19 Book Chapter. Elsevier publishers Ltd. 1–32pp.

[10] World Health Organization (2020) Global Update for COVID 19. https://www.worldhealthorganization.global.update.coivd-19, 2020.

[11] Cox E, Hooyberghs J, Pensaert MB. (1990). Sites of replication of a porcine respiratory coronavirus related to transmissible gastroenteritis virus. *Research in Veterinary Science* 48(2):165–9.

[12] deGroot RJ, Horzinek MC. (1995). Feline infectious peritonitis. In: Siddell SG, ed., *The Coronaviridae.* New York: Plenum Press. Pp. 293–315.
[13] Anonymous. (2003). Severe acute respiratory syndrome (SARS). *Weekly Epidemiological Record* 78:81–3.
[14] Ballesteros ML, Sanchez CM, Enjuanes L. (1997). Two amino acid changes at the N-terminus of transmissible gastroenteritis coronavirus spike protein result in the loss of enteric tropism. *Virology* 227(2):378–88.
[15] Baric RS, Fu K, Chen W, Yount B. (1995). High recombination and mutation rates in mouse hepatitis virus suggest that coronaviruses may be potentially important emerging viruses. *Advances in Experimental Medicine and Biology* 380:571–6.
[16] Ikai, A (1980) Thermostability and Aliphatic index globular ptoteins. Journal of Biochemistry 88(6): 1895–1988.
[17] Bonilla PJ, Gorbalenya AE, Weiss SR. (1994). Mouse hepatitis virus strain A59 RNA polymerase gene ORF 1a: heterogeneity among MHV strains. *Virology* 198(2):736–40.
[18] Bost AG, Prentice E, Denison MR. (2001). Mouse hepatitis virus replicase protein complexes are translocated to sites of M protein accumulation in the ERGIC at late times of infection. *Virology*285(1):21–9.
[19] BrianDA, HogueBG, KienzleTE. (1995). TheCoronavirusHemagluttinin Esterase Clycoprotein. In: Siddell SG, ed., *TheCoronaviridae*. New York: Plenum Press. Pp. 165–79.
[20] Brockway SM, Clay CT, Lu XT, Denison MR.(2003). Characterization of the expression, intracellular localization, and replication complex association of the putative mouse hepatitis virus RNAdependent RNA polymerase. *Journal of Virology* 77(19):10515–27.
[21] Whittaker M (2004). The role of bioinformatics in target validation. Drug Discovery To-Clinical trial registration: a statement from the International Committee of Medical Journal Editors. Medical Journal of Australia; 181: 293–4.
[22] Lengauer M (2002). Bioinformatics.From Genomes to Drugs.Wiley-VCH, Weinheim, Germany.
[23] Lipinski D (2004). Lead and drug-like compounds: the rule-of-five revolution. Drug Discovery Today: Technologies; 1(4): 337–341.
[24] Leeson P D, Davis A M, Steele J (2004). Drug-like properties: Guiding principles for design – or chemical prejudice? Drug Discovery Today: Technologies; 1(3): 189–195.
[25] Hou T. Xu X (2004). Recent development and Application of Virtual Screening in Drug Discovery: An Overview. Current Pharmaceutical Design; 10: 1011–1033.

[26] Klebbe G (2004). Lead Identification in Post-Genomics: Computers as a Complementary Alternative. Drug Discovery Today: Technologies; 1(3): 225–215.

[27] GisbertSchneider,Uli Fechner (2005). Computer-based de novo design of drug-like molecules.Nature. Reviews. Drug Discovery; 4(8): 649–663.

[28] Butte A (2011). The use and analysis of microarray data. Nature Reviews Drug Discovery, 1(12): 951–960.

[29] Richards W. G (1994). Computer-Aided Drug Design.*Pure and Applied Chemistry;* 6(68): 1589–1596.

[30] Kitchen D B. Decornez H. Furr J R. Bajorath J (2004). Docking and scoring in virtual screening for drug discovery: methods and applications. Nature reviews in drug discovery; 3: 935–949.

[31] DiMasi J A. Grabowski H G (2007). The cost of biopharmaceutical R&D: is biotech different? Managerial and Decision Economics; 28: 469–479.

[32] Hajduk PJ, Huth JR, and Tse C (2005). Predicting protein druggability. *Drug.Discov.Today*; 10: 1675–1682.

[33] Fauman EB, Rai BK, and Huang ES (2011) .Structure-based druggability assessment-identifying suitable targets for small molecule therapeutics.*Curr.Opin. Chem. Biol.*; 15: 463–468.

[34] Laurie AT, Jackson RM (2006). Methods for the prediction of protein-ligand binding sites for structure-based drug design and virtual ligand screening. *Curr.Protein.Pept. Sci*; 7: 395–406.

[35] Becker OM, Dhanoa DS, Marantz Y, Chen D, Shacham S, Cheruku S, Heifetz A, Mohanty P, Fichman M, Sharadendu A (2006). An integrated in silico 3D model-driven discovery of a novel, potent, and selective amidosulfonamide 5-HT1A agonist (PRX-00023) for the treatment of anxiety and depression. *J. Med. Chem*; 49: 3116–3135.

[36] Warner SL, Bashyam S, Vankayalapati H, Bearss DJ, Han H, Mahadevan D, Von Hoff DD, Hurley LH (2006). Identification of a lead small-molecule inhibitor of the Aurora kinases using a structure-assisted, fragment-based approach.*Mol. Cancer. Ther*; 5: 1764–1773.

[37] Budzik B, Garzya V, Walker G, Woolley-Roberts M, Pardoe J, Lucas A, Tehan B, Rivero RA, and Langmead CJ (2010). Novel N-substituted benzimidazolones as potent, selective, CNS-penetrant, and orally active M(1) mAChR agonists. *Med. Chem. Lett*; 1: 244–248.

[38] Buchan DW, Ward SM, Lobley AE, Nugent TC, Bryson K, and Jones DT (2010). Protein annotation and modelling servers at University College London.*Nucleic.Acids. Res*; 38: 563–568.

[39] Martí-Renom MA, Stuart AC, Fiser A, Sánchez R, Melo F, and Sali A (2000). Comparative protein structure modeling of genes and genomes. *Annu. Rev. Biophys. Biomol.Struct*; 29: 291–325.

[40] Schlitter J, Engels M, Krüger P (1994). Targeted molecular dynamics: a new approach for searching pathways of conformational transitions. *J. Mol. Graph*; 12: 84–89.

[41] Grubmüller H (1995). Predicting slow structural transitions in macromolecular systems: Conformational flooding. *Phys. Rev. E. Stat. Phys. Plasmas. Fluids.Relat.Interdiscip. Topics*; 52: 2893–2906.

[42] Abrams CF, Vanden-Eijnden E (2010). Large-scale conformational sampling of proteins using temperature-accelerated molecular dynamics. *Proc. Natl. Acad. Sci. U.S.A,*; 107: 4961–4966.

[43] Sugita Y, Okamoto Y (1999). Replica-exchange molecular dynamics method for protein folding. *Chem. Phys. Lett.,* 1999; 314: 141–151.

[44] Liu M, Wang SM. MCDOCK (1999): a Monte Carlo simulation approach to the molecular docking problem. J. Comput. Aided. Mol. Des; 13: 435–451.

[45] Jones G, Willett P, Glen RC (1995). A genetic algorithm for flexible molecular overlay and pharmacophore elucidation. J. Comput. Aided. Mol. Des; 9: 532–549.

[46] Halgren TA (1996). Merck molecular force field. 1. Basis, form, scope, parameterization, and performance of MMFF94. J. Comput. Chem; 17: 490–519.

[47] Böhm HJ (1992). The computer program LUDI: a new method for the de novo design of enzyme inhibitors. J. Comput. Aided. Mol. Des; 6: 61–78.

[48] Rarey M, Kramer B, Lengauer T, Klebe G (1996). A fast flexible docking method using an incremental construction algorithm. J. Mol. Biol; 261: 470–489.

[49] Jain AN (2003). Surflex: fully automatic flexible molecular docking using a molecular similarity-based search engine. J. Med. Chem; 46: 499–511.

[50] Shimada J, Ishchenko AV, Shakhnovich EI (2000). Analysis of knowledge-based protein-ligand potentials using a self-consistent method.Protein. Sci; 9: 765–775.

[51] Velec HFG, Gohlke H, Klebe G (2005). DrugScore (CSD)-knowledge-based scoring function derived from small molecule crystal data with superior recognition rate of near-native ligand poses and better affinity prediction. J. Med. Chem.; 48: 6296–6303.

[52] DeWitte RS, Shakhnovich E (1997). SMoG: De novo design method based on simple, fast and accurate free energy estimates. J. Am. Chem. Soc.; 119: 4608–4617.

[53] Mitchell JBO, Laskowski RA, Alex A, Forster MJ, Thornton JM (1999). BLEEP-Potential of mean force describing protein-ligand interactions: II. Calculation of binding energies and comparison with experimental data. J. Comput. Chem; 20: 1177–1185.
[54] Feher M (2006). Consensus scoring for protein-ligand interactions. Drug. Discov. Today; 11: 421–428.
[55] O'Boyle NM, Liebeschuetz JW, Cole JC (2009). Testing assumptions and hypotheses for rescoring success in protein-ligand docking. J. Chem. Inf. Model; 49: 1871–1878.
[56] Becker OM, Dhanoa DS, Marantz Y, Chen D, Shacham S, Cheruku S, Heifetz A, Mohanty P, Fichman M, Sharadendu A (2006). An integrated in silico 3D model-driven discovery of a novel, potent, and selective amidosulfonamide 5-HT1A agonist (PRX-00023) for the treatment of anxiety and depression. J. Med. Chem.; 49: 3116–3135.
[57] Johnson MA, Maggiora GM (1990). Concepts and Applications of Molecular Similarity, Wiley, New York.
[58] Stumpfe D, Bill A, Novak N, Loch G, Blockus H, Geppert H, Becker T, Schmitz A, Hoch M, Kolanus W (2010). Targeting multifunctional proteins by virtual screening: structurally diverse cytohesin inhibitors with differentiated biological functions. Chem. Biol., 5: 839–849.
[59] Cramer RD, Patterson DE, Bunce JD (1988).Comparative molecular field analysis (CoMFA). Effect of shape on binding of steroids to carrier proteins. J. Am. Chem. Soc; 110: 5959–5967.
[60] Kiaris H, Spandidos DA. (1995) Mutations of Ras Genes in Human Tumors. International Journal of Oncology; 7(3): 413–421.

# 16

# XAI in the Hybrid Classification of Brain MRI Tumor Images

**S. Akça, F. Atban, Z. Garip, and E. Ekinci**

Computer Engineering Department, Faculty of Technology, Sakarya University of Applied Sciences, Turkey
Email: saidakca@hotmail.com; furkanatban@subu.edu.tr; zbatik@subu.edu.tr; ekinekinci@subu.edu.tr

## Abstract

The brain is one of the most important organs of humans. Tumors in the brain occur with the abnormal development of cells in the brain tissue. Brain tumors seriously affect people's lives and can cause death. Accurate and early detection of tumors in the brain is very important for treatment. Magnetic resonance imaging (MRI) method is frequently used today for the detection of brain tumors. Tumor regions can be distinguished by using magnetic resonance (MR) images such as texture, brightness, and contrast. In this study, it is aimed to classify glioma, meningioma, pituitary brain tumors, and healthy category by creating a hybrid model with deep learning (DL) and machine learning (ML) algorithms. In the model, feature maps are created from MR images using the VGG-16 model, which was previously trained for the ImageNet dataset, and classification is made with ML algorithms. As classification algorithms, linear regression (LR), support vector machines (SVM), *k*-nearest neighbor (KNN), decision trees (DT), random forest (RF), AdaBoost, naive Bayes (NB), and multilayer perceptron (MLP) are used. When their performances are compared, MLP gives the highest performance score with an accuracy of 0.973 and an $F1$-score of 0.971. Since DL methods work with the black-box approach, reliability problems occur. In order to express the transparency and intelligibility of the model, visualization is performed by applying the gradient weighted class activation map (Grad-CAM) algorithm to the VGG-16 last layer, one of the convolutional neural networks (CNNs) used for feature extraction.

## 16.1 Introduction

Normal and abnormal developmental processes can both be found in a cell. The cell is functional during normal development; however, during abnormal development, the cell reduces its functionality and impedes its growth [1]. Irregular cell groups occur as a result of abnormal development. This fact emerges the formation of tissues called tumors [2].

According to the definition of brain tumor reclassified by the World Health Organization (WHO) in 2016, a brain tumor is a type of tumor that affects the central nervous system. In general, brain tumors are defined as a group of abnormally growing brain cells [3]. One of the most serious and urgent diseases is cancer of the brain tumor. Brain tumor cancer was determined in around 23,000 patients in the USA in 2015 [4]. In 2018, there were about 80,000 new primary brain tumor cases reported. Meningioma in the membrane region is 36.3% (29,320), glioma in the spinal cord region is 26.5% (21,200), pituitary tumors in the pituitary gland region are approximately 16.2% (13,210), and the remaining cases include other types of tumors [5–9].

Early or timely detection of brain tumors is one of the most important considerations for the treatment of the disease. Tumor treatment is considered according to the type of tumor, observation at the time of examination, and the result obtained from the pathology [10]. Manual classification of brain tumor MR images with similar appearances or structures involves a challenging task associated with the radiologist's expertise in determining and classifying brain tumors. Two types of brain tumors were classified by radiologists, the first of which is related to determining whether brain MRI images are normal or abnormal. The latter includes classifying abnormal brain MR images as per different tumor types. Such a method is not an efficient way for classifying brain tumors due to the fact that it is non-reproducible and time-consuming for a large number of MRI data. Automated classification is a possible way to solve this issue, in which brain tumor MR images with minimal intervention are classified by radiologists [11].

Hashemzehi et al. developed a classification model with 3064 images from 233 patients. 708 images of 3064 pieces of data consist of meningioma, 1426 images of glioma, and 930 images of pituitary brain tumor. In this study, they reduced the 512 × 512 pixel resolution images to 64 × 64 pixels. For the model they created with CNNs, six-fold cross-validation and Adam optimization were used. They obtained an accuracy value of 95% with the model they proposed [12]. Nazir et al. developed a model using feedforward artificial neural networks to classify MR images. The proposed model consists of three stages: image processing, feature extraction, and classification. There are 25 normal and 45 abnormal images in the dataset, which consists of a total of 70 MR images. The model they proposed reached 94.9% validation and 94.2% test accuracy [13]. Gumaei et al. used an MR image dataset of 3064 brain tumors. The dataset includes different images from 233 patients. MR images consist of 944 axials, 1025 sagittal, and 1045 coronal image types. The original size of the images in the dataset is 512 × 512. The proposed model works based on the hybrid feature extraction method. Accuracy performance in classification with regularized extreme learning machine was obtained as 94.233% [14]. Sajjada et al. developed a DL-based brain tumor classification model. Data augmentation was performed to increase the accuracy of the model. They performed the classification process with the pre-trained VGG-19 model. An accuracy value of 94.58% was obtained with the proposed model [15]. Cheng and colleagues used capsule networks to classify brain tumors. The model they created with capsule networks reached 93.5% accuracy [16]. While George et al. reached 91% accuracy with the model they created with deep neural networks using brain MRI images, the model they created with SVM reached 83% accuracy [17]. Bingöl et al. used DL architectures AlexNet, GoogleNet, and ResNet50 in their two-class study with brain tumor and no brain tumor. The highest accuracy value was obtained from the ResNet50 architecture, with an accuracy of 85.71% [18]. For the classification of brain tumors, Aslan created a two-category classifier as tumor presence and tumor absence, using MobilNetV2 from DL networks and KNN from ML algorithms. The accuracy value of the model was calculated as 96.44% [19]. Swati et al. formed a classification model in four categories as glioma, meningioma, and pituitary brain tumors and healthy class. They obtained the accuracy value of the model they created with transfer learning and ML as 94.82% [20].

Due to the input images and the output results being taken into account by DL algorithms, with no transparency of the underlying information flow in the network layers, DL still has limitations in biomedical applications. Understanding the logic underlying network prediction is essential to ensure that the model offers the correct prediction in brain classification applications. As a result, XAI has attracted a lot of attention to investigate "black-box" DL networks in the biomedical science. Through the application of XAI techniques, DL may be created that are transparent and can explain choices to people in a way that is understandable.

In this study, a hybrid system is proposed by combining DL and ML models. Features are extracted from the data using the VGG-16 model, which is previously trained with the ImageNet dataset. The extracted features are given to the ML algorithms and the classification process is carried out. VGG-16 model is made interpretable by using Grad-CAM algorithm. The performance metrics of the classifier models are evaluated and the models are compared. The highest performance is obtained with the MLP algorithm with an accuracy of 0.973 and an $F1$-score of 0.971.

## 16.2 Materials and Methods

### 16.2.1 Dataset

In this study, brain tumor MRI dataset, which is a combination of Sartaj, Figshare, and Br35H datasets,[1] consisting of four categories is used to train ML classification algorithms and measure their performance. The brain tumor MRI dataset has training and test sets. There are 5712 MRI data in the training set (1321 glioma, 1339 meningioma, 1457 pituitary, and 1595 healthy) and 1311 (300 gliomas, 306 meningioma, 300 pituitaries, and 405 healthy) MRI data in the test set. The samples from dataset are given in Figure 16.1.

In the dataset, there are MR images of each category with three different views, namely axial, coronal, and sagittal as shown in Figure 16.2.

### 16.2.2 Method

Image classification is a fundamental task in image processing. Identifying categories of brain tumor diseases from MRI scans is an image classification problem. CNN is a DL approach that has achieved great success in image classification. For this reason, feature extraction is performed using VGG-16 from CNNs in the presented study. The obtained features are given to the ML algorithms and the classification is made. The classical CNN consists of convolutional, pooling, and full-connection layers. In the hybrid method, convolution and pooling layers are used. The convolution layer is the basic component of the CNN architecture that performs feature extraction. Activation functions are used to determine which neuron will be active in the convolution layer with a non-linear transformation. The pooling layer is used after the convolution layer. The pooling layer performs down-sampling to reduce the number of next learnable parameters. It gives the next layer as input, reducing the size. There are no learnable parameters in the pooling layer [21].

[1] https://www.kaggle.com/datasets/masoudnickparvar/brain-tumor-mri-dataset

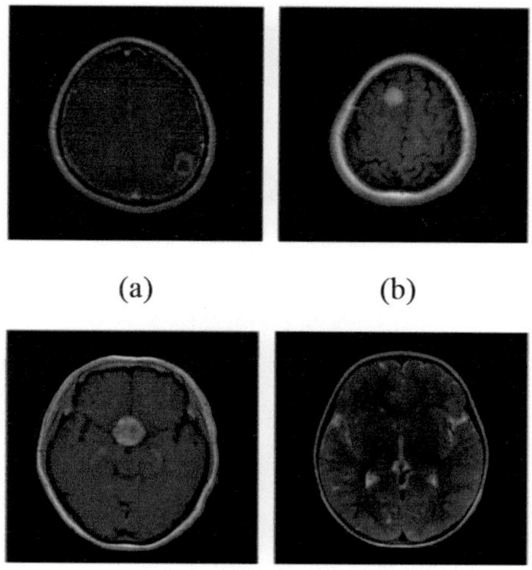

(a) (b) (c) (d)

**Figure 16.1** Brain tumor dataset classes. (a) Glioma. (b) Meningioma. (c) Pituitary. (d) Healthy.

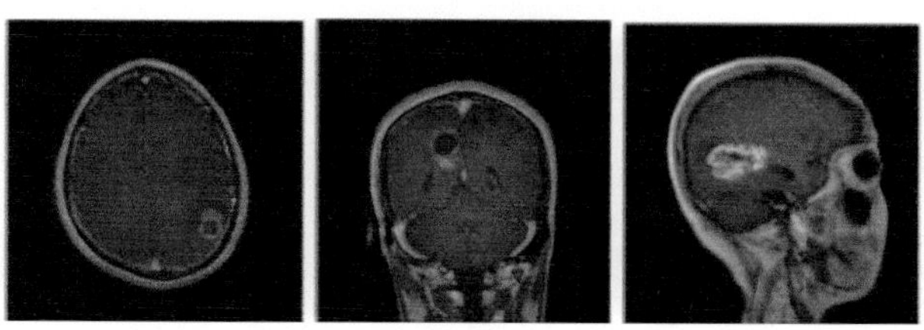

(a) (b) (c)

**Figure 16.2** Glinoma class images. (a) Axial. (b) Coronal. (c) Sagittal.

VGG-16 is a CNN developed by Simonyan and Zisserman from Oxford University [22]. This architecture achieved 92.7% accuracy on the ImageNet dataset containing more than 14 million images of 1000 classes. The input layer consists of 224 × 224 × 3 dimensions in RBG (red, blue, and green) format. The VGG-16 architecture was introduced in 2014. The VGG-16 architecture has 3 × 3 convolution filters and 2 × 2 pooling layers. The number 16 in the VGG-16 architecture indicates that it is a 16-layer deep neural network (VGGnet). The VGG-16 architecture is a very large network with more than 135 million parameters.

Selvaraju et al. proposed the Grad-CAM algorithm to demonstrate the reliability and transparency of their convolutional neural network based models. The purpose of the Grad-CAM algorithm is to visualize the regions

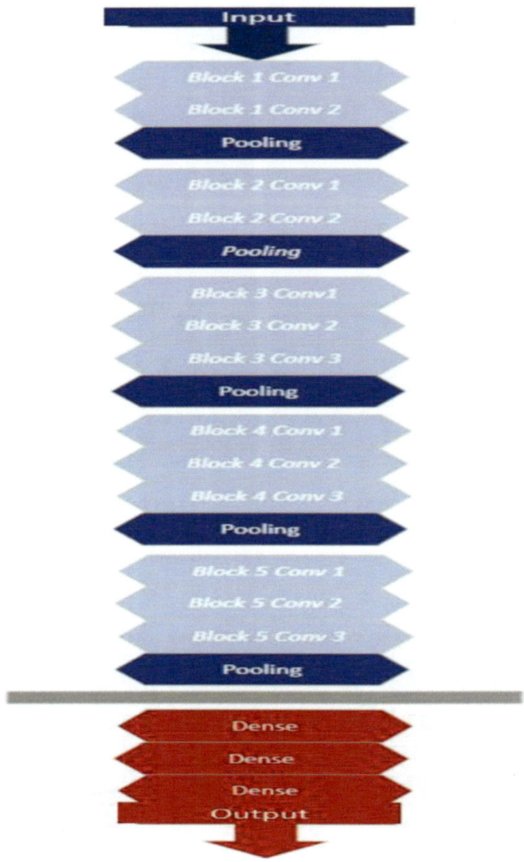


**Figure 16.3** Proposed VGG-16 architecture.

where the features determined for classification are concentrated in the last layer with a heat map [23].

The Grad-CAM algorithm is preferred to visualize the black box formed in the CNN part of the hybrid model proposed in this study. The Grad-CAM algorithm is applied to the Block 3 Conv 5 layer, which is the last layer of the VGG-16 architecture used for feature extraction of the hybrid model. The hybrid architecture is depicted in Figure 16.3.

The model is created by visualizing the features extracted in the Block 3 Conv 5 layer and is explained with the XAI method. In Figure 16.4, the Grad-CAM algorithm is applied to the brain MRI images of glioma, meningioma, pituitary tumors, and helty ones and where the features of the model are focused in the MRI images visualized with a heat map. The heat map is

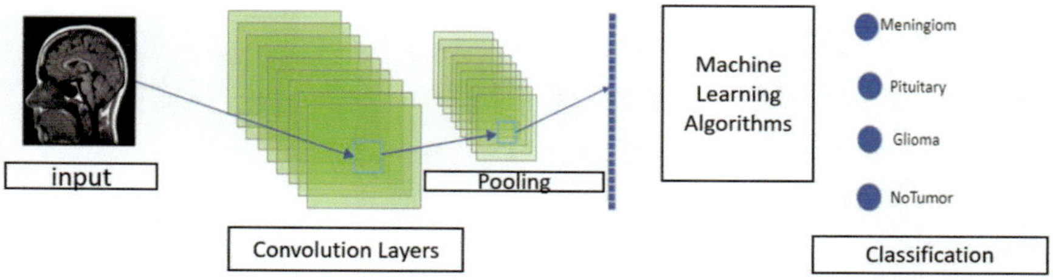


**Figure 16.4** Implementing Grad-CAM for glioma class label.

colored using the gradient values of Block 3 Conv 5 layers. In Figure 16.5, in the areas where Grad-CAM is applied, the red colored regions represent the regions where the model is most concentrated, while the blue colored regions represent the regions where the model is less focused. With the results obtained, the model has been explained and interpreted.

## 16.3 Results

### 16.3.1 Performance metrics and confusion matrix

Performance metrics are calculated to evaluate the success of the models. Accuracy refers to the ratio of correct predictions to total predictions. Accuracy can be defined as the ability to accurately predict the outcome of a situation [24]. The accuracy metric is calculated using eqn (16.1).

$$\text{Accuracy} = \frac{\text{TP} + \text{FP}}{\text{TP} + \text{FP} + \text{TN} + \text{FN}}. \tag{16.1}$$

If the above parameters are explained over a tumor class, we can say the following: TP (true positive) is the number of samples whose true labels and predicted labels are no tumor. FP (false positive) is the number of samples whose true labels and predicted labels are one of the glioma, meningioma, or pituitary. FN (false negative) is the number of samples, while true labels are no tumor, and predicted labels are one of the glioma, meningioma, or pituitary. TN (true negative) is the number of samples, while true labels are one of the glioma, and meningioma or pituitary predicted labels are no tumor.

Precision represents the ratio of correctly predicted positive samples to total predicted positive samples [24]. The precision value of the model is calculated by eqn (16.2).

$$\text{Precision} = \frac{\text{TP}}{\text{TP} + \text{FN}}. \tag{16.2}$$

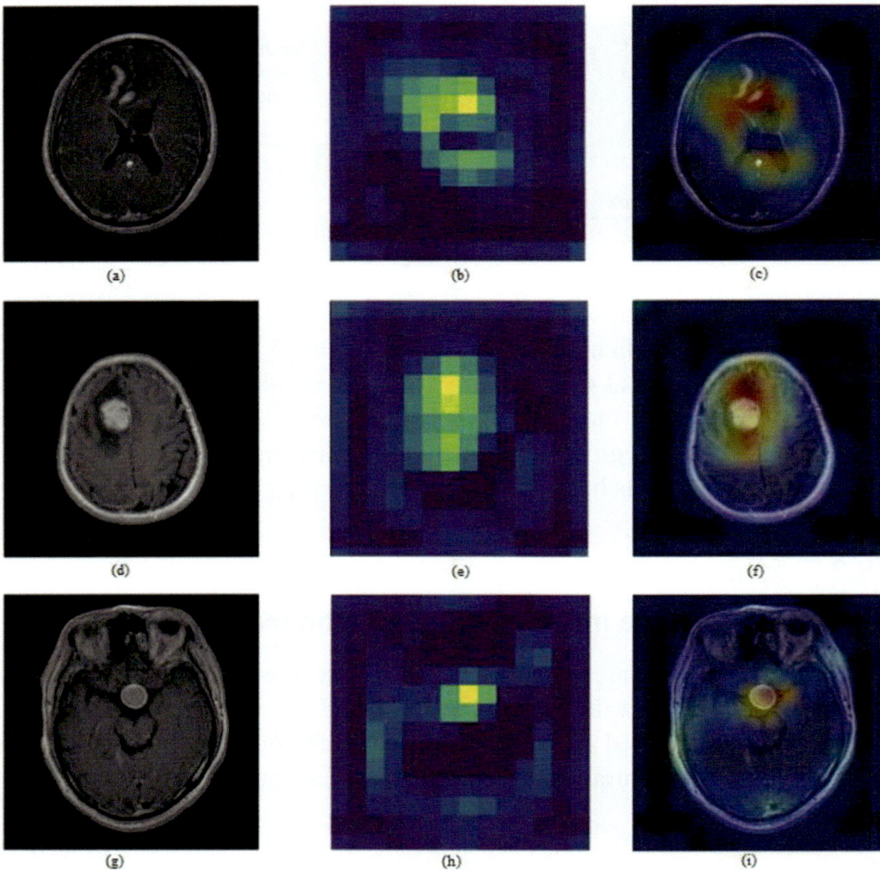


**Figure 16.5** Grad-CAM for brain MRI images. (a) Glinomo class images. (b) Block 3 Conv 5 layer Grad-CAM-glinoma. (c) Glinoma tumor Grad-CAM heat map. (d) Meningioma class images. (e) Block 3 Conv 5 layer Grad-CAM-meningioma. (f) Meningioma tumor Grad-CAM heat map. (g) Pituitary class images. (h) Block 3 Conv 5 layer Grad-CAM-pituitary. (i) Pituitary tumor Grad-CAM heat map.

Recall calculates the ratio of correctly predicted positive samples to the total number of samples in the class [24]. The recall metric is formulated with eqn (16.3).

$$\text{Recall} = \frac{\text{TP}}{\text{TP} + \text{FN}}. \tag{16.3}$$

The $F1$-score is the harmonic mean of precision and recall. The $F1$-score is calculated by eqn (16.4).

$$F1\text{-score} = \frac{2 \times \text{Precision} \times \text{Recall}}{\text{Precision} + \text{Recall}}. \tag{16.4}$$

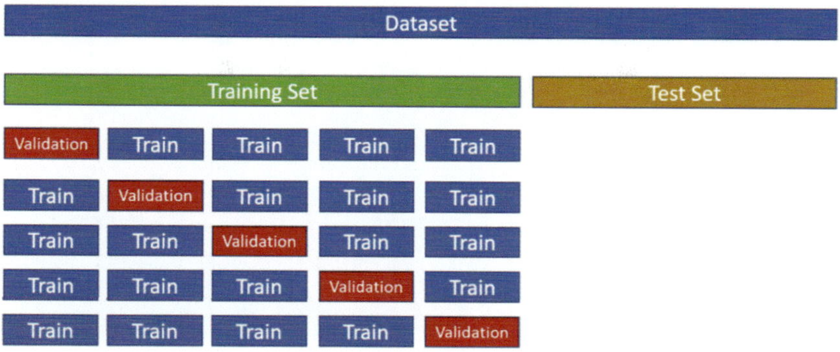


**Figure 16.6** Five-fold cross-validation.

### 16.3.2 *K*-fold cross-validation

A statistical technique known as cross-validation compares and evaluates learning algorithms by splitting data into two parts: one for training and the other for validation. The training and validation sets must overlap in subsequent rounds during a typical cross-validation so that every data point gets a chance to be validated against. The most basic form of cross-validation is *K*-fold cross-validation. The data are initially separated into *K* folds of equal size for *K*-fold cross-validation. Then, *K* iterations of training and validation are performed, using the remaining $K - 1$ folds for learning while holding out a different fold of the data for validation in each iteration.

Classification is performed using the *K*-fold cross-validation method. By taking $K = 5$, the training dataset is divided into five parts and the training phase is completed. The *K*-fold cross-validation is shown in Figure 16.6.

### 16.3.3 Results of simulation

First, features are extracted from the data with VGG-16, one of the pre-trained convolutional neural network architectures. After the attributes of the data are extracted, the training process of the model is performed and the classification process is carried out with ML algorithms. Figure 16.7 shows the accuracy graphs of the ML algorithms used in this study.

Considering the accuracy graphs of the models, while the accuracy is low in the early times of the training, the accuracy value rises above 0.9 toward the end of the training, reaching a successful result. During the testing phase, the models are given an MRI test set, which they have never seen before, and their accuracy is measured.

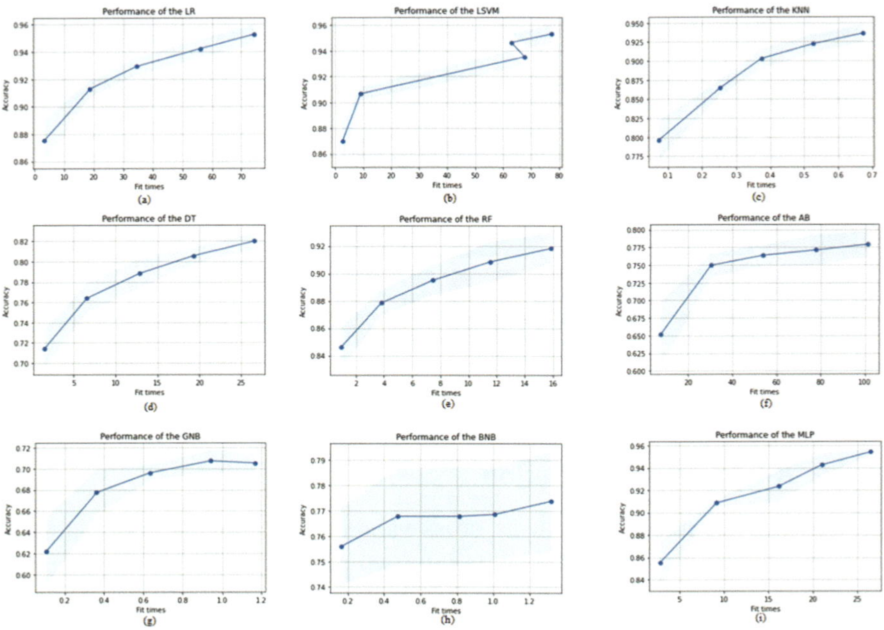


**Figure 16.7** Accuracy for each model. (a) LR. (b) Linear SVM. (c) KNN. (d) DT. (e) RF. (f) AdaBoost. (g) Gaussian NB. (h) Bernoulli NB. (i) MLP.

The highest performance results are achieved by MLP with an accuracy of 0.973, SVM with an accuracy of 0.965, and LR with an accuracy of 0.966, respectively.

The performances of the models are measured with accuracy, precision, recall, and $F1$-score and compared in Table 16.1. When the models are evaluated in terms of $F1$-score, MLP with 0.971 $F1$-score, LR with 0.963 $F1$-score, and SVM with 0.962 $F1$-score give the highest performances, respectively.

The confusion matrix is used to evaluate the performance of classification algorithms in which the predicted labels are compared with the actual labels. The confusion matrices of the models are shown in Figure 16.8.

### 16.3.4 Discussions

Considering the literature, 95% accuracy value was obtained in the CNN created with six-fold cross-validation and man optimization in four categories [12].

The accuracy value was reported as 94.9% [13] in the model created with the feed-forward artificial neural network, 94.233% [14] in the hybrid

**Table 16.1** Comparison of performance metrics of ML algorithms.

| Model | Class | Precision | Recall | *F*1-score | Accuracy |
|---|---|---|---|---|---|
| LR | | | | | 0.9664 |
| | Glioma | 0.9556 | 0.9333 | 0.9444 | |
| | Meningioma | 0.9256 | 0.9346 | 0.9301 | |
| | | 0.9975 | 1.0 | 0.9988 | |
| | Pituitary | 0.9769 | 0.9867 | 0.9818 | |
| | Macro Avg. | 0.9639 | 0.9637 | 0.9637 | |
| Linear SVM | | | | | 0.9657 |
| | Glioma | 0.9461 | 0.9367 | 0.9414 | |
| | Meningioma | 0.9281 | 0.9281 | 0.9281 | |
| | Healthy | 0.9975 | 1.00 | 0.9988 | |
| | Pituitary | 0.9801 | 0.9867 | 0.9834 | |
| | Macro Avg. | 0.9630 | 0.9629 | 0.9629 | |
| KNN | | | | | 0.9649 |
| | Glioma | 0.9467 | 0.9467 | 0.9467 | |
| | Meningioma | 0.9371 | 0.9248 | 0.9309 | |
| | Healthy | 0.9951 | 0.9975 | 0.9953 | |
| | Pituitary | 0.9703 | 0.9800 | 0.9751 | |
| | Macro Avg. | 0.9623 | 0.9623 | 0.9623 | |
| RF | | | | | 0.9268 |
| | Glioma | 0.9474 | 0.8133 | 0.8761 | |
| | Meningioma | 0.8303 | 0.8954 | 0.8616 | |
| | Healthy | 0.9951 | 1.0000 | 0.9975 | |
| | Pituitary | 0.9211 | 0.9733 | 0.9465 | |
| | Macro Avg. | 0.9312 | 0.9205 | 0.9205 | |
| AdaBoost | | | | | 0.7490 |
| | Glioma | 0.7103 | 0.7600 | 0.7343 | |
| | Meningioma | 0.4917 | 0.3856 | 0.4322 | |
| | Healthy | 0.8935 | 0.9111 | 0.9022 | |
| | Pituitary | 0.7923 | 0.8900 | 0.8383 | |
| | Macro Avg. | 7219 | 0.7367 | 0.7268 | |
| Gauss NB | | | | | 0.7124 |
| | Glioma | 0.5568 | 0.8167 | 0.6622 | |
| | Meningioma | 0.6553 | 0.4412 | 0.5273 | |
| | Healthy | 0.9135 | 0.7827 | 0.7670 | |
| | Pituitary | 0.7453 | 0.7900 | 0.7670 | |
| | Macro Avg. | 0.7177 | 0.7076 | 0.6999 | |
| Bernoulli NB | | | | | 0.7109 |
| | Glioma | 0.7751 | 0.6433 | 0.7031 | |
| | Meningioma | 0.98 | 0.3922 | 0.4580 | |
| | Healthy | 1.00 | 0.9086 | 0.8307 | |
| | Pituitary | 1.00 | 0.8367 | 0.7572 | |
| | Macro Avg. | 0.6955 | 0.6952 | 0.6872 | |

*Continued*

**Table 16.1** Continued

| Model | Class | Precision | Recall | *F*1-score | Accuracy |
|---|---|---|---|---|---|
| MLP | | | | | 0.9730 |
| | Glioma | 0.9723 | 0.9367 | 0.9542 | |
| | Meningioma | 0.9417 | 0.9510 | 0.9463 | |
| | Healthy | 0.9975 | 1.0000 | 0.9988 | |
| | Pituitary | 0.9739 | 0.9967 | 0.9988 | |
| | Macro Avg. | 0.9714 | 0.9711 | 0.9711 | |
| DT | | | | | 0.8452 |
| | Glioma | 0.7878 | 0.7300 | 0.7578 | |
| | Meningioma | 0.7304 | 0.7614 | 0.7456 | |
| | Healthy | 0.9344 | 0.9852 | 0.9591 | |
| | Pituitary | 0.8955 | 0.8567 | 0.8756 | |
| | Macro Avg. | 8445 | 0.8410 | | |

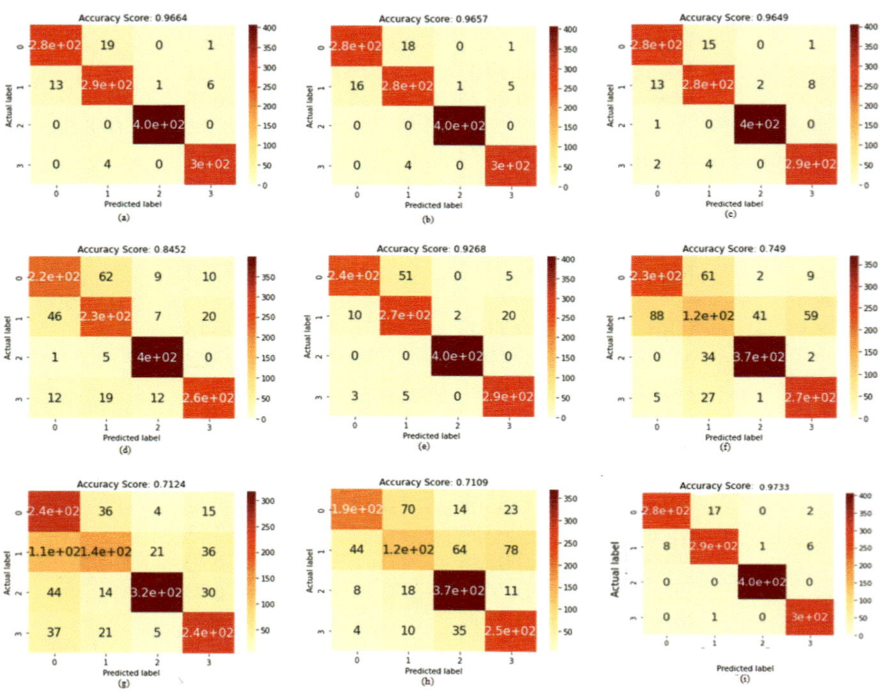


**Figure 16.8** Confusion matrix for ML algorithms. (a) LR. (b) Linear SVM. (c) KNN. (d) DT. (e) RF. (f) AdaBoost. (g) Gaussian NB. (h) Bernoulli NB. (i) MLP.

model created with four categories, and 94.58% [15] in the model created with the VGG-19 CNN.

The success rate was 93.5% [16] in the model created with capsule networks, 91% with deep neural networks, and 83% [17] in the ML.

In this study, a four-category classification model is proposed with ML algorithms by performing feature extraction with VGG-16 CNN. In the model created by using more categories than the studies in the literature, a higher accuracy value is obtained with 97.3% compared to the literature.

## 16.4 Conclusion

In this study, a hybrid model is proposed, in which features are extracted with VGG-16 CNN and classification is performed with ML algorithms. In the study, glioma, meningioma, pituitary brain tumors, and healthy tumors are classified using the hybrid model. The performances of ML classification algorithms are measured and compared with accuracy, precision, recall, and $F1$-score metrics. The complexity matrices of the classification algorithms are obtained and evaluated. In order to make CNNs more transparent and understandable, an XAI method is created by visualization in the last layer. With the Grad-CAM algorithm, the block 3 Conv 5 layer of VGG-16, one of the CNN architectures, is visualized and more reliable results are obtained by removing it from being a black box.

In hybrid models, LR 0.966 accuracy and 0.9637 $F1$-score, linear SVM 0.965 accuracy and 0.962 $F1$-score, KNN 0.964 accuracy and 0.962 $F1$-score, RF 0.926 accuracy and 0.920 $F1$-score, AdaBoost 0.749 accuracy and 0.726 $F1$-score, Gauss NB 0.712 accuracy and 0.699 $F1$-score, Bernoulli NB 0.966 accuracy and 0.9637 $F1$-score, MLP 0.973 accuracy and 0.971 $F1$-score, and DT 0.845 accuracy and 0.8345 $F1$-score are achieved.

## References

[1] I. Razzak, M. Imran, G Xu, 'Efficient brain tumor segmentation with multiscale two-pathway-group conventional neural networks', IEEE journal of biomedical and health informatics, 2018.

[2] A. Rehman, et. al., 'A deep learning-based framework for automatic brain tumors classification using transfer learning', Circuits, Systems, and Signal Processing, pp. 1–19,2019.

[3] WHO Statistics on Brain Cancer. Available online: http://www.who.int/cancer/en/ (accessed on 1 July 2019).

[4] R.L. Siegel, K.D. Miller, A. Jemal, Cancer statistics, CA Cancer J. Clin. 65(1), pp. 5–29, 2015.

[5] Brain tumor statistics, American Brain Tumor Association, URL: http://abta.pub30.convio.net/, (accessed on 26 October, 2019).

[6] BrainTumorBasics.Availableonline:https://www.thebraintumourcharity.org/ (accessed on 1 July 2019).

[7] Brain Tumor Diagnosis. Available online: https://www.cancer.net/cancer-types/brain-tumor/diagn osis (accessed on 1 July 2019).
[8] Litjens, Geert, et al., 'A survey on deep learning in medical image analysis. Medical image analysis 42,', pp. 60–88, 2017.
[9] M. Christine, et. al., 'Meningioma', Critical Reviews in Oncology/Hematology 67.2', pp.153–171, 2008.
[10] S. Deepak, P. M. Ameer, 'Brain tumor classification using deep CNN features via transfer learning" Computers in biology and medicine 111, p.103345, 2019'.
[11] Z.N.K. Swati, et al., 'Brain tumor classification for MR images using transfer learning and fine-tuning. Comput Med Imaging Graph', pp. 34–46, 2019.
[12] R. Hashemzehi, 'Detection of brain tumors from MRI images base on deep learning using hybrid model CNN and NADE', Biocybernetics and Biomedical Engineering 40 pp. 1225–1232, 2020.
[13] M. Nazir, 'A Simple and Intelligent Approach for Brain MRI Classification', pp. 1127–1135', 2015.
[14] A. Gumaei, et. al., 'A Hybrid Feature Extraction Method with Regularized Extreme Learning Machine for Braşb Tumor Classification', IEEE Access, vol 7, pp. 36266–36273, 2019.
[15] M. Sajjad, et al., 'Multi-grade brain tumor classification using deep CNN with extensive data augmentation.', Journal of Computational Science, 30, pp.174–182, 2019.
[16] Y. Cheng, et. al., 'ConvCaps: Multi-input Capsule Network for Brain Tumor Classification', International Conference on Neural Information Processing, pp. 524–534, 2019.
[17] N. George, M. Manuel, 'A Four Grade Brain Tumor Classification System Using Deep Neural Network,' 2019 2nd International Conference on Signal Processing and Communication (ICSPC)', pp. 127–132, 2019.
[18] H. Bingol, B. Alatas, 'Classification of Brain Tumor Images using Deep Learning Methods', Turkish Journal of Science and Technology, 16, vol. 1, pp. 137–143, 2021.
[19] M. Aslan, 'Derin Öğrenme Tabanlı Otomatik Beyin Tümör Tespiti', Fırat Üniversitesi Mühendislik Bilimleri Dergisi, 34, vol. 1, pp. 399–407, 2022.
[20] K.M. Macarthur, et. al., 'Detection of brain tumor cells in the peripheral blood by a telomerase promoter-based assay.' Cancer Research, 74.8, pp. 2152–2159, 2014.
[21] R. Yamashita, et. al., 'Convolutional neural networks: an overview and application in radiology'. Insights Imaging 9, pp. 611–629, 2018.

[22] K. Simonyan, A. Zisserman, 'Very Deep Convolutional Networks for Large-Scale Image Recognition.', arXiv preprint arXiv, 1409.1556, 2014.

[23] R. R. Selvaraju, et. al., 'Grad-CAM: Visual Explanations from Deep Networks via Gradient-Based Localization', IEEE International Conference on Computer Vision (ICCV), pp.618–626, 2017.

[24] R. Rajasekaran, V.K. Asari, V.Singh, 'A Deep Neural Network for Early Detection and Prediction of Chronic Kidney Disease', Diagnostics, 2022.

# 17

# Comparative Analysis of Breast Cancer Diagnosis Driven by the Smart IoT-based Approach

**Bhavya Mittal, Pranshu Sharma, Sushruta Mishra, and Sibanjan Das**

Kalinga Institute of Industrial Technology, Deemed to be University, India
Email: 20051819@kiit.ac.in; 20051821@kiit.ac.in;
sushruta.mishrafcs@kiit.ac.in; sibanjandas@gmail.com

## Abstract

The past few years have seen a growth in the occurrence of breast cancer in women, which has not only resulted in major health issues but has also taken away many lives. According to a survey in 2020, about 2.3 million women were diagnosed with breast cancer and 685,000 deaths were observed globally. The major challenge faced in the diagnosis of breast cancer is that it can occur in women at any age after puerty. It is extremely important to detect breast cancer as early as possible in order to increase the chances of survival for the patient. Efforts have been made in the IoT healthcare environment to diagnose breast cancer sooner and to provide more accuracy. Diagnostic systems based on machine learning have been proposed. In order to improve the performance of the classification system, the recursive feature selection algorithm has been used, which has selected the best features to bring out the best results of the applications of IoT in breast cancer diagnosis. In this chapter, we focus on comparing two different Internet of Things techniques for breast cancer diagnosis and analyzing their pros and cons through a comparative study of the chapters. We briefly go through machine learning and deep learning techniques and find out their pros and cons in the diagnosis of breast cancer. With the help of labeled diagrams and explanations, we try to understand both the techniques and then come to a conclusion regarding the same.

## 17.1 Introduction

Statistics have shown that breast cancer treatments can be immensely effective, provided it is diagnosed at an early and curable stage [1]. When a symptom such as a painless lump or abnormal thickening of the breast is detected, the patient awaits the doctor's final diagnosis. These words from the doctor are now responsible for the patient's future. Through this, we understand how delicate are the results of the diagnosis of this deadly disease, called breast cancer [2].

If one wonders what the possible risk factors that they can avoid to prevent the occurrence of breast cancer in them are, the answer is simple—nothing, except age and gender [3]. But the question that arises here is, "Is this information enough?"

The old saying, "Prevention is better than cure," unfortunately does not work in the case of breast cancer. One cannot prevent it but can definitely help themselves by getting it detected as early as possible. The survival probability of breast cancer treatments is about 90% if detected on time [4]. There are various treatments for breast cancer, including radiotherapy and mastectomy. Studies have shown that, in early stage breast cancers, radiotherapy or radiation can prove to be so important that a woman might not have to undergo mastectomy. However, if we calculate the effectiveness of a treatment, we need to be patient enough to wait for the entire course to be completed and not give a declaration mid-way [5].

We now understand why it is immensely important to detect breast cancer accurately and expeditiously. This is where the application of the Internet of Medical Things (IoMT) comes into action [6].

IoMT is a step ahead of other means of cancer diagnosis when it comes to providing a medical infrastructure that would ensure a timely diagnosis and, further, a treatment that would ensure recovery. Cancer needs rapid results, rapid diagnosis, and further rapid treatment. Today, studies are being conducted in the artificial intelligence (AI) and machine learning (ML) fields to build a healthcare environment such that no patient loses their life because of a delay [7]. There are innumerable studies that have been conducted keeping in mind the challenges that breast cancer throws at us. Through machine learning algorithms, we wish to build such diagnostic systems that can proficiently differentiate malignant and benign patients in the environment of IoMT. Figure 17.1 shows how the detection takes place with training, processing the data, and through feature extraction, creating a machine learning model [8].

In this chapter, we aim at comparing different models and then analyzing them. The first analysis is a study of breast cancer detection using deep learning and IoT technologies, while the second study is about feature

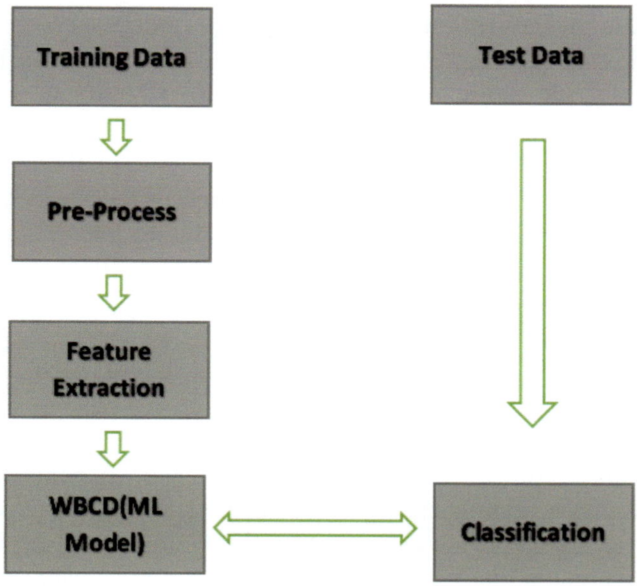


**Figure 17.1** Stages in diagnosis of breast cancer using machine learning.

selection and classification in breast cancer prediction using IoT and machine learning. Through a comparative study of the chapters, we briefly go through machine learning and deep learning techniques and find out their pros and cons in the diagnosis of breast cancer. With the help of labeled diagrams and explanations, we try to understand both the techniques and then come to a conclusion regarding the same. This chapter takes us through a section-wise study of the two techniques we have compared. The machine learning algorithm gives us a good accuracy with three phases involved in it. After seeing the result of this analysis, we move forward with our next technique, that is, the deep learning technique. With proper analytical and comparative study, we try to find out why deep learning is a better technique than machine learning for the diagnosis of breast cancer. With the help of various categories for differentiation including aim of work, methods used, results obtained, and pros and cons, we frame a table: deep learning v/s machine learning. Moving ahead in the chapter, we draw a comprehensive review of the machine techniques, which gives us the information about the benefits and limitations of various other techniques that come under machine learning like computer aided diagnostics (CAD) system, the nonlinear machine learning algorithm comparison, comparison of SVM and ANN, optimization of algorithms through genetics programming technique, and, lastly, comparative analysis of data mining classifier for cancer prediction and detection. However accurate these modern techniques are, challenges exist everywhere. We take a deeper look at what the challenges faced by techniques can be, such as mammography, ultrasound, and breast MRI. Every technique is developed with the aim of more accuracy, early detection, and better efficiency. After completing this chapter, our research for an even better method does not end. We wish to overcome any challenges that come in the way of a patient's healthy and cancer-free life. Losing one's life due to late diagnosis should not be acceptable in today's world, which is full of brilliant techniques like the Internet of Things and that is why the research for the betterment of the society and its people never ends.

### 17.1.1 Objective

The out of control growth of cells is called cancer, and when this occurs in the breasts, it results in breast cancer. This can be on one or both breasts. Majorly women are at a greater risk of getting this dangerous disease as compared to men, who are at a much lower ratio of risk [9]. Breast cancer can start in different parts of the breast. In women, this organ produces the milk for the newborns, and it is biologically possible using different parts of the breasts which further with no luck can be the victims of cancer and act as the cancer carrying medium of the breasts; therefore, breast cancer is further divided into different categories based on the part of it holding tumor (cancer). If the cancer is in the glands (lobules) that make breast milk, it is called lobular cancer. If it is in the ducts that come out of the lobules and carry milk to the nipple, it is called ductal cancer, and this is the most common place of all. Similarly, there are other kinds of cancer that further categorize breast cancer [10]. The causes of breast cancer are mostly unknown, resulting from two factors, i.e., lifestyle-related and those factors that cannot be changed. Lifestyle factors would include many things, such as alcohol, obesity, physical inactivity, not breastfeeding, birth control, menopausal hormone therapy, etc. However, the risk factors that cannot be changed are being a female, growing older, inheriting genes, having a history of breast cancer in family or personal, being tall, dense breast tissues, certain benign breast conditions, etc. Such vast factors that one way or the other could lead to cancer make it very hard to take any kind of precautions [11].

The main objective of this chapter will be to provide the solution and direct individuals toward the best possible set of precautions that could be taken if the risk of having breast cancer is higher and also to those individuals who are already at some stage of fighting it with the aim of being cured completely. Minimizing the risks that originate from one's life style and the factors which cannot be changed for individuals with a specific condition can help in finding solutions to this problem. At the same time, it can help people with different stages of breast cancer accordingly throughout the cycle [12]. From detecting the risk, preventing the causes that could lead toward this road and then screening if needed, for any individual, there is a possible model that could help in all these conditions and ultimately act as the efficient medium for bringing down the rate of breast cancer in women and hence bringing down the mortality rate to the lowest possible number with the help of IoMT (Internet of Medical Things) technology is the utmost priority. In this chapter, we study the two most efficient methods of IoT, which are the machine learning and the deep learning methods. We do an analysis of both the techniques, keeping in mind various criteria and going through past research chapters and their outcomes. A very detailed comparative analysis has been done in this chapter for both the techniques, which would help budding researchers to go ahead and study deeper and bring in better ways to diagnose breast cancer before it becomes fatal for one.

We are aware of the outcomes that any form of cancer can have in a patient, the ultimate being taking one's life. Our concern is to come up with such technologies that prevent the loss of one's life due to a very curable form of cancer that is breast cancer if only it is diagnosed on time. Researchers in the past have come up with such solutions that the rate of deaths due to breast cancer has now taken a dip, which can be decreased even more with further studies. With this chapter, we wish that more students and budding researchers and scientists find it easier to study the techniques broadly and in an organized way.

## 17.2 Analysis of Computational Techniques for Breast Cancer Diagnosis using IoT

In this section, a brief analysis and comparison is done between two different computational approaches for breast cancer assessment using smart IoT-enabled techniques.

### 17.2.1 Smart breast cancer diagnosis using machine learning

The purpose of this study is to propose a methodology using the Internet of Things that would conduct early diagnosis of breast cancer. With 98% of precision, 97% of recall, and 96% of *F*-measure, the study in this chapter has resulted in 98% of accuracy. This research work focuses on reducing the dimension of the dataset by selecting appropriate features for proper

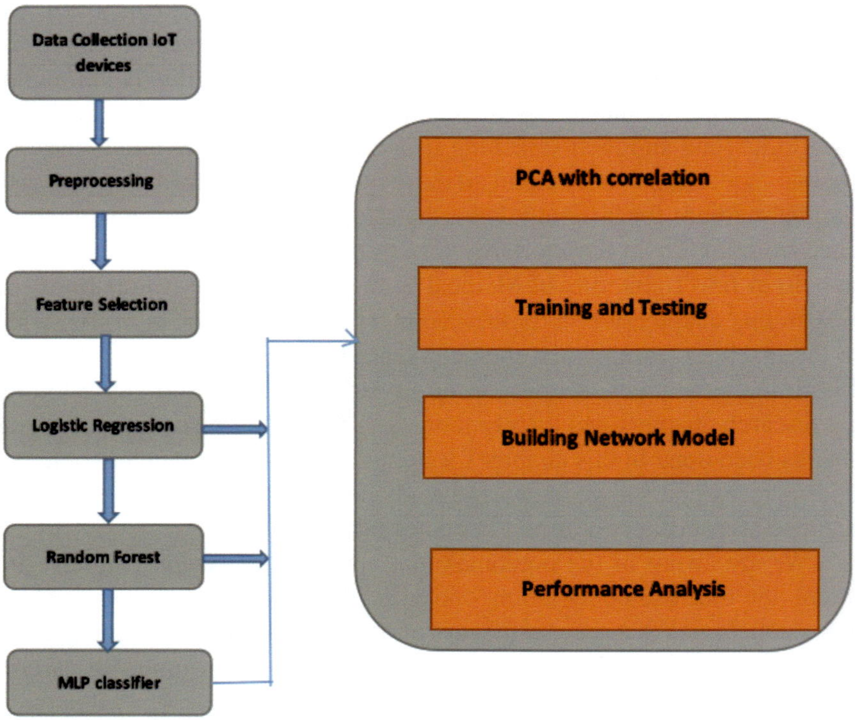


**Figure 17.2** Architecture model for breast cancer classification.

diagnosis using principal component analysis (PCA) with random forest (RF) and multi-layer perceptron (MLP) classifiers. The chapter aims at reducing the mortality rate and detecting tumors in their early stages.

The first phase of the chapter includes data preprocessing; the second has feature selection; and the last phase includes classification analysis [13]. (See Figure 17.2)

The methodology proposed in this chapter aims toward using machine learning techniques to make model tools that would identify the cancer gene pattern in all the stages. The physiological parameters are sensed with the help of IoT devices. The tumor cells in the breasts are detected with the help of microwave sensors.

- **First phase (preprocessing):**

  The Wisconsin Breast Cancer dataset, where preprocessing is carried out with 569 instances and 32 attributes, is introduced in this section. Then, by using the random RBF model in the WEKA tool, the data are

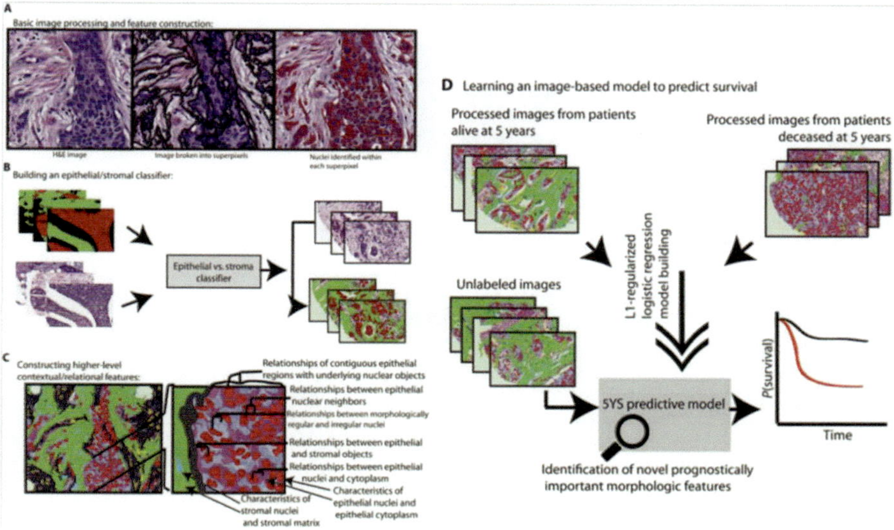


**Figure 17.3** A classic machine learning based system.

filtered and normalized. Figure 17.3 shows a classic machine learning based system.

- **Second phase (feature selection using correlation function):**

  The PCA-based attribute evaluator is used for feature selection with correlation-based feature selection (CFS) that selects the features by the ranking method. The concept is: the subsets that have a higher correlation matrix corresponding to their class label are ranked higher than the remaining features in the selection process. The work of the attribute evaluator is to exclude the duplicate or irrelevant features within the dataset. The problem of over-fitting is also solved by the PCA by removing the extra variables or substitutes that may be considered as a collection of two or more variables. It chooses the redundant variables to be eliminated on the basis of the scale ranging from 0 to 1, which makes the model more accurate and effective. The principal component analysis (PCA) is deployed to analyze features by evaluating the scatter plot of breast cancer cells. The process is then carried out with the training and test datasets using the correlation function.

- **Third phase (classification analysis):**

  Three different types of classification analysis have been used. Random forest, logistic regression, and MLP classifiers are examples of models

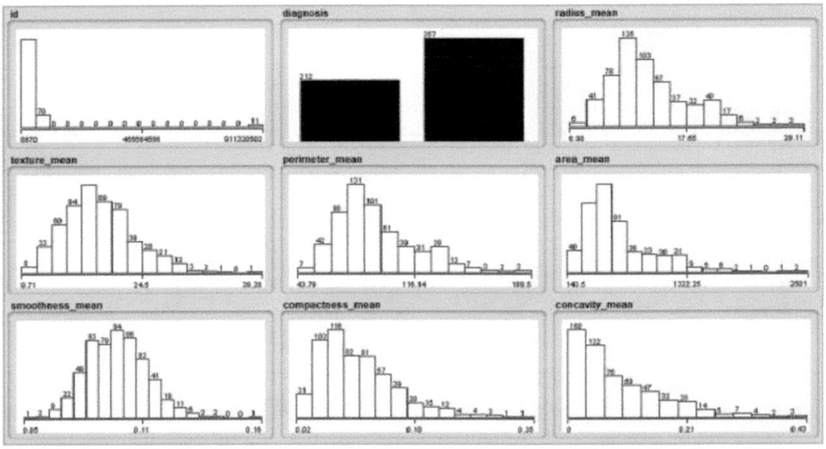


**Figure 17.4** Mean value cases.

that have been built for classification analysis, along with ten cross-fold methods [14]. The data samples of cancer that are collected are divided into two sets: training and testing. These results are then validated using the three models, and the MLP classifier is purposely used to generate the output as a combination of two covariance variables that will produce the correlation function.

#### 17.2.1.1 Result of the model

As we can see in Figure 17.4 and 17.5, the features are divided into seven mean cases and nine worst cases and are then analyzed using microwave sensors to detect tumors that are malignant.

In the next section, we will see how deep learning is better than machine learning for breast cancer diagnosis [15].

### 17.2.2 A deeper analysis of how deep learning is a step ahead of machine learning

There are some key features of both machine learning and deep learning that differentiate both of them and point toward how deep learning is better in the detection of breast cancer. So, starting from a basic level, in machine learning, there is a need for a human to identify, analyze, and code accordingly for the data under consideration, whereas a deep learning system does not need the involvement of a human to analyze the situation to build a feature. The training of the model needs the rendering of enormous amounts of data for the detection of breast cancer. Machine learning needs data analysis from time to time to check the results of the model, while in deep learning, with

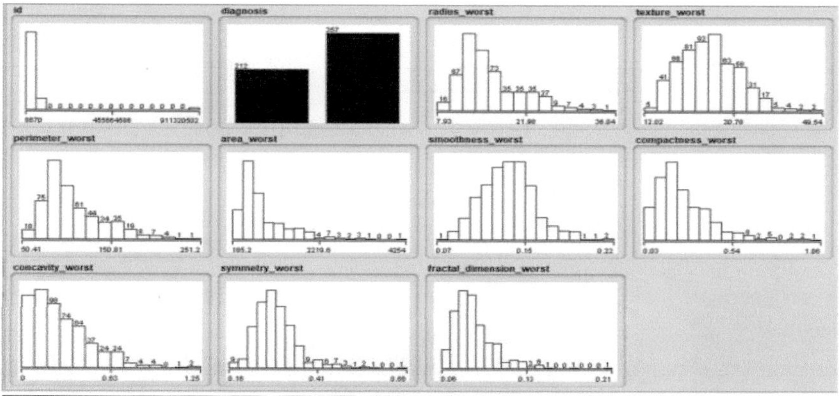


**Figure 17.5** Worst feature cases.

time, the program or model trains itself using neural networks without the need for a human. This also increases the probability of accurate results as the data are getting trained in real time with regular input of new data. The dataset in use for the detection of breast cancer is a huge one; so at an initial stage, the time taken by machine learning to process the data is going to be less than what would be needed by a deep learning model. But as the size of the dataset increases, the efficiency of the model will also increase with time and increase in data. Though deep learning may take more time sometimes, it will provide better accuracy as the model is trained with new data. Algorithms in use in machine learning distribute data into parts, and then these parts combine to give results. As seen in the model of machine learning under consideration above, it involves dividing the data into parts and then performing different operations (preprocessing, feature selection with correlation function, and classified analysis) to then combine and give results. Since the image acts as the dataset in the model for detection of breast cancer, the machine learning model detects and then recognizes the data for training purposes, whereas deep learning works on the entire dataset at one time and gives the result using the algorithm in use, which for the chapter we are going to discuss is the CNN algorithm, which gives the result and declares if the provided data (image) are benign or malignant. Figure 17.6 shows how the deep learning model provides results from taking images as data, augmenting data, and rendering the model layer by layer to provide accuracy in results.

Hence, deep learning can provide better and more efficient results with higher accuracy in the detection of breast cancer, and with fast and remote access to the model, detection of cancer can be done with ease and in less time.

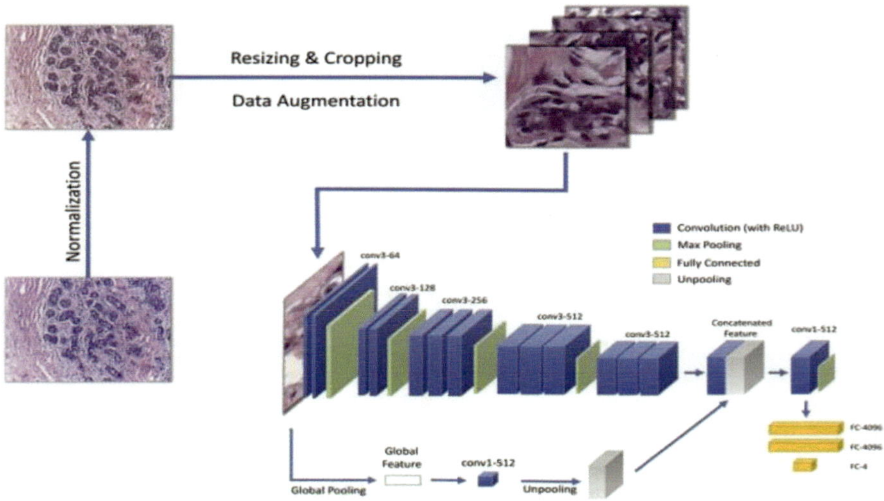


**Figure 17.6** Breast cancer diagnosis with deep learning.

### 17.2.3 Breast cancer diagnosis using deep learning and IoT

This study deals with the process of detection of breast cancer with the help of deep learning and IoT. It is using the CNN algorithm through the microcomputer Raspberry PI. As known already, the CNN algorithm helps with the image processing using an IR (infrared) image taken by the sensor connected to the microcomputer. Here, images act as the dataset for the algorithm to determine the given set of images as benign or malignant. Further, the model uses a WI-FI module and RFID reader with the microcomputer to send the concluded data and the set of images directly into consideration, as shown in Figure 17.7, to the doctor through the cloud for further actions, while the reader helps with keeping the patient's data secure and easy to log in if needed again.

The dataset as the image is divided into three categories, training category for using images as the training data, validation to validate the model, and the testing category for testing the trained model. The dataset is then partitioned into negative and positive images and the improvement of the model is done by adding more negative and positive images to the training dataset.

The CNN (convolutional neural network) basically classifies the visual data using images as the dataset. The images are in the form of tensor or matrix of higher dimensions. It applies weight to the image to further bias to differentiate it with others, which will be divided into the various layers of

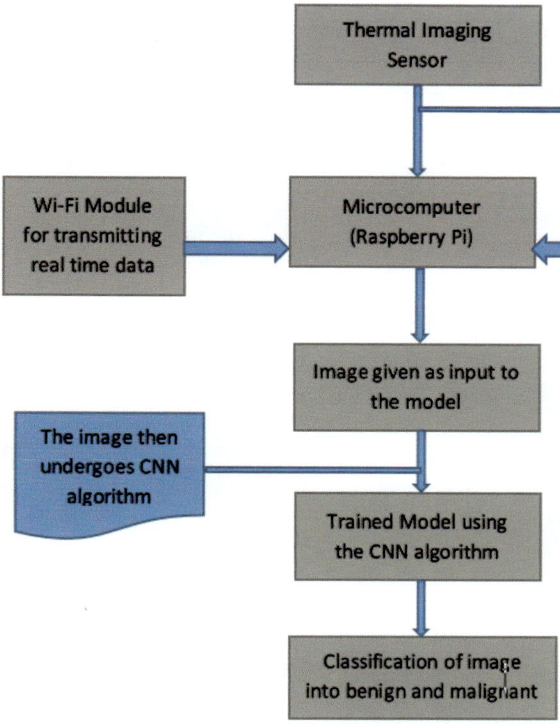


**Figure 17.7** CNN algorithm in deep learning for breast cancer diagnosis.

CNN. Different layers of the network work with different resolutions of the image being processed.

The CNN algorithm takes the image and renders it through different layers serially, as shown in Figure 17.8, from the input to the ReLu layer through the convolutional and pooling layers. The input layer changes the input picture into a network of shapes denoted by the matrix [32 × 32 × 3] of RGB channels. The convolutional layer results in providing a spatial degree of network, which is called the open field of the neurons that are associated with the information. To diminish the size of the spatial degree of network obtained in the convolutional layer, there are three parameters that take into account of going to the next and last layer that is depth, stride, and zero padding. It checks the usage of filters and its sliding on the input images to validate the padding of zeroes along the edges of input. There is the next layer called the pooling layer, which converts the picture into sets of non-covering square shapes. Figure 17.9 shows the images taken as data. Now the next layer, the ReLu layer, removes all the negative numbers from the picture to set it to 0 by

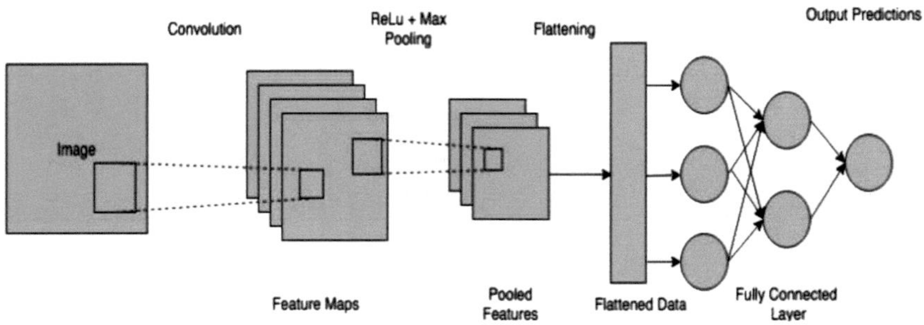


**Figure 17.8** CNN architecture.

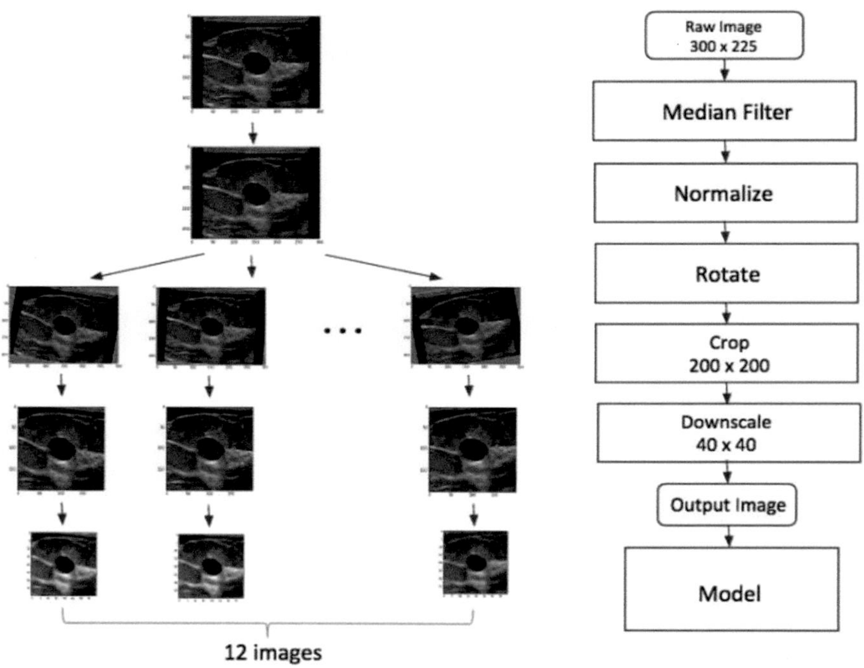


**Figure 17.9** Images (data) for the diagnosis.

using the non-saturating function, without affecting the convolutional layer. Figure 17.10 shows the positive and negative images that the model differentiates to give a result as malignant or benign.

### 17.2.3.1 Result of the model

This model achieves 91% accuracy with the help of images in the dataset, with the majority (80%) as the training data for the algorithm and the remaining 10% each for validation and testing.

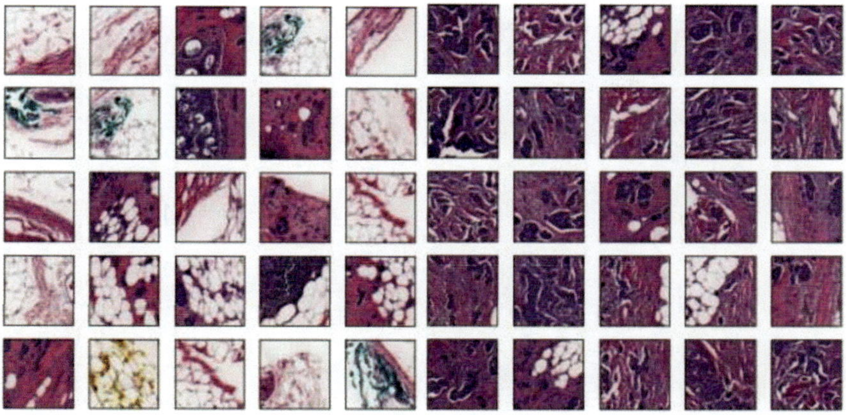

**Figure 17.10** Negative and positive images of a patient's data.

### 17.2.4 Challenges of breast cancer diagnosis using modern techniques

- Techniques like mammography, ultrasound, and breast MRI are used for the detection of breast cancer, which takes time to give results.
- Mammography, being the primary method in the detection of breast cancer, lacks reliability in providing results [22].
- MRI has its own problems as it has low specificity and the interpretation is complex with no standardization, which forces it to only be recommended to women with higher risks [23].
- The major challenge in prevention of breast cancer is to detect it at an early stage and then act on the results; some of the modern techniques provide with early detection, but then it lacks accuracy and efficiency.

### 17.2.5 Future scope and application

Tables 17.1 and 17.2 give us a brief comparison and review on the various machine techniques. Any chance to eradicate or lessen the effects of this fatal disease must always be taken with a precautionary mind. The fact that any woman can be affected by breast cancer unknowingly is terrifying as it has such a great number of factors that can lead to this. This makes the detection of breast cancer a leading priority for prevention. Many methods are being developed as new technologies for the detection of breast cancer and other types of cancer as well, all with one common aim: to reduce the death rate caused by this dreadful disease. Detection of breast cancer with the help of

**Table 17.1** Comparison of various machine techniques.

| **Categories for Differentiation** | **Deep learning model** | **Machine learning model** |
|---|---|---|
| Aim of work | Determining the presence of breast cancer and classifying it into benign or malicious using deep learning, IoT technologies and dataset of images. | Reducing the dimensions of the dataset using different classifiers and also the detection of tumors at an early stage, thus reducing the mortality rate. |
| Methods used | • The CNN algorithm is used in the machine learning model to train images in the dataset and taking that image as the input, determine if the image is benign or malignant.<br>• A thermal imaging sensor is used for capturing images of cancer cells.<br>• A microcomputer (Raspberry PI) is used for computation of the training model with images as the input.<br>• The Wi-Fi module is used for the transfer of images to the doctor for further consultation.<br>• An RFID reader is used for better organization of patients' data and images. | • Based on 11 attributes that were extracted using PCA (principal component analysis), a determination of the dataset is made.<br>• The WEKA tool is used for filtering and normalizing data using RandomRBF, the multifactor method, and then PCA for analysis.<br>• Classified analysis is done using three models, including random forest, logistic regression (LR), and MLP classifier, which are used to give an output in the combination of two variables to form the correlation function. |
| Results obtained | This chapter helps the need for real-time health and behavior detection using sensors to provide inputs that are then taken up for computation by the training model to give results as benign or malignant for that particular set of data inputs as images. Using IoT and machine learning; it detects breast cancer effectively and with ease, even in remote places. | This model is classifying the breast cancer instances using the MLP model, which is reducing the error rate with high accuracy compared to other classifiers. A ranking method is used to increase the accuracy, and hence the MLP model performs best in the prediction of breast cancer cells. |

| | | |
|---|---|---|
| Pros | • The dataset is built by real-time images, which test the algorithm and the model accurately to give the results, which can be further used in real-time computations.<br>• The CNN algorithm used provides a good accuracy of 91% overall.<br>• This model helps in the determination of breast cancer with ease and can be easily implemented in remote areas since it uses a Wi-Fi module to contact doctors for data transfer and consultation. | • The MLP classifier used for the classification of breast cancer is providing good and efficient results.<br>• It is also reducing the error rate in the classification of breast cancer.<br>• Hidden layers of cells and alpha–beta values are found using MLP to validate metrics like precaution, recall, $F1$-score, etc., for the correlation function, which again increases the efficiency of the model.<br>• This model helps the objective of diagnosing breast cancer at an early stage using machine learning and IoT to ultimately reduce the mortality rate. |
| Cons | • This model uses predefined images as datasets and needs the exposure for real-time acquiring of images and processing of the data for better accuracy and efficiency.<br>• The CNN algorithm removes the negative parameters of its ReLU layer with a non-saturating function, which can reduce the possibility of increasing accuracy by considering the nonlinearity as well.<br>• For further implementation, a larger dataset is needed to determine the training data. | • The research is done on a specific dataset, which limits the scope of the proposed model and is needed to expand the scope by experiments on different datasets to achieve higher accuracy and implementation.<br>• Since more experimentation is needed for this model with different datasets, real-time implementation of the research will take time.<br>• This chapter lacks the information needed to implement the model in real time using sensors and microcomputers. |

**Table 17.2** Comprehensive review of the machine techniques.

| **Technique** | **Description** | **Benefits** | **Limitations** | **Year and reference** |
|---|---|---|---|---|
| Computer aided diagnostics system (CAD) for breast cancer prediction. | Comparative analysis of algorithms like *K* nearest neighbors, support vector machine, random forest, and gradient boosting was performed. | Both classification and regression method random forest algorithm provided the highest accuracy. It is a mixture of many training models that provides the predictions about different training classifiers. | Expected probabilities of occurrence and non-occurrence are calculated through *K* fold cross-validation, which is a more expensive task. Data preprocessing stage took too much time as it converted raw data into valuable form. | 2019 [16] |
| Performance comparison of classification algorithm on WEKA and Spark. | Classification models such as support vector machine, decision tree, and random forest were considered for the evaluation of three types of data that consist of DM, GE, and a combination of both. | Support vector machine based on parallel computation has strength to analyze the multiple data at same time; it provides the highest accuracy rate on two different tools. | Gene expression data collection is one of the difficult tasks. To achieve a good accuracy result, precision, and sensitivity of data, a large number of samples were needed for computations. | 2019 [17] |
| Nonlinear machine learning algorithm comparison. | Comparison of MLP with nonlinear machine learning techniques: *K* nearest neighbor, CART, Naive Bayes, support vector machine, etc. | When datasets are linearly separable, it provides good accuracy level. | User was responsible to set the hidden layers for MLP algorithm. Setting some value sometimes provided under-fitting and sometimes over-fitting results. Without ten-fold cross-validation, it is impossible to predict the accuracy rate from training data models. | 2019 [18] |

| | | | | |
|---|---|---|---|---|
| Comparison of SVM and ANN for breast cancer prediction. | Evaluation of SVM and ANN was done through performance metrics such as accuracy, precision, recall, and ROC area. | After comparison, the most suitable technique for the prediction of breast cancer was found to be SVM because the classes are separated through hyper line that provides more accurate results than ANN. | Expected probabilities of occurrence and non-occurrence are calculated through *K* fold cross-validation. | 2019 [19] |
| Optimization of algorithms through genetics programming technique. | Data were in the form of digitized images, and feature selection and extraction methods were applied to get meaningful information. | Comparative analysis of different machine learning algorithms was performed after selecting some feature through polynomial features operator. | A lot of time was taken during the evaluation process and model training. GP algorithm was designed to solve the hyper-parameter problem, but the process time of the algorithm was too slow. | 2019 [20] |
| Comparative analysis of data mining classifier for cancer prediction and detection. | Classification algorithm random forest, bagging algorithm, random committee, simple CART, and IBK were analyzed through *K* fold cross-validation. | Random forest provided the highest accuracy during evaluation and it required less efforts. The random forest algorithm does not require the standardization and normalization of data and also can handle nonlinear data more efficiently. | A separate model was designed to check whether there is a tumor or not. This model took too much processing time. *K* fold cross-validation technique is applied for *n* number of iterations, just to get the desired result. Each iteration took a lot of time. | 2019 [21] |

IoT in combination with machine learning and deep learning has been ahead in this race to find the best possible method with the most accurate and efficient results. Now in the future, this model can help a lot of people with the time taken for detection of breast cancer and probably with the precautions that should be taken to prevent further problems while this model is already there. Detection using deep learning and IoT has the capacity to accurately detect and give results in less time. With more data input and training, this model will keep getting better and better in accuracy, and with remote access of this model with the help of IoT, it will help in more time-saving and early detection of breast cancer.

This model can be applied and used to make a device that can detect and share the results with the patient and doctor directly, saving a lot of time. The accuracy will increase with more and more use of this model with training of the available new data and previous ones. It can be made into a proper working tool to support other types of detection in the health sector using the data and application of the model. It can be made into a proper working tool to support other types of detection in the health sector with slight changes in the algorithm needed for that particular type of detection using the data and application of the model. Finally, this is going to help in the common goal of reducing the death rate across the globe.

## 17.3 Conclusion

There are several new techniques formed for the detection for breast cancer, but the ones being the most efficient and technology friendly are the ones going forward with the implementation phase, showing great results in the purpose of detecting breast cancer. Availability of technology everywhere is the biggest tool that is helping us to reach the remote areas of the planet and help those in need; the studies of different models to prevent breast cancer can be widely used once tested, with the help of the reachability of technology almost everywhere, and IoT is playing the major role in it. Implementation of these techniques by making it more and more efficient with the data and testing can help us cure the purpose of detecting breast cancer in early stages. Machine learning and deep learning are having the major role to achieve our purpose, building more secure and efficient database for testing and upgrading the models. Complex behavior of images while breaking it into different layers for detection is done efficiently by the algorithms of machine learning and deep learning.

After extensive research on the chapters of machine learning and deep learning applications in the detection of breast cancer using IoT, we chose the above two chapters to compare the results and conclude how deep learning acts as the better method for the detection. We also considered some modern techniques in use for the same and their challenges, which makes it even more important to develop a mindset to look at this problem from a deep learning aspect, which can overcome the challenges by providing early detection, more efficient and accurate results, and remote access to the technology for maximum reach to the people facing this risk. The main purpose is to solve these problems, which are a threat to a lot of women, at a higher rate so that the mortality rate due to breast cancer is reduced to the lowest possible number.

## Acknowledgements

We would like to thank the authors of the two research papers used in studying this chapter and "ScienceDirect" for providing us with the study on the basis of which this study had a conclusion toward the problem of breast cancer detection. A great thanks to the librarian at the University who helped us with finding the errors in the language of the chapter and helped us correcting it to the most. We would also like to show our gratitude to the IIT University for sharing their pearls of wisdom with us during the course of this research.

## References

[1] Anand, P.; Kunnumakara, A.B.; Sundaram, C.; Harikumar, K.B.; Tharakan, S.T.; Lai, O.S.; Sung, B.; Aggarwal, B.B. Cancer is a Preventable Disease that Requires Major Lifestyle Changes. Pharm. Res. 2008, 25, 2097–2116.

[2] De Martel, C.; Ferlay, J.; Franceschi, S.; Vignat, J.; Bray, F.; Forman, D.; Plummer, M. Global burden of cancers at-tributable to infections in 2008: A review and synthetic analysis. Lancet Oncol. 2012, 13, 607–615.

[3] Kim, W.; Kim, K.S.; Lee, J.E.; Noh, D.Y.; Kim, S.W.; Jung, Y.S.; Park, M.Y.; Park, R.W. Development of novel breast cancer re-currence prediction model using support vector machine. J. Breast Cancer 2012, 15, 230–238.

[4] Mishra, S., Tripathy, H. K., & Panda, A. R. (2018). An improved and adaptive attribute selection technique to optimize dengue fever prediction. Int J Eng Technol, 7, 480-486. 1.

[5] Ahmad, L.G.; Eshlaghy, A.T.; Poorebrahimi, A.; Ebrahimi, M.; Razavi, A.R. Using three machine learning techniques for predicting breast cancer recurrence. J. Health Med. Inf. 2013, 4, 3.

[6] Mishra, S., Raj, A., Kayal, A., Choudhary, V., Verma, P., & Biswal, L. (2012). Study of cluster based routing protocols in wireless sensor networks. International journal of scientific and engineering research, 3(7). 2.

[7] Rajinikanth, V.; Kadry, S.; Taniar, D.; Damasevicius, R.; Rauf, H.T. Breast-cancer detection using thermal images with marinepredators-algorithm selected features. In Proceedings of the 2021 IEEE 7th International Conference on Bio Signals, Images and Instrumentation, Chennai, India, 25–27 March 2021. ICBSII 2021.

[8] Azeez, N.A.; Towolawi, T.; Van der Vyver, C.; Misra, S.; Adewumi, A.; Damaševiˇcius, R.; Ahuja, R. A fuzzy expert system for diagnosing and analyzing human diseases. In Advances in Intelligent Systems and Computing; Springer Nature: Berlin, Switzerland, 2019; pp. 474–484.

[9] Parah, S.A.; Kaw, J.A.; Bellavista, P.; Loan, N.A.; Bhat, G.M.; Muhammad, K.; de Albuquerque, V.H.C. Efficient Security and Authentication for Edge-Based Internet of Medical Things. IEEE Internet Things J. 2020, 8, 15652–15662.

[10] Mishra, S., Jena, L., & Pradhan, A. (2012). Fault tolerance in wireless sensor networks. International Journal, 2(10), 146–153.

[11] Al-Turjman, F.; Zahmatkesh, H.; Mostarda, L. Quantifying uncertainty on the internet of medical things and big-data services using intelligence and deep learning. IEEE Access 2019, 7, 115749–115759.

[12] Alzubi, J.A.; Manikandan, R.; Alzubi, O.; Qiqieh, I.; Rahim, R.; Gupta, D.; Khanna, A. Hashed Needham Schroeder industrial IoT-based cost-optimized deep secured data transmission in the cloud. Measurement 2019, 150, 107077.

[13] Zebari, D.A.; Ibrahim, D.A.; Zeebaree, D.Q.; Haron, H.; Salih, M.S.; Damaševiˇcius, R.; Mohammed, M.A. Systematic review of computing approaches for breast cancer detection based computer aided diagnosis using mammo-gram images. Appl. Artif. Intell. 2021, 35, 2157–2203

[14] Mishra, S., Mahanty, C., Dash, S., & Mishra, B. K. (2019). Implementation of BFS-NB hybrid model in intrusion detection system. In Recent developments in machine learning and data analytics (pp. 167-175). Springer, Singapore.

[15] Sahoo, S., Das, M., Mishra, S., & Suman, S. (2021). A hybrid DTNB model for heart disorders prediction. In Advances in electronics, communication and computing (pp. 155–163). Springer, Singapore.

[16] M. K. Keles, "Breast cancer prediction and detection using data mining classification algorithms: A comparative study," Tehnički Vjesnik, vol. 26, no. 1, pp. 149–155, 2019.

[17] S. Alghunaim and H. H. Al-Baity, "On the scalability of machinelearning algorithms for breast cancer prediction in big data context," IEEE Access, vol. 7, pp. 91535–91546, 2019.

[18] E. A. Bayrak, P. Kirci, and T. Ensari, "Comparison of machine learning methods for breast cancer diagnosis," in Proc. Sci. Meeting Elect.-Electron. Biomed. Eng. Comput. Sci. (EBBT), Apr. 2019, pp. 1–3.

[19] A. A. Bataineh, "A comparative analysis of nonlinear machine learning algorithms for breast cancer detection," Int. J. Mach. Learn. Comput., vol. 9, no. 3, pp. 248–254, Jun. 2019.

[20] M. S. Yarabarla, L. K. Ravi, and A. Sivasangari, "Breast cancer prediction via machine learning," in Proc. 3rd Int. Conf. Trends Electron. Informat. (ICOEI), Apr. 2019, pp. 121–124.

[21] H. Dhahri, E. Al Maghayreh, A. Mahmood, W. Elkilani, and M. Faisal Nagi, "Automated breast cancer diagnosis based on machine learning algorithms," J. Healthcare Eng., vol. 2019, pp. 1–11, Nov. 2019.

[22] Hajiabadi, H.; Babaiyan, V.; Zabihzadeh, D.; Hajiabadi, M. Combination of loss functions for robust breast cancer prediction. Comput. Electr. Eng. 2020, 84, 106624.

[23] Shravya, C.; Pravalika, K.; Subhani, S. Prediction of breast cancer using supervised machine learning techniques. Int. J. Innov. Technol. Explor. Eng. 2019, 8, 1106–1110.

# Index

**A**
ADT (Android development tools) 293
AI (artificial intelligence) 3, 4, 7, 15, 17–19, 22, 28, 30, 31, 33–39, 42, 43, 45–51, 55–56, 76, 81–83, 88, 89, 93–98, 124, 126, 127, 130, 132, 133, 136–139, 145, 162, 164, 169, 170, 186, 201, 203, 209, 211, 213–217, 219, 222–224, 230, 234–237, 239, 243, 266, 281, 282, 291, 303, 304, 354
animal field 34
API 57, 74
artificial intelligence 4, 16–18, 31, 33–41, 45, 50–56, 67, 80, 82, 83, 95–97, 123, 132, 137, 139, 141, 155, 156, 164, 167, 169, 189, 190, 192, 193, 197, 198, 200–206, 208–218, 220, 226, 230–236, 239, 242, 265–272, 281, 282, 284, 287, 304, 307, 309, 311, 312, 330, 354
automatic segmentation 245, 247–250, 254–256, 258–259, 261–262

**B**
bioimaging 123, 124, 131
biomedical 36–37, 49–50, 79–83, 92–94, 98, 123–124, 131, 211, 239, 253, 264, 309–312, 315–318, 321, 324–325, 328–330, 339, 349
black-box 3, 6, 20, 22, 23, 28, 30, 35–36, 38, 46–47, 52, 80, 83, 87, 89, 93, 123–124, 126, 132, 136, 139, 282, 303, 337, 339
block-chain 145, 150–155, 160–161
brain tumor 338–340, 349–350
breast cancer diagnosis 130, 353, 357, 360, 363, 365, 373

**C**
class activation mapping 19, 123, 127, 130, 199, 210, 265, 283
classification 3, 9, 11, 13–15, 19–21, 26, 31, 35, 37, 56, 60–63, 81, 84, 92–93, 96, 103, 105–106, 112, 119, 121, 124–130, 132, 137–139, 142, 162, 167, 170–171, 179–180, 184–187, 199, 202–203, 208, 211, 219, 220, 237, 270, 278, 285, 337–340, 342, 345–346, 349–350, 353, 355, 358–360, 367–368, 373
CNN 7, 27, 48, 84, 90–91, 93, 124, 128, 130, 132–135, 156–157, 160–163, 169, 171–183, 199, 201–203, 249, 253, 255, 340–342, 346, 348–350, 361–364, 366, 367

convolutional neural network 7, 16, 56, 98, 119, 138, 140, 156, 167, 169, 176, 185–186, 202, 211, 238, 241, 249, 284, 341, 345, 362
COVID-19 17, 24, 31, 38, 52, 57–58, 60, 74–76, 134, 140, 147, 162, 210, 239, 307

**D**
dairy farmers 34, 39
data processing 156, 160, 214, 219, 281
deep learning 1, 3, 4, 9, 11, 16, 35, 38, 51, 54, 80, 94, 97, 123, 128, 138, 142, 145, 155, 157–158, 160–161, 167, 169, 170–171, 174, 176, 181, 185–186, 197–199, 203, 208, 210–219, 221–222, 225–228, 231–232, 234, 236–238, 241–242, 245, 247–250, 253–260, 263, 265–270, 273, 280–281, 286–287, 337, 349–350, 353–355, 357, 360–363, 366, 370–372
dental 129–130, 189–196, 200–208, 211–212
diseases 20, 35, 37–38, 40, 43, 50, 53, 80, 82–83, 101–102, 118, 120, 124, 129, 131–132, 163, 167–169, 177, 180–181, 184, 190–192, 195, 197, 200, 203, 219, 221, 245–247, 260, 267, 301, 303, 310–311, 325, 327, 330, 338, 340, 372
drug discovery 92–93, 98, 213–214, 216–217, 219, 221–222, 224, 226–228, 232, 234–240, 243, 265–267, 273–281, 286–287, 310–311, 333

**E**
endoscopy 2, 7, 14, 16
explainable AI 4, 30, 47, 49, 56, 93, 95, 127, 136, 138–139, 145, 162, 164, 201, 203, 230, 235–236, 291, 303
Explainable AI 17, 31, 50–51, 95, 97, 145, 164, 209, 236, 303
explainable artificial intelligence 4, 33–35, 50, 52–53, 56, 95–96, 123, 139, 189, 200–201, 203–204, 212, 217–218, 226, 239, 265, 267, 269–270, 282, 312
explainable artificial intelligence (XAI) 4, 33–35, 50, 52–53, 56, 95–96, 123, 139, 189, 200–204, 212, 217–218, 226, 239, 265, 267, 269–270, 282, 312

**G**
Gastric cancer 1, 10
gray matter 245–246, 249–250, 260–261, 264

**H**
healthcare 3, 17–18, 20, 22, 36–38, 50–51, 54, 92–93, 98, 132, 138, 145–157, 160–167, 169, 215, 233, 289–293, 295–297, 299, 303–305, 307, 353–354
heart failure 101–105, 110, 114–121
hybrid model 65, 93, 166, 306, 337, 342, 346, 349–350, 372

**I**
Internet of Things 31, 39, 76, 145–146, 150, 156, 163, 165–166, 289, 303, 306, 353, 356–357
IoT in healthcare 145–146, 307

IoT (Internet of Things) 39, 76, 77, 145–157, 160–167, 289–290, 303, 305–307, 353, 354–355, 357–358, 362, 366–367, 370, 372

**L**

LIME 6, 17, 19–29, 31, 81, 84, 133–135, 141, 162, 265, 270–273

**M**

machine learning 3, 6, 15, 17, 33–38, 41, 46, 49–55, 60, 64–65, 67, 80, 90, 96–98, 101, 103–106, 113, 116–120, 123, 131, 138, 140, 156–157, 160, 163–164, 166–167, 197–199, 201, 208–209, 213, 215–220, 223, 229, 235–241, 243, 247, 252, 266–267, 269, 281, 284–287, 306–307, 337, 353–361, 366–368, 369–370, 372–373

magnetic resonance 141, 169, 245, 261–262, 337

major and minor genes 310–317, 319–321, 324, 326–328, 330

medical imaging 33, 84, 123–124, 130–132, 163, 184, 208, 247

mutation 57, 60, 332

**O**

Omicron 57–60, 74–75

**P**

poultry farmers 34

prediction 6, 12–13, 17, 20–21, 24–28, 35–37, 41–42, 46, 48–49, 51, 53–54, 62–64, 82, 84, 91–92, 96, 98–99, 103–104, 106, 112–113, 115, 117–121, 126, 137–139, 163, 166, 171, 175, 200, 209, 216, 221–222, 224–229, 231–232, 234–239, 241–242, 265–267, 273–276, 279–280, 284, 286–287, 306–307, 333–334, 339, 355, 366, 368–369, 371–373

privacy 37, 45, 51, 81, 149, 156, 157, 159–161, 164, 165, 272

Python 57, 60, 254

**S**

security 44, 90, 94, 129, 145–148, 150–153, 156–157, 159–162, 164, 166–167, 198, 295

sentiments 74

SHAP values 6, 21, 113–115

smart healthcare 150, 156, 160–162, 164, 291, 303, 307

Spinal cord 195, 245, 250–251, 260–261

**T**

transfer learning 7, 84, 93, 132, 185–186, 202, 230, 339, 349–350

**U**

U-Net 128, 142, 202, 245–246, 248–250, 252–260, 263–264

**V**

variant 57–60, 75, 229

veterinary 33–34, 45, 46, 50, 55

**X**

XAI 4, 5, 15, 17–22, 26, 30–31, 33–40, 42, 45–56, 79–88, 89–90, 92–99, 123, 126–127, 130, 133, 136–139, 162–164, 167, 198–199, 201, 203, 213–217, 222, 224–227, 231–232, 265–270, 273–282, 290–292, 303–304, 313–321, 324, 326–328, 337, 339, 342, 349

# About the Editors

**Dr. Utku Kose** received the B.S. degree in computer education from Gazi University, Turkey in 2008 as a faculty valedictorian. He received the M.S. degree in the field of computer from Afyon Kocatepe University, Turkey in 2010 and the D.S./Ph.D. degree in the field of computer engineering from Selcuk University, Turkey in 2017. Between 2009 and 2011, he has worked as a Research Assistant with Afyon Kocatepe University. Following that, he has also worked as a Lecturer and Vocational School – Vice Director with Afyon Kocatepe University between 2011 and 2012, as a Lecturer and Research Center Director with Usak University between 2012 and 2017, and as an Assistant Professor with Suleyman Demirel University between 2017 and 2019. Currently, he is an Associate Professor with Suleyman Demirel University, Turkey. He has more than 200 publications including articles, authored and edited books, proceedings, and reports. He is also in the editorial boards of many scientific journals and serves as one of the editors of the *Biomedical and Robotics Healthcare* book series by CRC Press. His research interest includes artificial intelligence, machine ethics, artificial intelligence safety, biomedical applications, optimization, the chaos theory, distance education, e-learning, computer education, and computer science.

**Dr. Deepak Gupta** received the B.Tech. degree from the Guru Gobind Singh Indraprastha University, Delhi, India in 2006. He received the M.E. degree from Delhi Technological University, India, in 2010, and the Ph.D. degree from Dr. APJ Abdul Kalam Technical University (AKTU), Lucknow, India, in 2017. He completed his Post-Doc from the National Institute of Telecommunications (Inatel), Brazil, in 2018. He has co-authored more than 207 journal articles, including 168 SCI papers and 45 conference articles. He has authored/edited 60 books, published by IEEE-Wiley, Elsevier, Springer, Wiley, CRC Press, DeGruyter, and Katsons. He has filled four Indian patents. He is the convener of the ICICC, ICDAM, ICCCN, ICIIP, and DoSCI Springer conferences series. He is an Associate Editor for *Computer & Electrical Engineering*, *Expert Systems*, *Alexandria Engineering Journal*, and *Intelligent Decision Technologies*. He is the recipient of the 2021 IEEE System Council Best Paper Award. He has been featured in the list of top 2% scientist/researcher databases worldwide. In India, he holds Rank 1 as a researcher in the field of healthcare applications (as per Google Scholar citation) and Rank 78 in India among Top Scientists 2022 by Research.com. He is also working toward promoting Startups and also serving as a Startup Consultant. He is also a series editor of *Elsevier Biomedical Engineering* at Academic Press, Elsevier, *Intelligent Biomedical Data Analysis* at De Gruyter, Germany, and *Explainable AI (XAI) for Engineering Applications* at CRC Press. He is appointed as a Consulting Editor at Elsevier. He has accomplished productive collaborative research with grants of approximately $144,000 from various international funding agencies, and he is Co-PI in an International Indo-Russian Joint project of INR 1.31CR from the Department of Science and Technology.

**Dr. Xi Chen** received the Ph.D. degree in the field of bioinformatics from the University of Kentucky, USA in 2019. Between 2013 and 2019, he worked as a Graduate Research Assistant with the Department of Biochemistry, University of Kentucky. He was also a Research Collaborator with the Department of Statistics, University of Kentucky, USA, between 2017 and 2019. He was University Ambassadors/Deep Learning Institute (DLI) Certified Instructor at the Nvidia Deep Learning Institute between 2018 and 2021. In 2019, he worked as a Data Scientist and Machine Learning Engineer for the Verb Surgical, USA. Following that, he was a Computational Biologist/ML Engineer Lead with the Juvena Therapeutics, USA (2019–2021). Currently, he is working as a Senior Software Engineer (ML Data Foundation) with the Meta, USA. His research interest includes artificial intelligence, machine/ deep learning, biomedical, genomics, data science, and image processing.

For Product Safety Concerns and Information please contact our EU representative GPSR@taylorandfrancis.com Taylor & Francis Verlag GmbH, Kaufingerstraße 24, 80331 München, Germany